Drug Discovery

Drug Discovery

A Casebook and Analysis

By

Robert A. Maxwell

The Wellcome Research Laboratories
Research Triangle Park, North Carolina

and

Shohreh B. Eckhardt

University of Vermont College of Medicine,
Burlington, Vermont

Humana Press • **Clifton, New Jersey**

© 1990 The Humana Press Inc.
Crescent Manor
PO Box 2148
Clifton, New Jersey 07015

Printed in the United States of America.

Library of Congress Cataloging-in-Publication Data

Maxwell, Robert A., 1927–
    Drug discovery : a casebook and analysis / by Robert A. Maxwell and
  Shohreh B. Eckhardt.
        p. cm.
    Includes bibliographical references.
    Includes index.
    ISBN 0-89603-180-2
    1. Drugs—Design. 2. Pharmacy—Technological innovations.
I. Eckhardt, Shohreh B.   II. Title.
    [DNLM: 1. Drug Design.   QV 744 M465d]
RS420.M38   1990
615'.19—dc20
DNLM/DLC
for Library of Congress   90-4915
                                                                              CIP

Preface

This treatise had its origins in the authors' strong opinion that the discovery of new drugs, especially of innovative therapeutic agents, really does not happen as a spontaneous sequel to investigative research, no matter how penetrating such research may be. Rather, it seemed to us that the discovery of innovative therapeutic agents was a very active process, existing in and of itself, and demanding full attention—it was not simply a passive, dependent by-process of investigative research. And yet, many researchers—some close confreres of the authors, others more distant—believed otherwise. We felt that their view reflected unrealistic thinking and that reality probably lay closer to what Beyer* maintained:

> We are taught to believe that if we can understand a disease it should be easy enough to figure out, say, the molecular configuration of a definitive receptor mechanism somewhere along the line and to design a specific drug....And so we start out to understand the disease but never get around to doing much about therapy.

The authors very soon realized that there was essentially no quantitive information available on just where and how innovative therapeutic agents were discovered. There were only anecdotal accounts, and these were able to be selected and presented in ways that could be used to defend any point of view. We felt that to clarify the issue raised above (as well as for several other reasons), we would develop, insofar as it was possible, quantitative information about the drug discovery process and then see what this information would tell us about its nature. This volume represents our best efforts at doing so, and will, we hope, prove illuminating for all those working in the field in the years ahead.

Robert A. Maxwell
Shohreh B. Eckhardt

*Beyer, K. H. Jr.: *Discovery, Development and Delivery of New Drugs,* SP Medical & Science, New York, 1978.

Acknowledgments

The authors gratefully acknowledge the exceptional support for this project that was extended by the management of Burroughs Wellcome Co., especially Howard Schaeffer and David Barry of the Wellcome Research Laboratories. In addition, one of the authors (R.A.M.) gives very grateful acknowledgments to William Riker, Chairman of the Department of Pharmacology at the Oregon Health Sciences University, and to the University, for honoring him with a Visiting Adjunct Professorship and for the associated use of the medical library and office space during his three-year leave from the Wellcome Research Laboratories. Thanks are also extended (by S. B. E.) to John Bevan, Chairman of the Department of Pharmacology at the University of Vermont, College of Medicine, for understanding the need for the extensive time and effort expended on this project.

We thank Arletta Allan and Gabrielle Orzell of the University of Vermont for typing early drafts of some sections of the manuscript. We especially wish to acknowledge the invaluable help of Colleen Engle at OHSU for her patient, rapid, and excellent typing and retyping of the endless drafts of all the manuscript chapters—a veritable herculean task. We also gratefully acknowledge Judy McDuffie of Burroughs Wellcome Co. for her careful monitoring of reference citations and references, and for her general shepherding of the manuscript through other hurdles, including arrangments for the preparation of the figures. Thanks also to her associate, Mary Jane Adams, for photocopying some of the references used by the authors.

Additional acknowledgments are extended to the following people at Burroughs Wellcome Co. for their able help: Ildiko Trombitas and the members of the Technical Information Department who identified articles, obtained elusive publications, arranged translations, and verified our list of references for accuracy against standard sources; Linda Byrd and her staff for preparing the figures;

and Susan Young and Julian Wooldridge for designing and carrying out the computer analyses used in the text.

Finally, thanks are extended to all of those clinician-scientists who were kind enough to answer our queries regarding their choice of innovative drugs, and to those scientists, many of them participants in the drug discoveries described by us, who were kind enough to read pertinent parts of our manuscript and offer constructive criticism and suggestions.

Contents

Psychiatry Group

Neurology Group

Rheumatology Group

Anesthesiology Group

Pulmonary Group

Gastrointestinal Group

Analysis and Interpretation

Introduction

The present communication is our attempt at an analytical survey of research since World War II that led to innovative therapeutic agents. An innovative therapeutic agent is defined as a chemical whose use in a given indication had little or no precedent before its introduction and whose use also represented a very significant improvement over, or a very significant supplement to, available drugs (occasionally, only the latter conditions are met).

There are many descriptions concerning drug discovery. These range in character from vignettes in journals (e.g., Shanks, 1984) to chapters in books (e.g., Parnham and Bruinvels, 1983) to complete books (e.g., Swazey, 1974; Sneader, 1985). Many of these accounts are written by people who are involved in discovering innovative drugs or who are specialists in the pharmacological or therapeutic area encompassing the new agent. Because these accounts are generally anecdotal and are written years after the discovery, they can inadvertently be subject to the vagaries of memory, to "sanitization" of history, and to other errors endemic to hindsight. Finally, although descriptions of the discovery of individual innovative drugs, especially by the discoverers, are highly instructive, they do not teach us anything about the process in general.

We felt that scrutiny of the original source papers for specific facts dealing with discovery, for a large number of such agents, would be as objective a way as possible to approach the subject and certainly one that was time-honored. The information generated would also serve as a source of genuine data with which to characterize some important aspects of drug discovery.

It is the authors' intent to produce a reference compendium that will be useful to all basic and clinical researchers interested in medically important drugs and their origins. It will also be useful to those people interested in a documented analysis of the interplay among academic, industrial, governmental, and other institutions in the area of drug discovery.

Each chapter is divided into four sections:

I.   A defense, from primary and other sources, of the choice of drug X as an innovative therapeutic agent.* Also included is a presentation of the agent's early, significant, clinical history.

II. A literature review, *from primary sources only,* describing the scientific contributions leading to drug X. This review is considered to be the intellectual history of the discovery of drug X.

III. Comments, from primary and other source material, on the facts presented in section II. The views presented in this section are not necessarily those of the authors, but are presented because they seem to the authors to be significant statements. The authors' opinions, in large part, are restricted to the final chapter.

IV. A description, from primary and other source material, covering related new drugs developed in the wake of therapeutic agent X. Also, comments from the literature on the impact of the discovered drug on basic and clinical research are included where appropriate.

The text is meant to be factual and concise. Each chapter presents (in section II) a terse, documented exposition of those scientific contributions associated with the discovery of an innovative therapeutic agent.[†] Most importantly, a tabulation (labeled Table 1) is presented that contains the key observations and ideas, and the variables that characterize them. The entries in Table 1 are meant to represent the "distilled" intellectual history of the discovery of drug X. The text in section II serves as the basis for, and justification of, the selected entries made in each Table 1. The information in each table is categorized as follows:

---

*Information regarding the clinical uses of the drugs discussed in each chapter is culled from the world literature and should not be taken as a guide for their proper therapeutic application in any specific country. For such guidance, official sources should be consulted.

[†]Those scientific contributions not written in English were translated into English by professional translators. All quotes from these sources have been made from the translations.

- The orientation in which the contribution was made—clinical or preclinical;
- The type of research institution with which the authors were affiliated—governmental, industrial, academic, hospital, other;
- The nature of the study—pharmacological, physiological, biochemical, other;
- The nature of the discovery—whether orderly or serendipitous;
- Whether screening of compounds was involved;
- And national origin of the research.

Detailed definitions are given in the next chapter, entitled "Definitions for Table 1."

In a penultimate chapter, the data from all the tables are analyzed to find those points of commonality and difference that exist in the drug-discovery enterprise. The information from each table has been entered into a data file and analyzed by computer using SAS, a statistical analysis program, to give numerical values for the various categories or combination of categories. These results are discussed in relation to what they can tell us about the nature of drug discovery, i.e., what the important variables are and how they may have changed with time. Finally, in the last chapter, the authors give their interpretation of the significance of all the previous chapters, and discuss what, if anything, can be predicted from the patterns displayed by the variables.

The specific agents to be analyzed were selected via an informal written poll of leading North American clinician-scientists from a variety of medical specialties, namely, cardiovascular and renal (including renal transplant), psychiatry, neurology, anesthesiology, rheumatology, pulmonary, and gastrointestinal. A minimum of 10 returns per specialty was required; any drug appearing in more than 50% of the returns was analyzed. Agents used to treat infectious diseases or cancer were not reviewed except as they also had other uses in the specialties listed. Antiinfective and anticancer agents will be the subject of a second volume.

The authors have elected not to take a panoramic historical approach in describing innovation, as has been done by Comroe and Dripps (1976), Swazey (1974) and Dorkins (1982), for example. Instead we have taken what may be termed a "topical" approach: present the innovative science in the context of its own time, rather than how it fits (frequently with the benefit of considerable hindsight and *post hoc* reasoning) into the broadest historical perspective. This topical approach focuses on the time and events that were specific to the development of the innovative therapeutic agent and looks backward and forward from this vantage point. This approach is in no way meant to denigrate the obvious truth revealed by a broad historical perspective, that all innovation is indebted more or less heavily to the past, but to suggest that there may be another useful, supplemental, and complementary way to view developments. Thus, it is clearly understood that current drug-discovery research could not even take place but for the contributions of countless scientists—physiologists, biochemists, pharmacologists, chemists, clinicians, and others—who, over centuries, established their disciplines and generated the vast and varied knowledge that is now the stock-in-trade of drug discovery. The debt is enormous and is recognized.

However, how does one manage to recognize a contribution (or series of contributions) as distinct from its framework of past contributions and not as the inevitable consequence of it? We conclude that this is done, in any given instance, by tacitly categorizing much precedent research as permissive and not directly contributory: that is, as a necessary forerunner to the innovation but not directly involved in defining the specific innovation. Such work is classified by us as "background" research. A subsection of section II in each chapter recognizes some of the more immediate background research.

"Foreground" research, as we perceive it, takes the form of an *intellectually related* and *temporally related* series of research efforts that are responsible for, or helpful in, the discovery of an innovative compound or an innovative new use for a compound. A description of these research contributions forms the major part of section II. Intellectual relatedness means that the results or ideas in a given contribution speak directly to a pertinent theme(s), or progression of research, that can be recognized as developing in those contribu-

tions that were leading toward the innovation. Temporal relatedness means that the contribution under consideration was carried
out in reasonably close proximity in time to the other contributions
that were leading toward the innovation.‡ Both criteria had to be ful-
filled for placement into foreground research.

Finally, in making the important decision as to which of the
foreground studies were really crucial to the discovery, and, therefore, to be included in Table 1, we subjected all of them to the
following question: Would the discovery of the agent have been
materially delayed or not have taken place without this contribution? For inclusion in Table 1, our answer had to be yes.§

It should be noted that only those clinical studies that were

---

‡The temporal criteria we used were as follows: Any contribution that was
intellectually related to the body of contributions leading to the drug discovery and
had been published within five years before this body of contributions was auto-
matically considered as foreground work and included in the main part of section
II. If such intellectually related work was published 16 or more years earlier than the
main body of contributions, it was considered to be in the "scientific public domain"
and put into the background subsection of section II. Any intellectually related
contribution that was published 6–15 yr before the main body of contributions was
considered to be an "intergrade," and a judgment was made as to its status as
foreground or background research.

§In occasional instances, it was not possible to decide precisely whether a
contribution materially advanced the conceptions that lead to the innovative agent.
This indecisiveness occurred when a potentially significant, but essentially isolated,
contribution was found. These "indeterminate status" contributions were not
entered in Table 1.

In a few instances, several similar preclinical or clinical investigations, any one
of which could have served to lead on toward the innovative discovery, were carried
out independently and appeared in the literature within a short time of one another.
Since our ultimate goal was not the crediting of individual investigators, but the
gathering of quantitative information regarding the variables noted in the tables, we
chose only one of these contributions for entry into Table 1. Usually this was the
paper with a clear priority publication date, but on occasion it was the paper that
seemed to us, from the literature, to be the most germane to the scientific problem
at hand. The authors regret the necessity of being restricted to a single entry in order
not to distort the quantitative aspects of the tables.

directly involved in the discovery process were included in Table 1. Those clinical studies representing a straightforward, logical extension of the discovery to human use were not included in Table 1, since they, like background research, were considered as permissive, rather than germinal to the discovery. The early, important, permissive, clinical trials for each drug are described in section I under the subsection heading "Early Clinical Research History."

As one last item, we point out that, in our descriptions of the discoveries of innovative drugs (*see* section II of each chapter), our aim was to peruse all pertinent, documented, original literature. However, the authors recognize that, in an enterprise as extensive as the present one, it is conceivable that some omissions of information may have occurred and that such omissions could potentially lead to conclusions different from those arrived at by the authors. We believe this is very unlikely, but if any such omissions exist, they were inadvertent on the authors' part.

References

Comroe, J. H., Jr. and Dripps, R. D.: Scientific basis for the support of biomedical science. *Science* **192:** 105–111, 1976.

Dorkins, H. R.: Suxamethonium—the development of a modern drug from 1906 to the present day. *Med. Hist.* **26:** 145–168, 1982.

Parnham, M. J. and Bruinvels, J., eds.: *Discoveries in Pharmacology,* vol. 1, *Psycho- and Neuro-pharmacology.* Elsevier Science Publishers B.V., Amsterdam, 1983.

Shanks, R. G.: The discovery of beta-adrenoceptor blocking drugs. *Trends Pharmacol. Sci.* **5:** 405–410, 1984.

Sneader, W.: *Drug Discovery: The Evolution of Modern Medicines.* Wiley, Chichester, 1985.

Swazey, J. P.: *Chlorpromazine in Psychiatry; A Study of Therapeutic Innovation.* MIT Press, Cambridge, MA, 1974.

Definitions for Table 1

Orientation—The term "clinical" means that the research was carried out in humans or human material. The term "preclinical" means that the research was carried out in animals or animal material.

Nature of study —refers to the nature of the work carried out. It does not mean the name of the department in which the work happened to be conducted.

If chemical compounds were being utilized as tools to learn something about a particular physiological or biochemical (or other) system, the work was designated as physiology or biochemistry (or other), respectively. On the other hand, if a physiological or biochemical (or other) system was being used to characterize the biological activities of a chemical compound(s), the work was designated as pharmacology or, in some instances, as chemistry/pharmacology.

The chemistry/pharmacology designation amalgamates contributions from both medicinal chemistry and pharmacology, and is of special significance for industrial-based research, where the two disciplines are virtually inseparable in drug discovery. When the class of molecules being studied was known to have, or could be expected to have, the particular biological activity being sought, the entry was put as chemistry/pharmacology. If the occurrence of a particular activity in the molecules being studied was not at all predictable, but was found by the pharmacologist, the entry was put as pharmacology/chemistry. If attribution was unclear, the entry was left as chemistry/pharmacology. In all cases, the work necessarily was a fusion of both disciplines.

The clinical specialties entered into Table 1 are self-explanatory.

Research Institution—defines the type of research institution with which the investigator(s) was affiliated full-time when the work was done:

- Government—government research installation emphasizing pre-clinical and/or clinical research, e.g., NIH.
- Industry—industrial research laboratory.
- University—university affiliation; includes preclinical laboratories and hospitals that are part of a university.
- Hospital—any hospital that is not part of a university or of a government research installation. This term covers those hospitals, either private or government-operated, where health care delivery, and not research, is the sole or very paramount activity. Veterans Administration hospitals, which frequently have close affiliations with universities, are denoted as hospital (VA).
- Private—an institution that places heavy emphasis on research, encompassing preclinical laboratories and/or hospital facilities, but is not run by government, industry, or a university, e. g., Cleveland Clinic, Mayo Clinic.

National origin—means the country (or countries) in which the research was carried out, not the country of origin of the author(s).

Nature of discovery—The term "orderly" means that serendipitous events played no significant part in the work. The term "serendipitous" means, specifically, that a serendipitous event was an important factor in the work. Serendipity, as we use the term, is that form of good luck defined as the finding of valuable or agreeable things not sought for. However, all good luck is not serendipity, and a distinction between the two terms is maintained in the current treatise. Thus, for example, finding (during a clinical trial in tuberculous patients) that a compound synthesized as an antitubercular agent has marked antidepressant properties, or, similarly, finding by accident that a compound synthesized, and established, as an antimalarial agent is also an antirheumatic compound, were both considered serendipitous findings. On the other hand, for a chemist synthesizing *diuretics* to have an unexpected ring closure occur, which produces a very superior *diuretic*, was taken as good luck, not as a serendipitous event. Likewise, that a pharmacologist screening random compounds in a specific test finds an active agent in that test, was also taken to be good luck, not a serendipitous event.

The distinction in terms is important, because a major serendipitous finding represents an "intellectual discontinuity" with past research, and generally assigns the past work to background status, whereas this is not so for good luck, which is as ubiquitous in science as it is in other pursuits.

Screening involved—The term "screening" means the process of purposefully testing a specific chemical compound, for the first time, for a particular biological activity either in animals or in humans. It does not include any testing, either preclinical or clinical, that came as a logical sequel to earlier findings with that specific substance.

The term "screening" includes the following two categories:

1. *Targeted,* which means that, for the specific biological activity of interest, useful, positive knowledge was at hand regarding the effectiveness of compounds structurally related to the one(s) to be tested. In targeted screening, because of such knowledge, directed synthesis can be undertaken, with the compounds generated having a greater-than-chance probability of being active.
2. *Untargeted,* which means that, for the specific biological activity of interest, there was no useful, positive knowledge at hand regarding the effectiveness of compounds structurally related to the one(s) to be tested. In untargeted screening, since there is no guide as to what molecules to synthesize, chance largely determines if an active compound will be found. Untargeted screening is often carried out for a battery of biological activities, in which case it is usually termed "general screening."

It is possible that both targeted and untargeted screening may be carried out in the same study. This happens when, for example,

1. The same compounds are being screened for more than one biological activity, and structure–activity information is available for some, but not all, of the activites.
2. During the course of a targeted screen, an unsought-for activity is found (i.e., a serendipitous finding).
3. Early screening is untargeted, but as a result of new information, the screening can be targeted.

Cardiovascular and Renal Group (Including Renal Transplantation)

Propranolol

Captopril

Calcium Antagonists:

Verapamil
Nifedipine
Diltiazem

Chlorothiazide

Furosemide

Azathioprine

Cyclosporine

Propranolol

I. Propranolol as an Innovative Therapeutic Agent

Adrenergic receptor blocking drugs, both alpha and beta, selectively inhibit the effects of norepinephrine, the agonist secreted by adrenergic nerve terminals, and those of epinephrine, the agonist secreted by the adrenal medulla. The dampening of the physiological activities subserved by these endogenous agonists, especially those involving beta agonism, has had considerable and continuing therapeutic significance.

Propranolol, the first beta-adrenergic blocking drug to have broad therapeutic use, was initially introduced in the 1960s for the treatment of classical angina pectoris of effort. The discomfort and pain of angina of effort is considered to result from an imbalance, brought about by coronary artery disease, between the myocardial oxygen supply and the demands of the heart for oxygen (Berkow, 1982; Lorimer, 1985). Atherosclerotic narrowing and rigidification of coronary arteries prevents them from delivering adequate blood flow (oxygen) during muscular effort, and, therefore, transient ischemia and pain occur. Propranolol alleviates angina by blocking cardiac beta receptors, with resultant reductions in heart rate, myocardial contractility, and blood pressure during effort—all effects that reduce myocardial demand for oxygen. Since its introduction, propranolol has been prescribed extensively for this indication (Lampe, 1986).

Prior to propranolol, the nitrates, especially glyceryl trinitrate, were the major drugs to alleviate anginal pain, and they continue to have important use in this indication. These agents relax coronary arteries, but in large part reduce myocardial oxygen requirements

3

by relaxing peripheral venous and arteriolar smooth muscle. The consequent pooling of blood in the veins and reductions in systemic resistance and blood pressure all lead to a diminution in cardiac work and, hence, oxygen demand. Unfortunately, side effects exhibited by these drugs may be marked and include postural hypotension, flushing, and headache. The development of partial tolerance to the effects of the nitrates is not uncommon. Sublingual glyceryl trinitrate is usually taken for quick relief during an anginal attack. Some longer acting nitrates, or nitrate preparations such as isosorbide dinitrate or topically applied glyceryl trinitrate, are also available (Berkow, 1982; Lorimer, 1985; Lampe, 1986).

Propranolol has proved most efficacious in the prophylactic treatment of angina and is frequently used in conjunction with a nitrate vasodilator. Propranolol and some of its successors are also important antihypertensive agents. In cases of mild and moderate hypertension, they are the second drug to be used following a thiazide diuretic (Berkow, 1982). However, in patients with symptomatic coronary artery disease (particularly after myocardial infarction), they are usually the first drug in the regimen, because they may reduce reinfarction rate and improve the life expectancy of patients who have survived an acute myocardial infarction (Bennett, 1983; Frishman et al., 1984).

In addition to having use in hypertension, propranolol and other beta blocking agents are also valuable antiarrhythmic agents. They are used in supraventricular and ventricular tachyarrhythmias as well as arrhythmias associated with increased sympathetic tone or circulating catecholamines. They reduce heart rate and myocardial contractility by lengthening A–V conduction time and suppressing automaticity (Bigger and Hoffman, 1985).

Finally, propranolol and other beta blocking agents are also used for early and prolonged treatment of myocardial infarction (β-Blocker Heart Attack Trial Research Group, 1982; Frishman et al., 1984).

Because of their antihypertensive, antiarrhythmic, antianginal, and even antiplatelet action, beta blocking drugs can be considered to be cardioprotective agents (Bennett, 1983).

The important side effects of propranolol (and related agents) are largely the result of beta-adrenergic receptor blockade (Frishman, 1984; Weiner, 1985). Heart failure can occur in patients whose myocardial function is subnormal, and cardiac arrest can occur in patients suffering from partial heart block. Propranolol, by blocking beta-receptor-mediated relaxation of bronchiolar smooth muscle, increases airways resistance, which can be a serious event in asthmatic patients, and it is therefore contraindicated in this disease. Propranolol also enhances the hypoglycemic effect of insulin by blocking the normal compensatory activation of the sympathetic nervous system, and it must be employed with care by insulin users or people subject to episodes of hypoglycemia.

At present, the FDA has approved propranolol for use in hypertension, angina, arrhythmias, myocardial infarction, glaucoma, and migraine headaches (Schultz, 1983). The cardiovascular and non-cardiovascular uses of beta blocking agents continue to grow: as examples, their study and use in hypertrophic cardiomyopathy, dissecting aneurysm, thyrotoxicosis, and anxiety states (Frishman, 1984).

Early Clinical Research History

Much of the groundwork for the clinical research investigation of propranolol was carried out with a precursor compound, pronethalol, that eventually proved to be toxic (pronethalol is discussed in section II).

Hamer et al. (1964) showed that intravenously administered propranolol, like its forerunner, pronethalol, increased exercise tolerance in patients with angina pectoris, and suggested that propranolol might be helpful in this disorder. Gillam and Prichard (1965) also thought that propranolol might be of value in angina, since it was closely related—chemically and pharmacologically—to pronethalol. Their experiments demonstrated that orally administered propranolol reduced the number of attacks of angina, the pain of angina, and the number of glyceryl trinitrate tablets consumed.

Prichard and Gillam (1964) reported that propranolol had a hypotensive action in 15 of 16 patients who had been taking orally administered propranolol for up to seven months. Acute intravenous administration did not lower blood pressure. Gillam and Prichard (1965) also noted that hypotension was an added benefit for anginal patients who also were hypertensive. According to Gillam and Prichard (1976), "These observations [of the effectiveness of propranolol in hypertension] were slow to be accepted, as besides a novel mode of action, most attempts to repeat the work failed to pay enough attention to adequate dosage." With appropriate attention to titrating doses, the conflict over the effectiveness of propranolol in hypertension disappeared.

Because studies had demonstrated that propranolol reduced cardiac output and ventricular contractility, investigators were hesitant to use propranolol in acute stages of myocardial infarction. However, based on reports that beta blockers brought about a more economical use of the available oxygen and suppressed or corrected certain types of arrhythmias, Snow (1965) used propranolol in the acute phase of myocardial infarction. Propranolol brought about a reduction in mortality and a lower incidence of recurrent cardiac pain. Snow recognized the significance of a reduced demand for oxygen and a more efficient utilization of available oxygen during the acute stage of myocardial infarction, and suggested that the risk of using propranolol was much less than had been feared. This concept was extremely slow in being accepted. Shand (1975) stated, "As of now, however, this approach must be considered experimental and further evaluation is required before its use can be recommended." However, Jewitt and Singh (1974), Mueller and Ayres (1977), Ross (1976), and, more recently, the β-Blocker Heart Attack Trial Research Group (1982) reported, *inter alia*, that propranolol was beneficial for the ischemic myocardium and that it could play an important role in treating acute myocardial infarction and in protecting the heart against further infarcts.

There have been many reviews and textbook treatments of the clinical history of propranolol (*see*, for example, Braunwald, 1966; Morrelli, 1973; Dollery and George, 1974; Nies and Shand, 1975, Hoffbrand, 1976; Lewis, 1976; Cruickshank and Prichard, 1987).

II. The Scientific Departure Leading to Propranolol: Dichloroisoproterenol (DCI)

Powell et al. (1956) reported on the screening of novel sympathomimetics in a search for a bronchodilator compound that was longer acting than epinephrine and more specific in its effect than ephedrine. Although a series of compounds related to epinephrine was synthesized and assayed by these investigators, the first compound of interest was the ortho monochloro analog of isoproterenol, isoprophenamine. This compound was an effective bronchodilator and was longer acting than epinephrine in relaxing pilocarpine-contracted bronchi isolated from the guinea pig. Powell and Slater (1958) noted that sometimes it was difficult to obtain complete relaxation with epinephrine after the tissue had been exposed to isoprophenamine. An additional group of phenylethylamines and phenylethanolamines with halogen substitutions on the phenyl rings were synthesized: 3'-chlorophenyl, 4'-chlorophenyl, 2',4'-dichlorophenyl, 2',5'-dichlorophenyl, and 3'4'-dichlorophenyl. All of these compounds, to varying degrees, prevented the complete relaxation of bronchi to epinephrine. 1-(3',4'-Dichlorophenyl)-2-isopropylaminoethanol (DCI), which was structurally very similar to isoproterenol (Fig. 1), exhibited unusual and interesting properties beyond those of isoprophenamine (Slater and Powell, 1957): it antagonized the spasmolytic action of epinephrine and isoproterenol on rabbit ileum; in anesthetized cats it enhanced the pressor response to epinephrine and antagonized the secondary depressor response to epinephrine; it reduced the depressor action of isoproterenol. The authors concluded that DCI did not seem to affect excitatory adrenergic sites, but probably combined with "certain inhibitory adrenergic receptor sites without having much physiological effect." Powell and Slater (1958) published their results with DCI in full and noted, *inter alia*, that in frog isolated heart, concentrations of DCI that blocked the inotropic and chronotropic effects of epinephrine also reduced both the force and rate of heart beat. They concluded that, "Because of the considerable decrease in heart rate and contractility... the specificity of this response remains in doubt." Powell and Slater (1958) saw DCI as a useful tool in the study of pharmacological problems related to adrenergic mechanisms. They felt that the postulated drug–receptor interaction of DCI had special relevance when considered in terms of drug–receptor theory, particularly as an example of the separation of affinity and intrinsic activity.

Moran and Perkins (1958) showed that DCI blocked the inotropic and chronotropic effects of adrenergic stimulation on the hearts of mammals—dogs and rabbits—but had no effect on the augmentation of contractile force brought about by cardiac glycosides, xanthines, and calcium chloride. They concluded, as suggested earlier

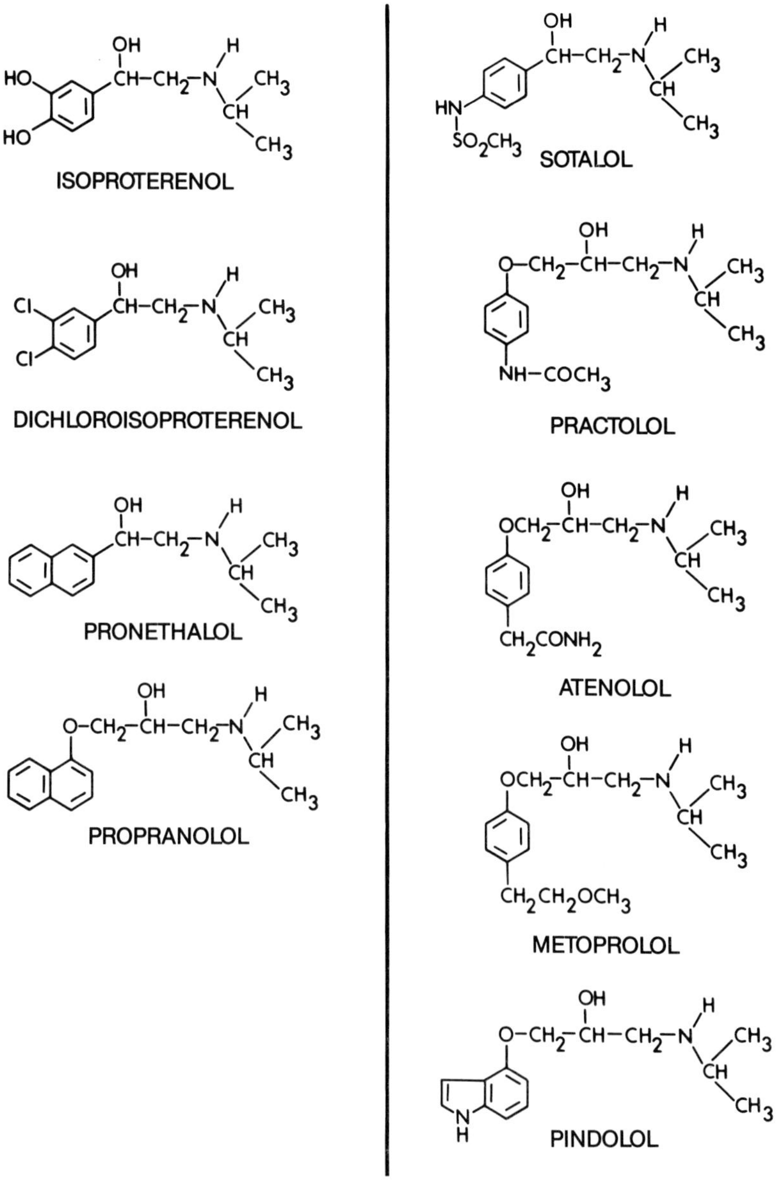

Fig. 1. The structures of propranolol and chemically and/or pharmacologically related substances.

by Ahlquist (1948), that cardiac adrenergic receptors were functionally homologous to the adrenergic-inhibitory receptors of other tissues. Moran and Perkins (1961) found no evidence that alpha-adrenergic blocking drugs antagonized the positive inotropic responses of mammalian heart to adrenergic stimuli, whereas DCI selectively blocked the inotropic response of the heart to adrenergic stimuli. DCI was labeled a beta-adrenergic blocking agent. Preliminary data (Moran and Perkins, 1958) indicated that DCI also inhibited the myocardial arrhythmogenic action of epinephrine and norepinephrine in the dog heart.

Moran and Perkins (1958), as well as other investigators, found DCI to have some stimulant activity (partial agonism or intrinsic sympathomimetic activity) in isolated hearts; furthermore, it was also noted to increase the heart rate of conscious and anesthetized dogs and cats.

Background Contributions Preceding DCI

The responses of organs and tissues to sympathetic stimulation and to sympathomimetic amines were known, on the basis of considerable work over decades, to fall into two broad categories—excitatory and inhibitory. Blockade of excitatory effects of pressor amines was reported for the ergot alkaloids (Dale, 1905) and for yohimbine (Hamet, 1925). In the 1930s and thereafter, synthetic agents, such as the benzodioxanes (Fourneau and Bovet, 1933), dibenamine (Nickerson and Goodman, 1947), and tolazoline (Chess and Yonkman, 1946), had been developed that selectively blocked most of the excitatory effects (a notable exception being cardiac stimulation). As late as the 1950s, however, there was no drug available that selectively blocked any of the inhibitory responses. Despite the absence of such an important pharmacological tool, Ahlquist (1948) suggested, as a consequence of his studies of the orders of potencies of a series of sympathomimetic amines in many tissues and organs, that there were only two kinds of adrenergic receptors, and dubbed them "alpha" and "beta." Alpha-receptor activation, he concluded, elicited the bulk of the excitatory effects and beta-receptor activation the inhibitory effects, with the controversial exception that cardiac excitation was evoked via a beta receptor.

Significant Events Following DCI

Black and Stephenson (1962) stated, "Since 1958 we have been trying to find an effective beta-receptor blocker which would be free from intrinsic sympathomimetic activity so that its possible therapeutic use could be explored in certain cardiac disorders...." They went on to describe a beta blocking agent that was free of intrinsic beta-agonist activity: pronethalol (nethalide). This agent can be viewed as DCI with the dichloro substitution in the phenyl ring replaced by a second phenyl ring, thereby producing a naphthalene ring system (Fig. 1). Pronethalol was the first beta blocking agent to become available after DCI. It reduced heart rate and the amplitude of inotropic responses to catecholamines, as well as creating some degree of bradycardia in animals. The authors hoped that pronethalol would be active enough to be used to block the effects of sympathetic nervous system excitation on atrial fibrillation and atrial and ventricular tachycardia. They also hoped that it could be of help to patients with angina pectoris by reducing myocardial demand for oxygen.

Clinical trials followed closely on the discovery of pronethalol. Dornhorst and Robinson (1962) showed that it decreased tachycardia of exercise in patients with angina pectoris. Alleyne et al. (1963) showed that pronethalol was effective in reducing both the number of attacks of pain and the consumption of glyceryl trinitrate tablets in patients with angina. Stock and Dale (1963), based on a limited number of patients, showed that pronethalol could have therapeutic value in cardiac arrhythmias. In atrial fibrillation it controlled ventricular rate, and when digitalis was used, the action of the two summated; also, it suppressed digitalis-induced arrhythmias. Prichard (1964) reported that pronethalol caused a considerable fall in blood pressure in anginal patients who had hypertension. No postural hypotension was observed. There was no consistent effect on blood pressure after intravenous administration; oral administration for a lengthy period was required to produce maximal hypotensive effect. Prichard (1964) concluded that, as a result of reports that pronethalol produced tumors in mice, this drug could no longer be used; however, he felt that a noncarcinogenic beta receptor blocking drug should be used in the treatment of hypertension.

Black et al. (1964) announced the development of a new beta blocking agent, propranolol. (These investigators noted that a large number of compounds were made and tested in an effort to find one with a wider therapeutic ratio than pronethalol and with no carcinogenic potential.) This new compound was structurally similar to pronethalol (Fig. 1) and had essentially the same pharmacological properties; however, its therapeutic ratio was ten times greater. Because propranolol was similar enough to pronethalol to be considered as an improved pronethalol, clinical studies were resumed with propranolol (*see* section I) where they had abruptly ended with the report of pronethalol's carcinogenic effect in mice.

Table 1 defines the critical scientific ideas and experiments leading to propranolol and categorizes their origin.

III. Comments on Events Leading to Propranolol

Black (1976) commented that, in the decade following the publication of Ahlquist's paper in 1948, Ahlquist's work was largely ignored. This is substantiated by the fact that only very passing mention of Ahlquist's work can be found in those chapters of the standard pharmacology reference (second edition) by Goodman and Gilman (1955) dealing with the autonomic nervous system, sympathomimetic drugs, and adrenergic blocking agents, although the fact that certain autonomic structures were stimulated by epinephrine and others were inhibited was clearly recognized. The terms "alpha" and "beta" do not appear as modifiers of the terms "adrenergic drugs" or "adrenergic blocking drugs," nor do they appear in the index. However, in the third edition (Goodman and Gilman, 1965) the terms "adrenergic receptors, alpha and beta types" as well as "alpha- (and beta-) adrenergic blocking agents" appear in the index. Ahlquist's theory is also given prominent discussion. The discovery of DCI was important in that, as the first selective antagonist of adrenergic-inhibitory responses, its use in concert with already available agents for blocking excitatory responses allowed notions about the nature of adrenergic receptors to be rigorously explored. This included the proof by Moran and Perk-

Table 1
Profile of Observations and Ideas Crucial to the Development of Propranolol[a]

Sequence: Departure compound* to innovative drug**	Orient- ation	Nature of study	Research institution	National origin	Nature of discovery	Screening involved	Crucial ideas or observations
DCI*							
Powell et al. (1956)	Pre- clinical	Pharma- cology/ chemistry	Indus- try	USA	Seren- dipitous	Targeted, untar- geted	The bronchodilator monochloro analog of isoproterenol, isoprophenamine, suppresses the bronchodilating action of epinephrine.
Powell and Slater (1958)	Pre- clinical	Chem- istry/ pharma- cology	Indus- try	USA	Orderly	Targeted	The dichloro analog of isoproterenol, DCI, blocks inhibi- tory adrenergic sites.
Moran and Perkins (1958)	Pre- clinical	Pharma- cology	Univer- sity	USA	Orderly	No	DCI selectively blocks adrenergic stimulation of the heart.
Pronethalol							
Black and Stephenson (1962)	Pre- clinical	Chem- istry/ pharma- cology	Indus- try	UK	Orderly	Targeted	A DCI analog, pronethalol, devel- oped; a beta blocker without intrinsic activity; potential for control of tachy- cardia and angina recognized (eventu- ally proved to be toxic).
Propranolol**							
Black et al. (1964)	Pre- clinical	Chem- istry/ pharma- cology	Indus- try	UK	Orderly	Targeted	A pronethalol ana- log, propranolol, developed.

*Taken from section II. Entries are those contributions without which the discovery of the agent (or additionally, in some cases, a relevant clinical application) would not have taken place or would have been materially delayed.

ins (1958) that excitatory adrenergic cardiac receptors were, indeed, beta in nature. At the same time, this proof of the beta nature of car- diac receptors, and the availability of a beta blocking agent, initiated a program of chemical synthesis that would eventually lead to a clinically useful beta blocking agent, propranolol.

Black (1976) emphasized that his work begun in 1958 would not have started but for the existence of Ahlquist's theory and, also, that "Powell and Slater's elegant use in 1958 of Ahlquist's hypothesis to classify the pharmacological properties of dichloroisoproterenol provided the turning point and the rapid acceptance of the idea of a dual receptor mechanism." Interestingly, Powell and Slater (1958) did not mention Ahlquist's theory but, as already noted, only referred to the empirically determined and commonly accepted notion of adrenergic inhibitory and excitatory sites, and instead mentioned the theories of Ariens (1954) and Stephenson (1956) concerning affinity and intrinsic activity. Somewhat later, Slater and Powell (1959) commented that, "the data [with DCI] seem to add support for the Ahlquist concept of alpha- and beta-adrenergic receptors...."

Shanks (1966, 1984) noted that Black (reference to personal communication) had the idea in the mid-1950s that it might be useful to try to reduce the myocardial demand for oxygen by blocking the action of adrenaline, and of sympathetic neuron activity, on the heart. According to Shanks (1984), Black was able to develop his ideas after moving from academia to Imperial Chemical Industries (ICI) in 1958. Shanks (1976) was of the opinion that the clinical significance of the discovery of DCI in 1958 was apparently recognized by very few people. This author felt that Black "...appreciated that DCI was the type of drug for which he was looking..." but, because of its partial agonist activity, he felt that he had to develop a similar drug devoid of this property. Cruickshank and Prichard (1987) seconded this point of view regarding Black's attitude toward DCI and felt that "[t]he major contribution of Black was to appreciate the possible clinical value of developing compounds to inhibit the sympathetic to the heart, and to then persuade, and then lead a team of scientists at ICI to translate the idea into reality." For his work leading to the discoveries of propranolol and cimetidine, Black shared in the 1988 Nobel Prize in Medicine.

As commented recently by Frishman (1984), "Twenty-five years ago the first beta adrenergic blocking drug dichloroisoprenaline (DCI) was synthesized....The finding that DCI selectively blocked... beta receptors has proven to be one of the most significant advances in human pharmacotherapy."

IV. Developments
Subsequent to Propranolol

DCI established the chemical basis for the progression to pronetholol and propranolol and beyond. Today there are 20 beta-blocking agents marketed worldwide; nine are available in the USA. The structures of several significant beta blocking agents developed subsequently to propranolol are shown in the right-hand column of Fig. 1.

A few years after its introduction, pronetholol was discovered to have local anesthetic activity (Vaughan Williams and Sekiya, 1963; Gill and Vaughan Williams, 1964) as was, later, propranolol as well. According to Shanks (1984), the Mead Johnson Co. had developed a new beta blocking agent, sotalol, in the early 1960s. Although this agent resembled DCI pharmacologically, it had no local anesthetic activity. Sotalol, and several novel derivatives of it, were then prepared at ICI (Shanks, 1984). The end result of this effort was ICI 50172. This compound, given the name practolol (Fig. 1), was devoid of local anesthetic activity but, more important, Dunlop and Shanks (1968) also reported that this compound was cardioselective in that it blocked beta receptors in the heart, but not those in the smooth muscle of blood vessels or of the respiratory tract.

During the same time-period that sotalol and practolol were evolving, a growing number of studies had emerged that showed some, but not all, beta receptor sites could be blocked with the blocking agents then available (Levy, 1964, 1966a,b). These observations suggested that beta receptors were not a homogeneous group and that there might be subgroups. Finally, Lands (1967), on the basis of his studies of the effects of a series of agonists on a number of organ systems, designated these subgroups "beta$_1$" and "beta$_2$." By this designation, practolol had selectivity for beta$_1$ over beta$_2$ receptors. Unfortunately, this drug eventually had to be withdrawn from clinical use because of toxicity. Atenolol and metoprolol, which are currently available, are relatively cardioselective drugs (Fig. 1). They have less tendency than propranolol to exacerbate asthmatic conditions or to aggravate vascular insufficiency.

Another property exhibited by some recently developed beta blockers is partial agonism. DCI, as already mentioned, exhibited this property, which was viewed at the time as a drawback. Black and Stephenson (1962) had labored to develop pronetholol because the intrinsic activity of DCI was considered to make it unacceptable for clinical use. Recently, beta blockers have again been developed that show partial agonism, e.g., pindolol. It has been suggested that, under certain circumstances (for example, in patients with severe bradycardia, asthma, or cardiac failure), some beta-receptor stimulation could be beneficial, although there is still much debate whether partial agonism is a therapeutic advantage or disadvantage (Frishman and Kostis, 1982).

References

Ahlquist, R. P.: A study of the adrenotropic receptors. *Am. J. Physiol.* **153:** 586–600, 1948.

Alleyne, G. A. O., Dickinson, C. J., Dornhorst, A. C., Fulton, R. M., Green, K. G., Hill, I. D., Hurst, P., Laurance, D. R., Pilkington, T., Prichard, B. N. C., Robinson, B. and Rosenheim, M. L.: Effect of pronethalol in angina pectoris. *Br. Med. J.* **2:** 1226,1227, 1963.

Ariens, E. J.: Affinity and intrinsic activity in the theory of competitive inhibition. Part I. Problems and theory. *Arch. Int. Pharmacodyn.* **99:** 32–49, 1954.

Bennett, D. R., ed.: *AMA Drug Evaluations,* 5th Ed., American Medical Association, Chicago, 1983.

Berkow, R., ed.: *Merck Manual,* Merck Sharp & Dohme Research Laboratories, Rahway, NJ, 1982.

β-Blocker Heart Attack Trial Research Group: A randomized trial of propranolol in patients with acute myocardial infarction: 1. Mortality results. *JAMA* **247:** 1707–1714, 1982.

Bigger, J. T. and Hoffman, B. F.: Antiarrhythmic drugs, in *The Pharmacological Basis of Therapeutics,* 7th Ed., A. G. Gilman, L. S. Goodman, T. W. Rall, and F. Murad, eds., pp. 748–805, Macmillan, New York, 1985.

Black, J. W.: Ahlquist and the development of beta-adrenoceptor antagonists. *Postgrad. Med. J.* **52:** (Suppl. 4) 11–13, 1976.

Black, J. W. and Stephenson, J. S.: Pharmacology of a new adrenergic beta-receptor-blocking compound (Nethalide). *Lancet* **2:** 311–314, 1962.

Black, J. W., Crowther, A. F., Shanks, R. G., Smith, L. H., and Dornhorst, A. C.: A new adrenergic beta-receptor antagonist. *Lancet* **1**: 1080,1081, 1964.

Braunwald, E., ed.: Symposium on beta adrenergic receptor blockade. *Am. J. Cardiol.* **18**: 303–459, 1966.

Chess, D. and Yonkman, F. F.: Adrenolytic and sympatholytic actions of priscol (benzyl-imidazoline). *Proc. Soc. Exp. Biol. Med.* **61**: 127–130, 1946.

Cruickshank, J. M. and Prichard, B. N. C.: *Beta-blockers in Clinical Practice*, Churchill Livingstone, Edinburgh, 1987.

Dale, H. H.: The physiological action of chrysotoxin. *J. Physiol.* (London) **32**: lviii–lx, 1905.

Dollery, C. T. and George, C.: Propranolol—ten years from introduction. Cardiovascular drug therapy, in *Cardiovascular Clinics*, K. L. Melmon, ed., pp. 255–268, Davis, Philadelphia, 1974.

Dornhorst, A. C. and Robinson, B. F.: Clinical pharmacology of a beta-adrenergic-blocking agent (Nethalide). *Lancet* **2**: 314–316, 1962.

Dunlop, D. and Shanks, R. G.: Selective blockade of adrenoceptive beta receptors in the heart. *Br. J. Pharm. Chemother.* **32**: 201–218, 1968.

Fourneau, E. and Bovet, D.: Recherches sur l'action sympathicolytique d'un nouveau dérivé du dioxane. *Arch. Int. Pharmacodyn.* **46**: 178–191, 1933.

Frishman, W. H.: *Clinical Pharmacology of the Beta-Adrenoceptor Blocking Agents*, 2nd Ed., Appleton-Century-Crofts, Norwalk, Connecticut, 1984.

Frishman, W. H. and Kostis, J.: The significance of intrinsic sympathomimetic activity in beta-adrenoceptor blocking drugs. *Cardiovasc. Rev. Reports* **3**: 503–512, 1982.

Frishman, W. H., Furberg, C. D., and Friedewald, W. T.: β-Adrenergic blockade for survivors of acute myocardial infarction. *N. Engl. J. Med.* **310**: 830–837, 1984.

Gill, E. and Vaughan Williams, E. M.: Local anaesthetic activity of the beta-receptor antagonist, pronethalol. *Nature* **201**: 199, 1964.

Gillam, P. M. S. and Prichard, B. N. C.: Use of propranolol in angina pectoris. *Br. Med. J.* **2**: 337–339, 1965.

Gillam, P. M. S. and Prichard, B. N. C.: Discovery of the hypotensive effect of propranolol. *Postgrad. Med. J.* **52**: (Suppl. 4): 70–75, 1976.

Goodman, L. S. and Gilman, A., eds.: *The Pharmacological Basis of Therapeutics*. 2nd Ed., Macmillan, New York, 1955.

Goodman, L. S. and Gilman, A., eds.: *The Pharmacological Basis of Therapeutics*. 3rd Ed., Macmillan, New York, 1965.

Hamer, J., Grandjean, T., Melendez, L. and Sowton, G. E.: Effect of propranolol (Inderal) in angina pectoris: Preliminary report. *Br. Med. J.* **2:** 720–723, 1964.

Hamet, R.: Sur un nouveau cas de'inversion des effets adrénaliniques. *Compt. Rendu.* **180:** 2074–2077, 1925.

Hoffbrand, B. I., ed.: Ten years of propranolol. *Postgrad. Med. J.* **52:** (Suppl. 4), 1–192, 1976.

Jewitt, D. E. and Singh, B. N.: The role of beta-adrenergic blockade in myocardial infarction. *Prog. Cardiovasc. Dis.* **16:** 421–438, 1974.

Lampe, K. F., ed.: *Drug Evaluations,* 6th Ed., American Medical Association, Chicago, 1986.

Lands, A. M., Arnold, A., McAuliff, J. P., Luduena, F. P., and Brown, T. G.: Differentiation of receptor systems activated by sympathomimetic amines. *Nature* **214:** 597,598, 1967.

Levy, B.: Alterations of adrenergic responses by *N*-isopropyl-methoxamine. *J. Pharmacol. Exp. Ther.* **146:** 129–138, 1964.

Levy, B.: The adrenergic blocking activity of *N*-tert-butylmethoxamine (butoxamine). *J. Pharmacol. Exp. Ther.* **151:** 413–422, 1966a.

Levy, B.: Dimethylisopropylmethoxamine: A selective beta-receptor blocking agent. *Br. J. Pharm. Chemother.* **27:** 277–285, 1966b.

Lewis, P.: The essential action of propranolol in hypertension. *Am. J. Med.* **60:** 837–852, 1976.

Lorimer, A. R.: Medical management, in *Angina Pectoris,* D. G. Julian, ed., pp. 164–187, Churchill Livingstone, Edinburgh, 1985.

Moran, N. C. and Perkins, M. E.: Adrenergic blockade of the mammalian heart by a dichloro analogue of isoproterenol. *J. Pharmacol. Exp. Ther.* **124:** 223–237, 1958.

Moran, N. C. and Perkins, M. E.: An evaluation of adrenergic blockade of the mammalian heart. *J. Pharmacol Exp. Ther.* **133:** 192–201, 1961.

Morrelli, H. F.: Propranolol. Diagnosis and treatment drugs: Five years later. *Ann. Intern. Med.* **78:** 913–917, 1973.

Mueller, H. S. and Ayres, S. M.: The role of propranolol in the treatment of acute myocardial infarction. *Prog. Cardiovasc. Dis.* **19:** 405–412, 1977.

Nickerson, M. and Goodman, L.: Pharmacological properties of a new adrenergic blocking agent: *N,N*-dibenzyl-b-chloroethylamine (dibenamine). *J. Pharmacol. Exp. Ther.* **89:** 167–185, 1947.

Nies, A. S. and Shand, D. G.: Clinical pharmacology of propranolol. *Circulation,* **52:** 6–15, 1975.

Powell, C. E. and Slater, I. H.: Blocking of inhibitory adrenergic receptors by a dichloro analog of isoproterenol. *J. Pharmacol. Exp. Ther.* **122:** 480– 488, 1958.

Powell, C. E., Gibson, W. R., and Swanson, E. E.: The pharmacological action of l-0-chlorophenyl-2-isopropylaminoethanol (isoprophenamine) a bronchodilator. *J. Am. Pharm. Assoc.* **45:** 785–787, 1956.

Prichard, B. N. C.: Hypotensive action of pronethalol. *Br. Med. J.* **1:** 1227, 1228, 1964.

Prichard, B. N. C. and Gillam, P. M. S.: Use of propranolol (Inderal) in treatment of hypertension. *Br. Med. J.* **2:** 725–727, 1964.

Ross, Jr., J.: Beta adrenergic blockade for prophylaxis against recurrent myocardial infarction and sudden death. *Ann. Intern. Med.* **84:** 486, 487, 1976.

Schultz, H. W.: Beta-adrenergic blocking agents. *Pharm Index* **April:** 8–15, 1983.

Shand, D. G.: Propranolol. *N. Engl. J. Med.* **293:** 280–285, 1975.

Shanks, R. G. : The pharmacology of beta sympathetic blockade. *Am. J. Cardiol.* **18:** 308–316, 1966.

Shanks, R. G.: The properties of beta-adrenoceptor antagonists. *Postgrad. Med. J.* **52:** (Suppl. 4), 14–20, 1976.

Shanks, R. G.: The discovery of beta-adrenoceptor blocking drugs. *Trends Pharmacol.* **5:** 405–409, 1984.

Slater, I. H. and Powell, C. E.: Blockade of adrenergic inhibitory receptor sites by 1-(3',4'-dichlorophenyl)-2-isopropylaminoethanol hydrochloride. *Fed. Proc.* **16:** 336, 1957.

Slater, I. H. and Powell, C. E.: Some aspects of blockade of inhibitory adrenergic receptors or adrenoceptive sites. *Pharmacol. Rev.* **7:** 462,463, 1959.

Snow, P. J. D.: Effect of propranolol in myocardial infarction. *Lancet* **2:** 551–553, 1965.

Stephenson, R. P.: A modification of receptor theory. *Br. J. Pharmacol.* **11:** 379–393, 1956.

Stock, J. P. P. and Dale, N.: Beta-adrenergic receptor blockade in cardiac arrhythmias. *Br. Med. J.* **2:** 1230–1233, 1963.

Vaughan Williams, E. M. and Sekiya, A.: Prevention of arrhythmias due to cardiac glycosides by block of sympathetic beta receptors. *Lancet* **1:** 420,421, 1963.

Weiner, N.: Drugs that inhibit adrenergic nerves and block adrenergic receptors, in *The Pharmacological Basis of Therapeutics*, 7th Ed., A. G. Gilman, L. S. Goodman, T. W. Rall, and F. Murad, eds., pp. 181–214, Macmillan, New York, 1985.

Captopril

I. Captopril as an Innovative Therapeutic Agent

Captopril was the first inhibitor of angiotensin-converting enzyme (ACE) to be effective by the oral route. ACE catalyzes the conversion of angiotensin I, a weakly active product of renin activity, to angiotensin II, a potent vasoconstrictor agent and stimulator of aldosterone secretion (Fig. 1). It is generally agreed that captopril represents a significant therapeutic advance as well as a tool for defining the control mechanisms for sodium balance, extracellular volume maintenance, and blood-pressure regulation. Moreover, some clinicians believe that it is the most significant advance yet in the diagnosis and management of hypertension (Laragh, 1984).

In 1981, the FDA approved the use of captopril in patients who did not respond to other forms of therapy, in patients who had severe or advanced cases of hypertension, and in patients on multidrug regimens consisting of beta blockers, diuretics, and vasodilators (Ferguson and Vlasses, 1981). In view of the occurrence of frequent side effects, including renal toxicity and neutropenia, captopril was not approved for use in mild or moderate hypertension. However, with additional clinical experience, it became evident that the drug doses being given were too high and that the drug was effective at lower doses with consequent minimalization of side effects. Some studies (e.g., Heel et al., 1980) have shown that patients taking captopril alone did as well as those on a standard multidrug regimen. Captopril can be as effective as beta blockers (or other drugs interfering with sympathetic control) in lowering blood pressure, but has practically no CNS side effects, does not cause impotence, and can be used in patients with congestive heart failure,

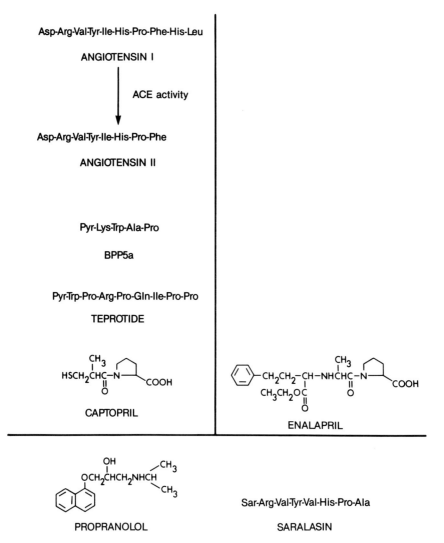

Fig. 1. The structures of captopril and chemically and/or pharmacologically related substances.

coronary insufficiency, diabetes, and asthma. Unlike diuretics, captopril does not cause hypokalemia or hyperuricemia. For patients who are on joint captopril and diuretic therapy, captopril potentiates the action of the diuretic and prevents hypokalemia; hence, potassium supplements are not necessary. Patients taking captopril have a feeling of well-being that Laragh (1984) attributes to captopril improving blood flow to vital organs. Other investigators attribute some of the sense of well-being to the discontinuance of the antihypertensive drugs that had heretofore been sustaining the patients.

Captopril has also made an important contribution to our understanding of hypertension. A single dose of this drug is used for a fast evaluation of the renin profile; depending on the response to captopril, the physician can choose the course of antihypertensive therapy necessary (Laragh, 1984; Müller et al., 1986). All forms of hypertension that result from increased activity of the renin–angiotensin system, such as malignant and renovascular hypertension, respond well to captopril (Ferguson and Vlasses, 1981).

A more recent FDA-approved use for captopril is in the treatment of chronic congestive heart failure (Ferguson et al., 1984). Patients with severe or drug-resistant heart failure show improved cardiac performance and decreased myocardial oxygen consumption (Romankiewicz et al., 1983).

Early Clinical Research History

Much of the early clinical work that defined ACE inhibition in humans was done with the peptide teprotide. Teprotide is a clinically effective drug for lowering blood pressure; however, because it is not effective by the oral route, its use is limited. This compound will be discussed in a later section.

Initial clinical trials with captopril were conducted by Ferguson et al. (1977). They used the drug in 14 normal male volunteers. Blood pressure was elevated by the administration of angiotensin I. Fifteen minutes after an oral dose of captopril, the blood-pressure response to angiotensin I was antagonized with no adverse side effects. There was no effect on the pressor response to angiotensin II. Ferguson and coworkers concluded that, "SQ 14,225 [captopril] represents an advance in the development of specific inhibitors of the renin–angiotensin system. It offers the advantage of safety, potency and oral efficacy." Gavras et al. (1978), who had also done clinical trials with teprotide, used captopril in 12 hypertensive patients. They noted a maximal decrease in blood pressure in patients, all of whom had been "...refractory to usual medical treatment in the past." The drug had excellent antihypertensive effects, and it was considered that an inhibitor of ACE that was suitable for long-term oral treatment of hypertension appeared to have an excellent therapeutic potential. Numerous clinical trials followed: Case et al. (1978), Brunner et al. (1979, 1980), Swales et al. (1982), Vlasses et al. (1982b), Drayer and Weber (1983), and Groel et al. (1983) are examples. Although captopril is a relatively new drug, a very large number of articles have been published concerning its development, therapeutic uses, and mode of action (see, for example, Atkinson and Robertson (1979), Ferguson and Vlasses (1981), Vidt et al. (1982), Vlasses et al. (1982a,b), Antonaccio (1982), Cohn and Levine (1982), Johnston et al. (1984), Williams (1988), Gavras (1988).

II. The Scientific Departure
Leading to Captopril: Teprotide

Ferreira and Rocha e Silva (1962) sought to prevent the rapid degradation of the peptide bradykinin in their experiments. Since Erdös (1962) had suggested that a carboxypeptidase, or an enzyme similar to it, was responsible for the rapid breakdown of bradykinin, Ferreira and Rocha e Silva (1962) used several metal binding agents that were known to inhibit carboxypeptidases by binding to their functional zinc atom. Bradykinin was potentiated by these agents, and its degradation was prevented. Subsequently, Ferreira (1965), while studying the effect of these metal chelating agents on endogenous bradykinin released from tissues by the venom of the Brazilian snake, *Bothrops jararaca*, discovered serendipitously that the venom itself potentiated the effect of bradykinin on guinea pig ileum. This finding prompted the partial purification of the bradykinin potentiating factor (BPF). The hypotensive effects of bradykinin were potentiated by BPF in dogs and cats.

Ferreira and Vane (1967) studied the disappearance of bradykinin in the pulmonary circulation and in other vascular beds. At the same time Ng and Vane (1967) were comparing the conversion rate of angiotensin I to angiotensin II in the blood with that in the pulmonary circulation. The results indicated that the lung and the pulmonary circulation were the most important sites for both biotransformations. With further experiments, Ng and Vane (1968) suggested that it was "...possible that the inactivation of bradykinin and the formation of angiotensin II from angiotensin I in the lungs were caused by the same enzyme." They speculated that the pulmonary enzyme was not an endopeptidase, but a carboxypeptidase. Bakhle (1968), working in Vane's laboratory, found that BPF made by Ferreira from *Bothrops* venom was a competitive inhibitor of converting enzyme from dog lung and that it also protected bradykinin against inactivation.

Ferreira et al. (1970b) isolated 22 fractions from *Bothrops jararaca* venom and tested each as an inhibitor of ACE, using rat colon, and as an inhibitor of bradykininase, using guinea pig ileum. In general, the fractions that were potent inhibitors of ACE were also potent potentiators of bradykinin. Fraction IV-1-D was the most potent. Nine biologically active peptides were isolated, and their amino acid compositions were determined. The amino acid sequence of the smallest peptide was determined, and this peptide was synthesized (Ferreira et al., 1970a). This was Bradykinin-Potentiating Peptide 5a (BPP5a) (Fig. 1). All nine peptides potentiated the action of bradykinin on guinea pig ileum, and they also inhibited the actions of partially purified ACE from dog lung. BPP5a decreased the pulmonary destruction of bradykinin and potentiated the hypotensive effects of injected bradykinin as well. Both of these actions were of short duration. BPP5a was also tested in several other systems (Stewart et al., 1971). It had little or no hypotensive effect in dogs, cats, or rabbits, but potentiated the hypotension evoked by bradykinin in all three species. When administered to rats in vivo, increasing amounts of angiotensin I were required in order to obtain a standard pressor response, indicating that the converting enzyme was being inhibited. Krieger et al. (1971) found that BPP5a produced hypotension in those hypertensive rats in which the angiotensin system was likely to be overactive.

Ondetti et al. (1971) independently followed up on the report of Bakhle (1968) that BPF blocked ACE. These authors reported the isolation from *Bothrops* venom of the peptides that were inhibiting the renin–angiotensin system. Six peptides were isolated, and their amino acid sequences were identified. All of these peptides were synthesized. The properties of the natural and synthetic peptides were the same, and they were similar or identical to the bradykinin-potentiating peptides reported by Ferreira (1970a,b). Ondetti et al. (1971) observed that the peptides with longer amino acid chains were potent as well as longer acting. Bakhle (1971) tested three of these peptides and reported that SQ 20, 881 was the most potent in inhibiting ACE of dog lung and of superfused guinea pig lung. SQ 20,881 was similar to Ferreira's fraction IV-1-D and eventually was named teprotide (Fig. 1). Engel et al. (1972, 1973) studied Ondetti's six peptides as well as SQ 20,475 (BPP5a) in different models of renovascular hypertension. SQ 20,881 was more effective in lowering blood pressure than SQ 20,475. Collier et al. (1973) administered teprotide to six male volunteers. A single intravenous dose reduced blood pressure that had been elevated by angiotensin I, but did not consistently alter the effects of angiotensin II. It was concluded that the new drug could be useful in elucidating the causes of hypertension as well as in its treatment. Gavras et al. (1974), Johnson et al. (1975), Case et al. (1977), and Williams and Hollenberg (1977) tested teprotide in hypertensive patients. The drug proved to be an excellent antihypertensive; safe, specific, fast-acting, and free of any observable toxicity. However, the usefulness of teprotide was limited because it was not active by the oral route.

Background Contributions Preceding Teprotide

Rocha e Silva et al. (1949) discovered the peptide bradykinin while studying the physiological actions of snake venoms, including that of *Bothrops jararaca*. Snake poisoning was known to produce a fall in blood pressure, shock, and frequently as a sequela, death. Bradykinin was found to be the vascularly active agent released from blood and from tissues by snake venoms, and Rocha e Silva suggested that it could be responsible for the observed symptoms. Ferreira's serendipitous discovery of the bradykinin-potentiating factor of *Bothrops jararaca* venom, as described earlier, occurred in Rocha e Silva's laboratory (Ferreira and Rocha e Silva, 1962).

The concept that oversecretion of renin (the enzymatic activity of which releases angiotensin I from angiotensinogen) could be the cause of human hypertension was the contribution of Goldblatt and associates (1934,1948) and was extensively explored by Braun-

Menendez and by Page and their associates in the succeeding decades (e.g., Page, 1939,1951; Braun-Menendez et al., 1940; Braun-Menendez and Page, 1958; Page and Bumpus, 1961; Page et al., 1965).

ACE was discovered by Skeggs et al. in 1954. They showed that hypertensin I (now known as angiotensin I) was rapidly converted to hypertensin II (now angiotensin II) and that the enzyme for this conversion was in the plasma. They also concluded that either or both hypertensins were important in hypertension, because both hypertensins elevated blood pressure when injected into volunteers. Helmer (1955,1957) reported that rabbit aortic strips responded to hypertensin II, but not to I. Skeggs et al. (1956) found that hypertensin I only became pressor after interacting with the converting enzyme.

Significant Work Following Teprotide

Cushman and Cheung (1971) devised a simple spectrophotometric assay for ACE. This assay was more reliable than the methods used before that time. Their experiments indicated that ACE (from rabbit lung) was a chloride ion activated metalloenzyme—a dipeptidyl carboxypeptidase—and that zinc was probably the metal ion involved. Cushman et al. (1973) carried out structure–activity studies with the *Bothrops jararaca* peptides and analogs. They concluded that peptidal inhibitors from venom bind to at least two sites on the ACE: competitively at the active site for substrates (that is, at the c-terminal tripeptide) and, in addition, at a site removed from the active site. The venom peptides were bound at least 50-fold more tightly to ACE than were their c-terminal tripeptide fragments, indicating that very significant binding occurred away from the active site.

In the six-year interval from the development of teprotide (SQ 20,881) by Ondetti et al. (1971) to the initial report on captopril (SQ 14,225) (Ondetti et al., 1977; Cushman et al., 1977), many nonpeptidic compounds were tested by these investigators, but only a small fraction were potent and very few were specific. In 1973, Byers and Wolfenden discovered that L-benzylsuccinic acid was a potent, competitive inhibitor of bovine carboxypeptidase A. Ondetti et al. (1977)

found that succinyl L-proline was a weak inhibitor of ACE. They proceeded to explore the length and substitution of the acyl moiety. Methyl substitution in the succinyl group enhanced potency approximately tenfold. Replacement of the succinyl carboxyl with a mercapto group increased potency very considerably (approximately 2400-fold). Ondetti and coworkers (1977) rationalized their work with a model for a three-point attachment to the active site of ACE—based on analogy to the active site of bovine carboxypeptidase that had been developed by Byers and Wolfenden (1973) with L-benzylsuccinic acid. The most potent compound was eventually given the name captopril. It was tested on guinea pig ileum to show inhibition of angiotensin I and potentiation of bradykinin, as well as in two animal models of hypertension. Oral administration produced moderate to maximal lowering of blood pressure. Ondetti et al. (1977) and Cushman et al. (1977) felt that their approach had led to the development of an antihypertensive agent that could have great potential in therapeutics.

Table 1 defines the critical scientific ideas and experiments leading to captopril and categorizes their origin.

III. Comments on Events Leading to Captopril

Laragh (1984) considered the converting enzyme inhibitors to be "...one of the landmark discoveries for understanding and treatment of hypertension." He placed captopril within a broader framework. It was the most specific and useful of the small group of compounds that had been identified as being both antihypertensive and capable of blocking the activity of the renin system: propranolol, saralasin, and teprotide (Fig. 1). Propranolol and saralasin, although able to inhibit the renin system, had many other cardiovascular and CNS actions, or partial agonist activities, respectively, that marred their clinical usefulness and their conceptual value. Laragh felt that the conceptual value of ACE inhibitors is that they provide the rationale for their clinical use. Response or lack of response to these agents has diagnostic and, perhaps, nosological value. From a practical standpoint, these agents enable the physician "...to lower blood pressure with a single agent and, at the same time, increase blood flow to the heart, brain, and kidneys, and

Table 1
Profile of Observations and Ideas Crucial to the Development of Captopril[a]

Sequence: Departure compound* to innovative drug**	Orient- ation	Nature of study	Research institution	National origin	Nature of discovery	Screening involved	Crucial ideas or observations
Teprotide*							
Ferreira (1965)	Pre- clinical	Pharma- cology	Uni- versity	Brazil	Seren- dipitous	No	Snake venom (BPF) potentiates bradykinin.
Ferreira and Vane (1967)	Pre- clinical	Physi- ology	Uni- versity	UK	Orderly	No	Lung circulation most important site to inactivate brady- kinin.
Ng and Vane (1967)	Pre- clinical	Physi- ology	Uni- versity	UK	Orderly	No	Lung circulation most important to activate angiotensin I.
Ng and Vane (1968)	Pre- clinical	Physi- ology	Uni- versity	UK	Orderly	No	Possible that same enzyme inactivates bradykinin and acti- vates angiotensin I.
Bakhle (1968)	Pre- clinical	Bio- chem- istry	Uni- versity	UK	Orderly	No	BPF inhibits ACE and protects bradykinin from inactivation in vitro.
Ondetti et al. (1971)	Pre- clinical	Chem- istry/ pharma- cology	Industry	USA	Orderly	Targeted	Teprotide and other peptidal inhibitors of the renin-angiotensin system are isolated from BPF, sequenced, and synthesized.
Captopril**							
Byers and Wolfenden (1973)	Pre- clinical	Biochem- istry	Uni- versity	USA	Orderly	Targeted	L-Benzylsuccinic acid inhibits carboxypep- tidase A; model for attachment proposed.
Ondetti et al. (1977)	Pre- clinical	Chem- istry/ pharma- cology	Industry	USA	Orderly	Untar- geted, targeted	Captopril synthe- sized.

[a]Taken from section II. Entries are those contributions without which the discovery of the agent (or additionally, in some cases, a relevant clinical application) would not have taken place or would have been materially delayed.

probably to all tissues, including the skeletal muscle." Laragh's group started acquiring ACE inhibitors from Ondetti in 1972 for animal and clinical studies. There was so much doubt that these agents could have any value as drugs that no fiscal support was offered for Laragh's studies. Because of the negative opinions, their group was the only group to request these drugs (including teprotide) for experimentation for three or four years (Laragh, 1984) and the only group to evaluate and demonstrate their effectiveness in human hypertension (Gavras et al., 1974; Case et al., 1976,1977).

The degree of the scientific community's lack of acceptance of ACE inhibitors was reflected in an article by Gross (1982). He stated that seven years earlier, in predicting future ways of controlling hypertension, he did not even mention the possibility of using drugs to interfere with the renin–angiotensin system. This exclusion was based on the facts that an antagonist of angiotensin II (saralasin) was not very effective and teprotide was not orally active, and on the belief, past and present, that the renin–angiotensin system had little, if any, significance in the pathogenesis of essential hypertension.

Clinically, the peptidal ACE inhibitors were used by Laragh's group in 89 patients with essential hypertension (Case et al., 1977; Laragh, 1984). The drugs were used effectively for identification and quantification of the renin factor in essential hypertension. According to Laragh, on the strength of his findings, Ondetti and Cushman went ahead with the search for an analog of teprotide that was active by the oral route.

IV. Developments Subsequent to Captopril

Cushman et al. (1982), in a symposium on ACE inhibitors, stated that "...captopril is a very simple chemical structure with at least five well-defined chemical interactions with the active site of ACE." The interaction of the sulfhydryl group of captopril with the enzyme-bound zinc ion contributes greatly to its overall enzyme-binding affinity. However, captopril does not incorporate all the possible competitive interactions, making possible the development of many more drugs. To date this has involved varying the amino acid backbone or substituting the sulfhydryl group, which has led to the development of numerous compounds at various stages of development (Materson, 1984).

Certain side effects of captopril, for example, rashes and loss of taste, are similar to side effects of penicillamine. This suggested to Patchett et al. (1980) that perhaps the sulfhydryl group common to both drugs was responsible. They worked on developing compounds that lacked a mercapto function and that were weak chelating agents. Enalapril (Fig. 1) emerged from this effort. It has the following advantages over captopril: less incidence of rashes and taste disturbances, better absorption, and, perhaps, longer action (Davies et al., 1984).

Many analogs of captopril, and especially of enalapril, have been synthesized in the hopes of improving upon these two agents (Brunner et al., 1985; Kostis, 1989). Williams (1988) noted that 16 such agents appeared in the literature between 1983 and 1987, and found that the most widely mentioned, besides captopril and enalapril, were lisinopril, pentopril, ramipril, and alacepril. A bright future was predicted for ACE inhibitors by Edwards and Padfield (1985): they will be more extensively prescribed for patients with less severe forms of hypertension as their side effects are better understood, and because the euphoria and feeling of well-being that ACE inhibitors produce is probably not from any central actions, but from stopping other drugs.

Kostis (1989) noted that ACE is present, and may have functional significance, in many tissues, e.g., blood vessels, brain, heart, kidney, testis, and adrenals. The synthesis of a large number of ACE inhibitors, some with differing patterns of tissue distribution, is providing tools that may be useful in elucidating such functional significance (Cushman et al., 1989).

References

Antonaccio, M.-J.: Angiotensin converting enzyme (ACE) inhibitors. *Annu. Rev. Pharmacol. Toxicol.* **22:** 57–87, 1982.

Atkinson, A. B. and Robertson, J. I. S.: Captopril in the treatment of clinical hypertension and cardiac failure. *Lancet* **2:** 836–839, 1979.

Bakhle, Y. S.: Conversion of angiotensin I to angiotensin II by cell-free extracts of dog lung. *Nature* **220:** 919–921, 1968.

Bakhle, Y. S.: Inhibition of angiotensin I converting enzyme by venom peptides. *Br. J. Pharmacol.* **43:** 252–254, 1971.

Braun-Menendez, E. and Page, I. H.: Suggested revision of nomenclature—angiotensin. *Science* **127:** 242, 1958.

Braun-Menendez, E., Fasciolo, J. C., Leloir, L. F. , and Muñoz, J. M.: The substance causing renal hypertension. *J. Physiol.* (London) **98**: 283–298, 1940.

Brunner, H. R., Nussberger, J., and Waeber, B.: The present molecules of converting enzyme inhibitors. *J. Cardiovasc. Pharmacol.* **7**: S2–S11, 1985.

Brunner, H. R., Gavras, H., Waeber, B., Textor, S. C., Turini, G. A., and Wauters, J. P.: Clinical use of an orally acting converting enzyme inhibitor: Captopril. *Hypertension* **2**: 558–566, 1980.

Brunner, H. R., Gavras, H., Waeber, B., Kershaw, G. R., Turini, G. A., Vukovich, R. A., McKinstry, D. N., and Gavras, I.: Oral angiotensin-converting enzyme inhibitor in long-term treatment of hypertensive patients. *Ann. Intern. Med.* **90**: 19–23, 1979.

Byers, L. D. and Wolfenden, R.: Binding of the by-product analog benzyl-succinic acid by carboxypeptidase A. *Biochemistry* **12**: 2070–2078, 1973.

Case, D. B., Atlas, S. A., Laragh, J. H., Sealey, J. E., Sullivan, P. A., and McKinstry, D. N.: Clinical experience with blockade of the renin-angio-tensin-aldosterone system by an oral converting-enzyme inhibitor (SQ 14,225, Captopril) in hypertensive patients. *Prog. Cardiovasc. Dis.* **21**: 195–206, 1978.

Case, D. B., Wallace, J. M., Keim, H. J., Weber, M. A., Sealey, J. E., and Laragh, J. H.: Possible role of renin in hypertension as suggested by renin-sodium profiling and inhibition of converting enzyme. *N. Engl. J. Med.* **296**: 641–646, 1977.

Case, D. B., Wallace, J. M., Keim, H. J., Weber, M. A., Drayer, J. I. M., White, R. P., Sealey, J. E., and Laragh, J. H.: Estimating renin participation in hypertension. Superiority of converting enzyme inhibitor over Saralasin. *Am. J. Med.* **61**: 790–796, 1976.

Cohn, J. N. and Levine, T. B.: Angiotensin-converting enzyme inhibition in congestive heart failure: The concept. *Am. J. Cardiol.* **49**: 1480–1483, 1982.

Collier, J. G., Robinson, B. F., and Vane, J. R.: Reduction of pressor effects of angiotensin I in man by synthetic nonapeptide (BPP9a or SQ 20,881) which inhibits converting enzyme. *Lancet* **1**: 72–74, 1973.

Cushman, D. W. and Cheung, H. S.: Spectrophotometric assay and properties of the angiotensin-converting enzyme of rabbit lung. *Biochem. Pharmacol.* **20**: 1637–1648, 1971.

Cushman, D. W., Cheung, H. S., Sabo, E. F., and Ondetti, M. A.: Design of potent competitive inhibitors of angiotensin-converting enzyme. Car-boxyalkanoyl and mercaptoalkanoyl amino acids. *Biochemistry* **16**: 5484–5491, 1977.

Cushman, D. W., Cheung, H. S., Sabo, E. F., and Ondetti, M. A.: Develop-ment and design of specific inhibitors of angiotensin-converting enzyme. *Am. J. Cardiol.* **49**: 1390–1394, 1982.

Cushman, D. W., Wang, F. L., Fung, W. C., Harvey, C. M., and DeForrest, J. M.: Differentiation of angiotensin-converting enzyme (ACE) inhibitors by their selective inhibition of ACE in physiologically important target organs. *Am. J. Hypertension* **2:** 294–306, 1989.

Cushman, D. W., Pluscec, J., Williams, N. J., Weaver, E., Sabo, E. F., Kocy, O., Cheung, H. S., and Ondetti, M. A.: Inhibition of angiotensin-converting enzyme by analogs of peptides from *Bothrops jararaca* venom. *Experientia* **29:** 1032–1035, 1973.

Davies, R. O., Irvin, J. D., Kramsch, D. K., Walker, J. F., and Moncloa, F.: Enalapril worldwide experience. *Am. J. Med.* **77:** 23–35, 1984.

Drayer, J. I. M. and Weber, M. A.: Monotherapy of essential hypertension with a converting-enzyme inhibitor. *Hypertension* **5** (Suppl. III): 108–113, 1983.

Edwards, C. R. W. and Padfield, P. L.: Angiotensin-converting enzyme inhibitors: Past, present, and bright future. *Lancet* **1:** 30–34, 1985.

Engel, S. L., Schaeffer, T. R., Gold, B. I., and Rubin, B.: Inhibition of pressor effects of angiotensin I and augmentation of depressor effects of bradykinin by synthetic peptides. *Proc. Soc. Exp. Biol. Med.* **140:** 240–244, 1972.

Engel, S. L., Schaeffer, T. R., Waugh, M. H., and Rubin, B.: Effects of the nonapeptide SQ 20,881 on blood pressure of rats with experimental renovascular hypertension. *Proc. Soc. Exp. Biol. Med.* **143:** 483–487, 1973.

Erdös, E. G.: Enzymes that inactivate polypeptides, in *Proceedings of 1st Int. Pharmacol. Meeting, Stockholm,* pp. 159–178, Macmillan, New York, 1962.

Ferguson, R. K. and Vlasses, P. H.: Clinical pharmacology and therapeutic applications of the new oral angiotensin converting enzyme inhibitor, captopril. *Am. Heart J.* **101:** 650–656, 1981.

Ferguson, R. K., Vlasses, P. H., and Rotmensch, H. H.: Clinical applications of angiotensin-converting enzyme inhibitors. *Am. Heart J.* **77:** 690–698, 1984.

Ferguson, R. K., Turini, G. A., Brunner, H. R., Gavras, H., and McKinstry, D. N.: A specific orally active inhibitor of angiotensin-converting enzyme in man. *Lancet* **1:** 775–778, 1977.

Ferreira, S. H.: A bradykinin-potentiating factor, (BPF) present in the venom of *Bothrops jararaca. Br. J. Pharmacol. Chemother.* **24:** 163–169, 1965.

Ferreira, S. H. and Rocha e Silva, M.: Potentiation of bradykinin by dimercaptopropanol (BAL) and other inhibitors of its destroying enzyme in plasma. *Biochem. Pharmacol.* **11:** 1123–1128, 1962.

Ferreira, S. H. and Vane, J. R.: The disappearance of bradykinin and eledoisin in the circulation and vascular beds of the cat. *Br. J. Pharmac. Chemother.* **30:** 417–424, 1967.

Ferreira, S. H., Bartelt, D. C., and Greene, L. J.: Isolation of bradykinin-potentiating peptides from *Bothrops jararaca* venom. *Biochemistry* **9**: 2583–2593, 1970a.

Ferreira, S. H., Greene, L. J., Alabaster, V. A., Bakhle, Y. S., and Vane, J. R.: Activity of various fractions of bradykinin potentiating factor against angiotensin I converting enzyme. *Nature* **225**: 379, 380, 1970b.

Gavras, H.: The place of angiotensin-converting enzyme inhibition in the treatment of cardiovascular diseases. *N. Engl. J. Med.* **319**: 1541–1543, 1988.

Gavras, H., Brunner, H. R., Laragh, J. H., Sealey, J. E., Gavras, I., and Vukovich, R. A.: An angiotensin converting-enzyme inhibitor to identify and treat vasoconstrictor and volume factors in hypertensive patients. *N. Engl. J. Med.* **291**: 817–821, 1974.

Gavras, H., Brunner, H. R., Turini, G. A., Kershaw, G. R., Tifft, C. P., Cuttelod, S., Gavras, I., Vukovich, R. A., and McKinstry, D. N.: Antihypertensive effect of the oral angiotensin converting-enzyme inhibitor SQ 14,225 in man. *N. Engl. J. Med.* **298**: 991–995, 1978.

Goldblatt, H.: *The Renal Origin of Hypertension,* Charles C. Thomas, Springfield, IL, 1948.

Goldblatt, H., Lynch, J., Hanzal, R. F., and Summerville, W. W.: Studies on experimental hypertension. *J. Exp. Med.* **59**: 347–379, 1934.

Groel, J. T., Tadros, S. S., Dreslinski, G. R., and Jenkins, A. C.: Long-term antihypertensive therapy with captopril. *Hypertension* **5**: 145–151, 1983.

Gross, F.: Angiotensin-converting enzyme inhibition: A developing therapeutic concept. *Am. J. Cardiol.* **49**: 1384, 1982.

Heel, R. C., Brogden, R. N., Speight, T. M., and Avery, G. S.: Captopril: A preliminary review of its pharmacological properties and therapeutic efficacy. *Drugs* **20**: 409–452, 1980.

Helmer, O. M.: A factor in plasma that enhances contractions produced by angiotensin in rabbit aortic strips. *Fed. Proc.* **14**: 225, 1955.

Helmer, O. M.: Differentiation between two forms of angiotensin by means of spirally cut strips of rabbit aorta. *Am. J. Physiol.* **188**: 571–577, 1957.

Johnson, J. G., Black, W. D., Vukovich, R. A., Hatch, F. E., Friedman, B. I., Blackwell, C. F., Shenouda, A. N., Share, L., Shade, R. E., Acchiardo, S. R., and Muirhead, E. E.: Treatment of patients with severe hypertension by inhibition of angiotensin-converting enzyme. *Clin. Sci. Mol. Med.* **48**: (Suppl. 2): 53S–56S, 1975.

Johnston, C. I., Arnolda, L., and Hiwatari, M.: Angiotensin-converting enzyme inhibitors in the treatment of hypertension. *Drugs* **27**: 271–277, 1984.

Kostis, J. B.: Angiotension-converting enzyme inhibitors. Emerging differences and new compounds. *Am. J. Hypertension* **2**: 57–64, 1989.

Krieger, E. M., Salgado, H. C., Assan, C. J., Greene, L. L. J., and Ferreira,

S. H.: Potential screening test for detection of overactivity of renin-angiotensin system. *Lancet* **1:** 269–271, 1971.

Laragh, J. H.: Concept of anti-renin system therapy. Historical perspective. *Am. J. Med.* **77:** 1–6, 1984.

Materson, B. J.: Monotherapy of hypertension with antiotensin-converting enzyme inhibitors. New concepts in hypertension therapy. *Am. J. Med.* **77:** 128–134, 1984.

Müller, F. B., Sealey, J. E., Case, D. B., Atlas, S. A., Pickering, T. G., Pecker, M. S., Preibisz, J. J., and Laragh, J. H.: The captopril test for identifying renovascular disease in hypertensive patients. *Am. J. Med.* **80:** 633–644, 1986.

Ng, K. K. F. and Vane, J. R.: Conversion of angiotensin I to angiotensin II. *Nature* **216:** 762–766, 1967.

Ng, K. K. F. and Vane, J. R.: Fate of angiotensin I in the circulation. *Nature* **218:** 144–150, 1968.

Ondetti, M. A., Rubin, B., and Cushman, D. W.: Design of specific inhibitors of angiotensin-converting enzyme: New class of orally active antihypertensive agents. *Science* **196:** 441–444, 1977.

Ondetti, M. A., Williams, N. J., Sabo, E. F., Pluscec, J., Weaver, E. R., and Kocy, O.: Angiotensin-converting enzyme inhibitors from the venom of *Bothrops jararaca.* Isolation, elucidation of structure, and synthesis. *Biochemistry* **10:** 4033–4038, 1971.

Page, I. H.: Production of persistent arterial hypertension by cellophane perinephritis. *J. Am. Med. Assoc.* **113:** 2046–2048, 1939.

Page, I. H.: The renin-angiotensin pressor system, in *Hypertension: A Symposium*, E. T. Bell, ed., University of Minnesota Press, Minneapolis, 1951.

Page, I. H. and Bumpus, F. M.: Angiotensin. *Physiol. Rev.* **41:** 331–390, 1961.

Page, I. H., Dustan, H. P., and Bumpus, F. M.: A commentary on the measurement of renin and angiotensin. *Circulation* **32:** 513, 514, 1965.

Patchett, A. A., Harris, E., Tristram, E. W., Wyvratt, M. J., Wu, M. T., Taub, D., Peterson, E. R., Ikeler, T. J., ten Broeke, J., Payne, L. G., Ondeyka, D. L., Thorsett, E. D., Greenlee, W. J., Lohr, N. S., Hoffsommer, R. D., Joshua, H., Ruyle, W. V., Rothrock, J. W., Aster, S. D., Maycock, A. L., Robinson, F. M., Hirschmann, R., Sweet, C. S., Ulm, E. H., Gross, D. M., Vassil, T. C., and Stone, C. A.: A new class of angiotensin-converting enzyme inhibitors. *Nature* **288:** 280–283, 1980.

Rocha e Silva, M., Beraldo, W. T., and Rosenfeld, G.: Bradykinin, hypotensive and smooth muscle stimulating factor released from plasma globulin by snake venoms and by trypsin. *Am. J. Physiol.* **156:** 261–273, 1949.

Romankiewicz, J. A., Brogden, R. N., Heel, R. C., Speight, T. M., and Avery, G. S.: Captopril: An update review of its pharmacological properties and therapeutic efficacy in congestive heart failure. *Drugs* **25:** 6–40, 1983.

Skeggs, L. T., Kahn, J. R., and Shumway, N. P.: The preparation and function of the hypertensin-converting enzyme. *J. Exp. Med.* **103:** 295–299, 1956.

Skeggs, L. T., Marsh, W. H., Kahn, J. R., and Shumway, N. P.: The existence of two forms of hypertensin. *J. Exp. Med.* **99:** 275–282, 1954.

Stewart, J. M., Ferreira, S. H., and Greene, L. J.: Bradykinin potentiating peptide PCA-Lys-Trp-Ala-Pro. An inhibitor of the pulmonary inactivation of bradykinin and conversion of angiotensin I to II. *Biochem. Pharmacol.* **20:** 1557–1567, 1971.

Swales, J. D., Bing, R. F., Heagerty, A., Pohl, J. E. F., Russell, G. I., and Thurston, H.: Treatment of refractory hypertension. *Lancet* **1:** 894– 896, 1982.

Vidt, D. G., Bravo, E. L., and Fouad, F. M.: Captopril. *N. Engl. J. Med.* **306:** 214–219, 1982.

Vlasses, P. H., Ferguson, R. K., and Chatterjee, K.: Captopril: Clinical pharmacology and benefit-to-risk ratio in hypertension and congestive heart failure. *Pharmacotherapy* **2:** 1–17, 1982a.

Vlasses, P. H., Rotmensch, H. H., Swanson, B. N., Mojaverian, P., and Ferguson, R. K.: Low-dose captopril: Its use in mild to moderate hypertension unresponsive to diuretic treatment. *Arch. Intern. Med.* **142:** 1098–1101, 1982b.

Williams, G. H.: Converting-enzyme inhibitors in the treatment of hypertension. *N. Engl. J. Med.* **319:** 1517–1525, 1988.

Williams, G. H. and Hollenberg, N. K.: Accentuated vascular and endocrine response to SQ 20,881 in hypertension. *N. Engl. J. Med.* **297:** 184–188, 1977.

Calcium Antagonists

I. Calcium Antagonists—Verapamil, Nifedipine, and Diltiazem—as Innovative Therapeutic Agents

The first drugs to become known as Ca antagonists* were four structurally unrelated substances: verapamil, nifedipine, diltiazem, and perhexiline. The synthesis, pharmacology and initial clinical testing of verapamil as an antianginal agent occurred several years before it was demonstrated to block Ca channels, and a similar sequence was apparently true for nifedipine, diltiazem, and perhexiline (Fleckenstein, 1983; Kendall and Okopski, 1986; Krikler, 1987; Winbury, 1984). Via the use of verapamil (and prenylamine, a weaker, less specific agent), the concept that a dual ionic carrier system existed in mammalian myocardial fibers (Reuter, 1967; Reuter and Beeler, 1969) was strongly substantiated, and the phenomenon

---

*For convenience, Ca^{2+} will be abbreviated as Ca. The term "Ca antagonist" was the one first applied by Fleckenstein et al. (1969, 1984) to define selective inhibition of the transport of Ca into the cell (*see also* Fleckenstein, 1984). The term was gradually broadened to include many compounds for which it was uncertain whether their actions depended predominantly on the mechanism defined by Fleckenstein or were the result of other possible intracellular interactions with Ca (Henry, 1980). It seems, however, that use of the less-specific term "Ca antagonist," even when discussing specific Ca-channel blockers, may be preferable (*see* Opie, 1984a; Fleckenstein, 1983). A broad definition has been proposed for the term "Ca antagonist" by Cohen et al. (1984): "Ca^{2+} antagonists may be defined as drugs which potentially inhibit Ca^{2+} dependent processes or regulatory mechanisms without exerting their primary effect at some other known sites, such as ion channels other than Ca^{2+} channels or receptors for neurotransmitters." Ca-channel blockers become a subcategory of Ca antagonists in this definition.

of Ca antagonism was first demonstrated (Fleckenstein et al., 1967, 1969; Fleckenstein, 1983; Kohlhardt et al., 1972). It became clear that, in addition to the well-known "fast" channel for the inward passage of Na, which accounted for the generation of the action potential spike, a "slow" channel existed for the inward movement of Ca. This slow Ca influx, which was initiated by the action potential spike, acted to trigger the contractile apparatus and thereby linked contraction with membrane excitation in the myocardium. The same process was later demonstrated to occur in vascular smooth muscle as well (see Fleckenstein, 1977 for refs.). Moreover, both normal and ectopic pacemaker activities (in sinoatrial and atrioventricular nodes) were shown to be linked to Ca transport through slow channels. Skeletal muscle fibers, on the other hand, contained large endoplasmic Ca pools, which made excitation–contraction coupling in this tissue relatively insensitive to transmembrane Ca conductivity (Fleckenstein, 1977). Thus, inhibition of cardiac force and automaticity could be obtained experimentally with Ca-channel blockers (resulting in reduced myocardial demand for O_2), while they simultaneously elicited coronary and peripheral vasodilation (which sent more O_2 to the myocardium and reduced afterload), but did not interfere with skeletal muscle function.

Prior to the appearance of the Ca antagonists, nitroglycerin and beta blocking agents were the major drugs for treating angina pectoris. Beta blocking agents are effective in the prophylactic treatment of exertional angina by reducing sympathetic drive to the heart. They are not helpful for Prinzmetal's variant (vasospastic) angina, presumably because of an increase in coronary resistance caused by unopposed action of catecholamines acting on vascular alpha receptors (Needleman et al., 1985). Beta blocking agents are also used in treating arrhythmias, hypertension, myocardial infarction, and other conditions. Nitroglycerin is effective in relieving both variant and exertional angina, but is short-acting and has numerous side effects, e.g., headache, postural hypotension, and tolerance to its effects.

Verapamil, diltiazem, and nifedipine have found important clinical use in cardiovascular disorders, particularly angina pectoris and cardiac dysrhythmias. In general, they are better tolerated than nitrates and beta blockers, and have proven to be safe. Their tendency to evoke more myocardial depression than might be desirable is usually offset by the reflex sympathetic drive induced by peripheral vasodilation (Krikler, 1987), because the sympathetic neurotransmitter norepinephrine, by enhancing the influx of Ca into cells, acts as a direct antagonist to Ca-channel blockers. All three agents are useful in hypertension (Opie and Singh, 1987).

Verapamil, because of its unusually potent effect on nodal conduction in vivo, is used for the termination and prevention of paroxysmal supraventricular tachycardias (Stone et al., 1980; Henry, 1980). Combining verapamil with beta blockers must be done with care, because both depress nodal conduction.

Nifedipine, which has little effect on nodal conduction in vivo, is effective in Prinzmetal's variant angina and in classic exertional angina and may be safely combined with a beta blocking agent (Stone et al., 1980; Opie and Singh, 1987). Nifedipine is also especially useful in patients with bronchospasm, left ventricular failure, or peripheral vascular disease, conditions in which beta blockade is contraindicated.

Diltiazem is used for the same spectrum of diseases as verapamil—angina pectoris, hypertension, and supraventricular arrhythmias (Opie and Singh, 1987). Perhexiline is effective for exertional angina, but its use is limited by its side effects and the availability of other agents (Stone et al., 1980).

Ca antagonists also hold out promise for effectiveness in other cardiovascular disorders and for greater understanding of the pathologic mechanisms underlying the disorders. They have been proposed to be of use for left ventricular failure, acute myocardial infarction, cardiac preservation, cardiomyopathy, and cerebral vasospasm (Karlsberg, 1982; Fleckenstein, 1983; Urthaler, 1986; Larach and Zelis, 1986; Lichtlen, 1986).

Stone et al. (1980) stated that the calcium antagonists "...are greatly expanding the cardiovascular therapeutic armamentarium." Singh et al. (1978) considered verapamil not only "...a significant agent in cardiovascular therapeutics but also....a powerful tool to examine the nature of some of the biophysical phenomena at the membrane of cardiac and other excitable tissues." Winbury (1984) was of the opinion that "...this is the decade of the calcium entry blockers."

Early Clinical Research History

Verapamil, nifedipine, and diltiazem, although their uses have broadened, all drew attention first as effective agents against stable (exertional) angina pectoris.

Verapamil

Verapamil exhibited antianginal effects in open studies in humans. Tschirdewahn and Klepzig (1963) gave verapamil to 16 patients with chronic stable angina pectoris and reported that 93% had subjective improvement and 50% had improvements in their electrocardiograms. Ten of 11 patients who were subsequently placed on placebo experienced increased pain. Hoffmann (1964) found positive results in an open study of 191 patients with symptomatic cardiac ischemia. In another open study of 72 patients, verapamil had a more-or-less pronounced effect on severe anginal pain in 59 patients (Hofbauer, 1966). This author recommended the use of verapamil for patients suffering from coronary insufficiency. Neumann and Luisada (1966) found, in 30 aged, anginal patients in a double-blind, placebo-controlled study, that verapamil significantly decreased the number of nitroglycerin tablets required over a six-week period. In 16 anginal patients in a double-blind, placebo-controlled study, verapamil produced a significant reduction in anginal frequency, nitroglycerin consumption, and exercise tolerance, and favorably affected ischemic S–T depression during exercise (Sandler et al., 1968). Interestingly, Luebs et al. (1966) noted that, although verapamil (and several other agents) increased myocardial flow in normal individuals, it failed to raise coronary flow in patients with coronary artery disease. They concluded that improvement in angina pectoris need not depend on an increase in coronary blood flow. Mignault (1966) also concluded that the clinical improvement that they observed in five patients must be explained by a mechanism that was independent of an influence on coronary flow.

Nifedipine

In a single-blind, placebo-controlled, crossover study, four out of five patients with angina of effort plus angina at rest became attack-free during the administration of nifedipine (Hayase et al.,

1971). The authors considered that nifedipine had outstanding "preventive" efficacy on the occurrence of anginal attacks. A double-blind, crossover study, in 17 patients with typical anginal attacks and ECG changes, measured the effect of nifedipine on anginal pain, exercise tolerance, and nitroglycerin consumption (Kimura et al., 1972). The investigators, using a sequential analysis, found that the probability of success was 80% for nifedipine and 30% for placebo. They concluded that nifedipine had an efficacy rate similar to isosorbide dinitrate and propranolol. Kobayashi et al. (1972), in an open study in 47 patients with angina of effort and/or at rest, measured subjective symptoms, blood pressure, heart rate, and ECG. Nifedipine corrected T-wave abnormalities and tended to lower blood pressure, and thereby was conducive to decreasing the number of anginal attacks. Nifedipine in a few cases "...proved indispensable for prevention of attacks of angina pectoris." Loos and Kaltenbach (1972) found that subjective improvement was elicited by nifedipine in 18 patients with angina of effort and that depression of the S–T segment was diminished by a mean of 48%. These workers expressed the opinion that "[t]he relatively long-lasting, nitroglycerin-like, anti-anginous effect may justify the clinical use of the substance." Nifedipine was also found to be effective in variant (vasospastic) angina (Hosada and Kimura, 1976).

Diltiazem

Diltiazem reduced objective measurements of heart function and reduced anginal attacks (Oyama et al., 1972). In a study by Mizuno et al. (1973), it improved subjective symptoms, ECG findings, and overall assessment of the angina provoked by effort.

Yasue et al. (1978a) demonstrated in eight of nine patients with Prinzmetal's variant angina that coronary arterial vasospasm and angina could be induced by hyperventilation and Tris-buffer infusion. In five of these patients, diltiazem prevented these evoked attacks. Yasue et al. (1978b) reported that, in 26 patients with angina at rest (including 13 with variant angina), diltiazem completely suppressed attacks in all cases.

Subsequent experimentation has confirmed and expanded this early work with verapamil, nifedipine, and diltiazem. Many reviews, text chapters, and books regarding the experimental and clinical effects of Ca antagonists are available (*see,* for example, Fleckenstein, 1971,1977,1983,1984; Kimura, 1978; Fleckenstein and Roskamm, 1980; Antman et al., 1980; Stone et al., 1980; Henry, 1980, 1983; Karlsberg, 1982; Spivack et al., 1983; Winbury, 1984; Opie, 1984b; Schneck, 1985; Crawford, 1985; Kendall and Okopski, 1986; Urthaler, 1986; Larach and Zelis, 1986; Frishman et al., 1986; Halperin and Cubeddu, 1986; Krikler, 1987; Scriabine, 1987).

II. The Scientific Work Leading to Verapamil, Nifedipine, and Diltiazem

Verapamil

Haas and Härtfelder (1962) reported verapamil (originally known as D365 or iproveratril) (Fig. 1) to be a marked dilator of the coronary artery in dogs and in hearts isolated from rabbits. They found the compound to be approximately 100 times more active than papaverine (Fig. 1). The oxygen content of the coronary sinus blood was increased, and coronary arteriovenous oxygen difference was decreased. In most instances coronary oxygen uptake was slightly reduced and reflected heart-rate changes. Negative inotropic effects were seen in isolated papillary muscles, but in the intact animal this effect was compensated for, with stroke volume actually increasing.

Melville et al. (1964) reported verapamil to be a potent coronary vasodilator and a depressant of the myocardium and conducting system in hearts isolated from rabbits. This same group concluded that verapamil was a competitive antagonist of norepinephrine in papillary muscle isolated from cat (Melville and Benfey, 1965), but that verapamil had no beta-adrenergic blocking action (Benfey et al., 1967).

Fleckenstein (1964) observed that verapamil, among other agents, produced negative inotropic effects that resembled calcium deficiency and, as already mentioned in section I, subsequently went on to define verapamil as the first specific Ca-channel blocking agent (Fleckenstein et al., 1969).

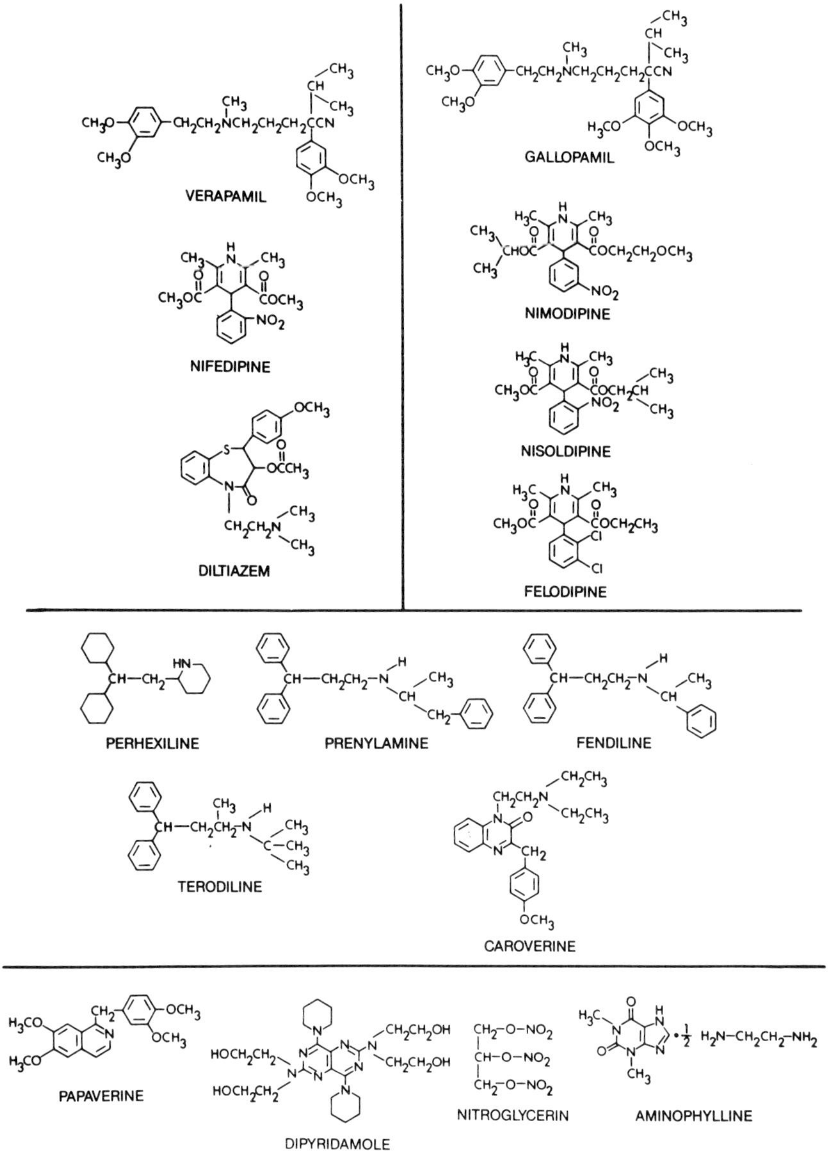

Fig. 1. The structures of verapamil, nifedipine, diltiazem, and chemically and/or pharmacologically related substances.

Nifedipine

Nifedipine (Fig. 1) was the result of a systematic search for new coronary active agents (Bossert and Vater, 1971). Among the large number of dihydropyridine compounds that were synthesized, Bay a 1040 (later called nifedipine) was especially effective. In anesthetized dogs, over a range of very low intravenous doses, oxygen saturation in the coronary sinus increased secondarily to increased perfusion of the coronary arteries. Nifedipine was active within minutes by the oral route and much more rapidly following sublingual application. The difference in arteriocoronary sinus lactate concentrations did not become positive, indicating that the flow was not increased as a consequence of increased myocardial work. Bossert and Vater (1971) noted that inhibition of excitation–contraction coupling by nifedipine, as demonstrated by Fleckenstein, was important in its mechanism of action.

Vater et al. (1972) presented a fuller accounting of the pharmacology of nifedipine. Fleckenstein et al. (1972) described the highly potent Ca-antagonist properties of nifedipine in mammalian myocardium, and Grün and Fleckenstein (1972) described a similar effect of the drug in vascular smooth muscle.

Diltiazem

During the course of a screening test in anesthetized dogs, certain benzothiazepine derivatives were found to exert a strong coronary vasodilator effect. Among the compounds tested, CRD-401 (later given the generic name diltiazem) was the most potent (Fig. 1) (Sato et al., 1971). It did not increase myocardial oxygen consumption, and heart rate was only slightly affected. Because of the two asymmetric carbon atoms in its structure, the molecule existed as four isomers. Diltiazem, the most potent isomer, had the *d-cis* configuration.

Nakajima et al. (1975) demonstrated that diltiazem, at a low concentration, decreased the contractile force of papillary muscle isolated from guinea pigs without significiantly altering the transmembrane resting and action potentials. The authors concluded that diltiazem was an excitation–contraction uncoupler in cardiac muscle.

Table 1 defines the critical scientific ideas and experiments leading to verapamil, nifedipine, and diltiazem, and categorizes their origin.

Background Contributions
Preceding Verapamil, Nifedipine, and Diltiazem

Compounds having coronary vasodilator properties in animal preparations have been known for many decades, and some of them have been useful as antianginal agents in humans, e.g., nitroglycerin, papaverine, theophylline ethylenediamine (aminophylline), and dipyridamole (Fig. 1). As a corollary to this knowledge, coronary-dilating action had long been considered *prima facie* evidence that a compound would have a useful antianginal application. As noted by Winbury (1984), more sophisticated concepts concerning cardiac function and the mode of action of antianginal drugs have been developed over the last three decades, and have tempered this assumption. Nonetheless, verapamil, nifedipine, and diltiazem were discovered during empirical searches for potent coronary dilating agents, albeit within this more sophisticated scientific atmosphere. A permissive attitude toward the negative inotropic effects seen experimentally with these newer coronary vasodilators had been established as a result of the successful clinical use of the anti-inotropic effect of beta blocking agents to reduce O_2 demands in the ischemic myocardium of anginal patients.

III. Comments on Events
Leading to Ca Antagonists

As noted by Winbury (1984), "We should not lose sight of the fact that verapamil—the first of these agents—has been with us since the early 1960s....later its calcium antagonism was demonstrated by Fleckenstein et al. (1969)." According to Kroneberg (1984) of the Bayer Co., after having seen the results with verapamil, he asked Fleckenstein in 1969 if a new compound (later to be named nifedipine), which had strong negative inotropic effects in isolated hearts and strong coronary dilator effects, could be a Ca antagonist agent. Kroneberg (1984) reported that, later in 1969, Fleckenstein told him

Table 1
Profile of Observations and Ideas Crucial to the Development
of Calcium Antagonists Verapamil, Nifedipine, and Diltiazem[a]

Sequence: Routes[b] to innovative drugs**	Orient- ation	Nature of study	Research institution	National origin	Nature of discovery	Screening involved	Crucial ideas or observations
Verapamil							
Haas and Härtfelder (1962)	Pre- clinical	Pharma- cology/ chemistry	Indus- try	West Germany	Orderly	Untargeted	A potent coronary vasodilator, verapa- mil, reported; cor- onary sinus O_2 in- creased; increased coronary perfusion not secondary to increased cardiac work.
Nifedipine							
Bossert and Vater (1971)	Pre- clinical	Pharma- cology/ chemistry	Indus- try	West Germany	Orderly	Untargeted	A potent coronary vasodilator, nifedi- pine, reported; coro- nary sinus O_2 in- creased; increased coronary perfusion not secondary to increased cardiac work.
Diltiazem							
Sato et al. (1971)	Pre- clinical	Pharma- cology/ chem- istry	Indus- try	Japan	Orderly	Untargeted	A potent coronary vasodilator, diltia- zem, reported; no in- crease in myocardial O_2 consumption; increased coronary perfusion not sec- ondary to increased cardiac work.

[a]Taken from section II. Entries are those contributions without which the discovery of the agent (or additionally, in some cases, a relevant clinical application) would not have taken place or would have been materially delayed.
[b]All three drugs were discovered independently.

that the compound was the most potent Ca antagonist he had ever investigated. Fleckenstein (1983) also commented,

The original reports on marked cardiodepressant influences of pren- ylamine..., verapamil..., and nifedipine did not offer an explanation of the specific mode of action. The same was true of the introductory paper on...perhexiline..., which also did not contribute to the understanding of the fundamental mechanism...

Diltiazem, as already noted, was introduced as an antianginal agent in 1971 and only identified as a Ca antagonist in 1975.

Verapamil bears some resemblance to a ring-opened papaverine molecule. Papaverine seems to have served as a conceptual starting point for verapamil's synthesis. The other agents appear to have had no obvious vasodilator progenitors.

The above comments suggest that the purely pragmatically based development of verapamil, nifedipine, and diltiazem as vasodilator drugs constituted very productive effort by the researchers involved: this effort had very important consequences.

Fleckenstein (1983) maintained that the introduction of nifedipine into coronary therapy profited from the research work with verapamil. Thus, in early 1970, clinical investigators could be informed that nifedipine was another highly potent Ca-channel blocker. This preliminary information "...was conducive to a better orientation of the clinical research projects on nifedipine, which were at that time already underway."

Medicinal chemists and pharmacologists entered the lists in force once the usefulness of verapamil, nifedipine, and diltiazem began to surface. This entry was further stimulated by the availability of a unifying concept regarding their mechanisms of action. Winbury (1984) expressed the opinion that Fleckenstein's contribution provided "...the impetus for this field." The consequences of the chemical effort are discussed in section IV.

IV. Developments Subsequent to Verapamil, Nifedipine, and Diltiazem

Verapamil is a benzeneacetonitrile, nifedipine a dihydropyridine, and diltiazem a benzothiazepine—all very distinct chemical structures (Fig. 1). Fleckenstein (1983) expressed the opinion that, because of the marked chemical differences, any attempt to attribute the Ca-channel blocking property to a distinct molecular configuration was probably in vain. Not only did these substances differ chemically, but also, to some extent (as noted in section I) pharmacologically and clinically. Krebs (1984) considered that the latter two differences resulted from the variation in potencies and specificities that these agents exhibit for various tissues and from the probability that they do not share a common site of action at the cellular level. There has been evidence for, and considerable discussion of, the existence of more than one action for Ca-channel blocking agents in altering Ca interactions in the cell (Church and Zsotér, 1980). This possibility in turn raised the possibility of synthesizing organic molecules that could very selectively manipulate Ca regulation.

Subsequently, gallopamil (D600) (Fig. 1), a chemical analog of verapamil, was introduced. Several chemical relatives of nifedipine were developed, e.g., nimodipine, nisoldipine, and felodipine (Fig. 1). In addition, two derivatives of prenylamine having significant activity were synthesized: terodiline and fendiline (Fig. 1). Caroverine (Fig. 1) also became available (Fleckenstein 1983,1984).

According to Krebs (1984), nimodipine was very effective in blocking contractions of the basilar artery to a variety of receptor agonists, whereas its effects on the response of the femoral arteries to the same agonists were very small, suggesting a selective effect on cerebral vessels. Towart (1981) postulated "...that the selective inhibition...of the basilar artery...is due to a selective inhibition by nimodipine of calcium movement through ROCs [receptor operated channels] in this vessel.... ROCs in peripheral blood vessels [do] not seem to be affected."

Nisoldipine, in contrast to nifedipine, was very effective in the portal vein, whereas the effects of both agents on the myocardium were approximately equal (Kazda et al., 1980). Nisoldipine appeared to be the first Ca antagonist for which an effect on the venous system could be seen at reasonable concentrations (Krebs, 1984). Kass (1982) considered nisoldipine to be a potent calcium current blocker, more specific than the standard Ca-channel blockers, and suggested that this drug might be a tool with experimental and therapeutic usefulness.

These examples indicate that the thrust of current chemical and pharmacological research is to develop agents that take advantage of what appears to be a range of sites for altering Ca transport and binding, in order to make new, more selective therapeutic agents. Scriabine (1987) made clear that there were potential new indications for Ca antagonists not only in the cardiovascular area, but also in disorders of respiration, central nervous system, uterus, gastrointestinal tract, and possibly even in cancer therapy.

It should be noted that Ca antagonists have had a large impact on the basic knowledge of Ca regulations in cells. As stated by Janis et al. (1987), "...a pharmacological dissection of Ca^{2+} channels from other ionic pathways did not become possible until the advent of the Ca^{2+} channel antagonists.... This class of agents...served to dramatically enhance our knowledge of Ca^{2+} channels."

References

Antman, E. M., Stone, P. H., Muller, J. E., and Braunwald, E.: Calcium channel blocking agents in the treatment of cardiovascular disorders. Part 1: basic and clinical electrophysiologic effects. *Ann. Intern. Med.* 93: 875–885, 1980.

Benfey, B. G., Greeff, K., and Heeg, E.: Evaluation of sympathetic beta-receptor blockade by recording the rate of ventricular pressure rise in cats. *Br. J. Pharmacol. Chemother.* 30: 23–29, 1967.

Bossert, F. and Vater, W.: Dihydropyridine, eine neue Gruppe stark wirksamer Coronartherapeutika. *Naturwissenschaften* 58: 578, 1971.

Church, J. and Zsotér, T. T.: Calcium antagonistic drugs. Mechanism of action. *Can. J. Physiol. Pharmacol.* 58: 254–264, 1980.

Cohen, C. J., Janis, R. A., Taylor, D. G., and Scriabine, A.: Where do calcium antagonists act?, in *Calcium Antagonists and Cardiovascular Disease*, L. H. Opie, ed., pp. 151–163, Raven, New York, 1984.

Crawford, M. H.: Effectiveness of diltiazem for chronic stable angina pectoris. *Acta Pharmacol. Toxicol.* 57 (Suppl. 2): 44–48, 1985.

Fleckenstein, A.: Die Bedeutung der energiereichen Phosphate für Kontraktilität und Tonus des Myokards. *Verh. Dtsch. Ges. Inn. Med.* 70: 81–99, 1964.

Fleckenstein, A.: Specific inhibitors and promoters of calcium action in the excitation–contraction coupling of heart muscle and their role in the prevention or production of myocardial lesions, in *Calcium and the Heart*, P. Harris and L. Opie, eds., pp. 135–188, Academic, London, 1971.

Fleckenstein, A.: Specific pharmacology of calcium in myocardium, cardiac pacemakers, and vascular smooth muscle. *Annu. Rev. Pharmacol. Toxicol.* 17: 149–166, 1977.

Fleckenstein, A.: *Calcium Antagonism in Heart and Smooth Muscle: Experimental Facts and Therapeutic Prospects.* Wiley, New York, 1983.

Fleckenstein, A.: Calcium antagonism: History and prospects for a multifaceted pharmacodynamic principle, in *Calcium Antagonists and Cardiovascular Disease*, L. H. Opie, ed., pp. 9–28, Raven, New York, 1984.

Fleckenstein, A. and Roskamm, H.: *Calcium-Antagonismus.* Springer-Verlag, Berlin, 1980.

Fleckenstein, A., Kammermeier, H., Döring, H. J., and Freund, H. J.: Zum Wirkungsmechanismus neuartiger Koronardilatatoren mit gleichzeitig Sauerstoff-einsparenden Myokard-Effekten, Prenylamin und Iproveratril. *Kreislaufforsch* **56:** part 1, 716–744; part 2, 839–858, 1967.

Fleckenstein, A., Tritthart, H., Döring, H. J., and Byon, K. Y.: Bay a 1040— ein hochaktiver Ca^{++}-antagonistischer Inhibitor der elektro-mechanischen Koppelungsprozesse im Warmblütter-Myokard. *Arzneimittelforsch.* **22:** 22–33, 1972.

Fleckenstein, A., Tritthart, H., Fleckenstein, B., Herbst, A., and Grün, G.: A new group of competitive Ca-antagonists (Iproveratril, D600, Prenylamine) with highly potent inhibitory effects on excitation–contraction coupling in mammalian myocardium. *Pflugers Arch.* **307:** R25, 1969.

Frishman, W. H., Charlap, S., and Michelson, E. L.: Calcium channel blockers in systemic hypertension. *Am. J. Cardiol.* **58:** 157–160, 1986.

Grün, G. and Fleckenstein, A.: Die elektromechanische Entkoppelung der glatten Gefässmuskulatur als Grundprinzip der Coronardilatation durch 4-(2'-Nitrophenyl)-2,6-dimethyl-1,4,dihydropyridin-3,5-dicarbonsäure-dimethyl-ester (Bay a 1040, Nifedipine). *Arzneimittelforsch.* **22:** 334–344, 1972.

Haas, H. and Härtfelder, G.: α-Isopropyl-α-[(N-methyl-N-homoveratryl)-γ-amino-propyl]-3,4-dimethoxyphenylacetonitril, eine Substanz mit coronargefässerweiternden Eigenschaften. *Arzneimittelforsch.* **12:** 549–558, 1962.

Halperin, A. K. and Cubeddu, L. X.: The role of calcium channel blockers in the treatment of hypertension. *Am. Heart J.* **111:** 363–382, 1986.

Hayase, S., Hirakawa, S., Hosokawa, S., Mori, N., Ito, H., Kondo, Y., Hiei, K., and Banno, S.: Basic and clinical studies on Bay a 1040 with special reference to its influence on the coronary, systemic resistance and capacitance blood vessels. *Jpn. Circ. J.* **35:** 903–914, 1971.

Henry, P. D.: Comparative pharmacology of calcium antagonists: Nifedipine, verapamil and diltiazem. *Am. J. Cardiol.* **46:** 1047–1058, 1980.

Henry, P. D.: Mechanisms of action of calcium antagonists in cardiac and smooth muscle, in *Calcium Channel Blocking Agents in the Treatment of Cardiovascular Disorders*, P. H. Stone and E. M. Antman, eds., pp. 107–154, Futura, Mount Kisco, NY, 1983.

Hofbauer, K.: Zur Behandlung stenokardischer Beschwerden mit Iproveratril. *Wien Med. Wochenschr.* **116:** 1155, 1156, 1966.

Hoffmann, P.: Behandlung koronarer Durchblutungsstörungen mit Isoptin in der Praxis. *Mediz. Klin.* **59**: 1387–1391, 1964.

Hosada, S. and Kimura, E.: Efficacy of nifedipine in the variant form of angina pectoris, in *3rd International Adalat" Symposium: New Therapy of Ischemic Heart Disease*, A. D. Jatene and P. R. Lichtlen, eds., pp. 195–199, Excerpta Medica, Amsterdam, 1976.

Janis, R. A., Silver, P. J., and Triggle, D. J.: Drug action and cellular calcium regulation. *Adv. Drug Res.* **16**: 309–591, 1987.

Karlsberg, R. P.: Calcium channel blockers for cardiovascular disorders. *Arch. Intern. Med.* **142**: 452–455, 1982.

Kass, R. S.: Nisoldipine: A new, more selective calcium current blocker in cardiac Purkinje fibers. *J. Pharmacol. Exp. Ther.* **223**: 446–456, 1982.

Kazda, S., Garthoff, B., Meyer, H., Schlossmann, K., Stoepel, K., Towart, R., Vater, W., and Wehinger, E.: Pharmacology of a new calcium antagonistic compound, isobutyl methyl 1,4-dihydro-2,6-dimethyl-4-(2- nitrophenyl)-3,5-pyridinedicarboxylate (nisoldipine, Bay k 5552) *Arzneimittelforsch.* **30**: 2144–2162, 1980.

Kendall, M. J. and Okopski, J. V.: Calcium antagonism—with special reference to diltiazem. *J. Clin. Hosp. Pharm.* **11**: 159–174, 1986.

Kimura, E., moderator: Panel discussion on the variant form of angina pectoris. *Jpn. Circ. J.* **42**: 455–476, 1978.

Kimura, E., Mabuchi, G., and Kikuchi, H.: The clinical effect of 4-(2'-nitrophenyl)-2,6-dimethyl-3-5-dicarbomethoxy-1,4-dihydropyridine (Bay a 1040) on angina pectoris evaluated by sequential analysis. *Arzneimittelforsch.* **22**: 365–367, 1972.

Kobayashi, T., Ito, Y., and Tawara, I.: Clinical experience with a new coronary-active substance (Bay a 1040). *Arzneimittelforsch.* **22**: 380–389, 1972.

Kohlhardt, M., Bauer, B., Krause, H., and Fleckenstein, A.: Differentiation of the transmembrane Na and Ca channels in mammalian cardiac fibres by the use of specific inhibitors. *Pflugers Arch.* **335**: 309–322, 1972.

Krebs, R.: Calcium antagonists: New vistas in theoretical basis and clinical use, in *Calcium Antagonists and Cardiovascular Disease*, L. H. Opie, ed., pp. 347–357, Raven, New York, 1984.

Krikler, D. M.: Calcium antagonists for chronic stable angina pectoris. *Am. J. Cardiol.* **59**: 95B–100B, 1987.

Kroneberg, G.: Angina and myocardial infarction—introduction, in *Calcium Antagonists and Cardiovascular Disease*, L. H. Opie, ed., pp. 205–207, Raven, New York, 1984.

Larach, D. R. and Zelis, R.: Advances in calcium blocker therapy. *Am. J. Surgery* **151**: 527–537, 1986.

Lichtlen, P. R., ed.: *6th International Adalat® Symposium: New Therapy of*

Ischaemic Heart Disease and Hypertension, Excerpta Medica, Amsterdam, 1986.

Loos, A. and Kaltenbach, M.: Die Wirkung von Nifedipine (Bay a 1040) auf das Belastungs-Elektrokardiogramm von Angina pectoris-Kranken. _Arzneimittelforsch._ **22:** 358–362, 1972.

Luebs, E. D., Cohen, A., Zaleski, E. J., and Bing, R. J.: Effect of nitroglycerin, intensain, isoptin and papaverine on coronary blood flow in man. _Am. J. Cardiol._ **17:** 535–541, 1966.

Melville, K. I. and Benfey, B. G.: Coronary vasodilatory and cardiac adrenergic blocking effects of iproveratril. _Can. J. Physiol. Pharmacol._ **43:** 339–342, 1965.

Melville, K. I., Shister, H. E., and Huq, S.: Iproveratril: Experimental data on coronary dilatation and antiarrhythmic action. _Can. Med. Assoc. J._ **90:** 761–770, 1964.

Mignault, J. de L.: Coronary cineangiographic study of intravenously administered isoptin. _Can. Med. Assoc. J._ **95:** 1252, 1253, 1966.

Mizuno, Y., Yasui, S., Sotohata, I., Nakagawa, K., Hashimoto, Y., Nagaya, A., Nonokawa, A., Horiba, Y., Aihara, N., Tsuchiya, T., Ishikawa, K., Ooishi, H., Uchiyama, O., Kuwuhara, M., and Kashiwagi, C.: Effect of CRD-401 on ischemic heart disease. _Jpn. J. Clin. Exp. Med._ **50:** 565–573, (in Japanese), 1973.

Nakajima, H., Hoshiyama, M., Yamashita, K., and Kiyomoto, A.: Effect of diltiazem on electrical and mechanical activity of isolated cardiac ventricular muscle of guinea pig. _Jpn. J. Pharmacol._ **25:** 383–392, 1975.

Needleman, P., Corr, P. B., and Johnson, E. M., Jr.: Drugs used for the treatment of angina: Organic nitrates, calcium channel blockers, and beta-adrenergic antagonists, in _The Pharmacological Basis of Therapeutics,_ 7th Ed., A. G. Gilman, L. S. Goodman, T. W. Rall, and F. Murad, eds., pp. 806–826, Macmillan, New York, 1985.

Neumann, M. and Luisada, A. A.: Double blind evaluation of orally administered iproveratril in patients with angina pectoris. _Am. J. Med. Sci._ **251:** 552–556, 1966.

Opie, L. H.: Calcium, calcium ions, and cardiovascular disease, in _Calcium Antagonists and Cardiovascular Disease,_ L. H. Opie, ed., pp. 1–8, Raven, New York, 1984a.

Opie, L. H., ed.: _Calcium Antagonists and Cardiovascular Disease,_ Raven, New York, 1984b.

Opie, L. H. and Singh, B. N.: Calcium channel antagonists (slow channel blockers) in _Drugs for the Heart,_ 2nd Ed., pp. 34–53, Grune and Stratton, Orlando, FL, 1987.

Oyama, Y., Akutsu, Y., Tsushima, N., and Iwamoto, M.: Clinical experience with CRD-401 in angina pectoris. _Jpn. J. Clin. Exp. Med._ **49:** 1954–1957, (in Japanese), 1972.

Reuter, H.: The dependence of slow inward current in Purkinje fibres on the extracellular calcium-concentration. *J. Physiol.* **192:** 479–492, 1967.

Reuter, H. and Beeler, G. W., Jr.: Calcium current and activation of contraction in ventricular myocardial fibers. *Science* **163:** 399–401, 1969.

Sandler, G., Clayton, G. A., and Thornicroft, S. G.: Clinical evaluation of verapamil in angina pectoris. *Br. Med. J.* **3:** 224–227, 1968.

Sato, M., Nagao, T., Yamaguchi, I., Nakajima, H., and Kiyomoto, A.: Pharmacological studies on a new 1,5-benzothiazepine derivative (CRD-401). *Arzneimittelforsch.* **21:** 1338–1343, 1971.

Schneck, D. W.: Calcium-entry blockers: A review of their basic and clinical pharmacology and therapeutic applications. *Ration. Drug Ther.* **19:** 1–6, 1985.

Scriabine, A.: Current and potential indications for Ca^{2+} antagonists. *Ration. Drug Ther.* **21:** 1–6, 1987.

Singh, B. N., Ellrodt, G., and Peter, C. T.: Verapamil: A review of its pharmacological properties and therapeutic use. *Drugs* **15:** 169–197, 1978.

Spivack, C., Ocken, S., and Frishman, W. H.: Calcium antagonists. Clinical use in the treatment of systemic hypertension. *Drugs* **25:** 154–177, 1983.

Stone, P. H., Antman, E. M., Muller, J. E., and Braunwald, E.: Calcium channel blocking agents in the treatment of cardiovascular disorders. Part 2: Hemodynamic effects and clinical applications. *Ann. Intern. Med.* **93:** 886–904, 1980.

Towart, R.: The selective inhibition of serotonin-induced contractions of rabbit cerebral vascular smooth muscle by calcium-antagonistic dihydropyridines. *Circ. Res.* **48:** 650–657, 1981.

Tschirdewahn, B. and Klepzig, H.: Klinische Untersuchung über die Wirkung von Isoptin und Isoptin S bei Patienten mit Koronarinsuffizienz. *Dtsch. Med. Wochenschr.* **88:** 1702–1707, 1963.

Urthaler, F.: Review: Role of calcium channel blockers in clinical medicine. *Am. J. Med. Sci.* **292:** 217–230, 1986.

Vater, W., Kroneburg, G., Hoffmeister, F., Kaller, H., Meng, K., Oberdorf, A., Puls, W., Schlossman, K., and Stoepel, K.: Zur Pharmakologie von 4-(2'-Nitrophenyl)-2, 6-dimethyl-1, 4-dihydropyridin-3, 5-dicarbonsäuredimethylester (Nifedipine, Bay a 1040). *Arzneimittelforsch.* **22:** 1–14, 1972.

Winbury, M. M.: Antianginal drugs, in *Discoveries in Pharmacology*, vol. 2, *Haemodynamics, Hormones and Inflammation*, M. J. Parnham and J. Bruinvels, eds., pp. 141–161, Elsevier, Amsterdam 1984.

Yasue, H., Nagao, M., Orote, S., Takizawa, A., Miwa, K., and Tanaka, S.: Coronary arterial spasm and Prinzmetal's variant form of angina induced by hyperventilation and tris-buffer infusion. *Circulation* **58:** 56–62, 1978a.

Yasue, H., Omote, S., Takizawa, A., Nagao, M., Miwa, K., Kato, H., Tanaka, S., and Akiyama, F.: Pathogenesis and treatment of angina pectoris at rest as seen from its response to various drugs. *Jpn. Circ. J.,* **42:** 1–10, 1978b.

Chlorothiazide

I. Chlorothiazide as an Innovative Therapeutic Agent

Edema is defined as "[a]n accumulation of an excessive amount of watery fluid in cells, tissues or serous cavities" (Stedman, 1982). It is an accompaniment to a variety of diseases, e.g., congestive heart failure, pulmonary heart failure, cirrhosis of the liver, and chronic renal diseases. It can cause serious respiratory symptoms, abdominal distress, and disabling swelling of limbs. The underlying abnormality in these edematous states involves a decreased rate of renal excretion of Na^+, the primary extracellular cation (Weiner and Mudge, 1985). Associated with this retention of Na^+ is the retention of extracellular anion (to maintain electroneutrality) and a volume of water adequate to maintain normal osmolality.

Diuretics have long been used to mobilize edema fluids. Before the advent of chlorothiazide, the most effective diuretics were the organic mercurials and the carbonic anhydrase inhibitors (primarily acetazolamide). Both of these classes of diuretics were clinically effective, but had serious shortcomings.

According to Modell et al. (1976), organic mercurials, although very effective diuretics, usually had to be given by intramuscular injection, and many were irritant to tissues. Moreover, because of their predominant effect on Cl^- excretion, the intensive, sustained use of organic mercurial agents tended to elicit serious hypochloremic alkalosis, since HCO_3^- concentration increased in the extracellular fluid to replace the lost Cl^-. This situation had the potential of leading to renal failure and uremia. Mercurials also, on occasion, produced cardiac toxicity and acute allergic reactions.

The therapeutic usefulness of acetazolamide in counteracting edema was limited by the metabolic acidosis that it produced and the rapid development of refractoriness to its effects (Modell, et al., 1976).

The appearance of the first benzothiadiazine diuretic, chlorothiazide, initiated the decline of the mercurial diuretics, which were soon to be rendered obsolete even though they had dominated the therapy of edema for over 30 years. It also relegated acetazolamide to very limited therapeutic use. Chlorothiazide was a potent, orally effective agent that reliably mobilized Na^+ and water in edematous states and did not lose potency with prolonged use.

Chlorothiazide and related drugs have become first-line drugs in the treatment of essential hypertension. Gifford (1976) considered the introduction of potent orally administered diuretics to be one of the most significant therapeutic milestones of this century.

Early Clinical Research History

Ford et al. (1957) compared the effects of orally administered chlorothiazide with mercurial diuretics in 20 patients with mild chronic congestive heart failure. They reported that, compared to the orally administered mercurial chlormerodrin, chlorothiazide produced adequate control of edema in 18 of 20 patients. It was a potent inhibitor of the renal tubular reabsorption of Na^+, and it did not produce metabolic acidosis or other physiological or pharmacodynamic side effects. Laragh (1958) studied the effect of chlorothiazide on edemas seen in a variety of illnesses, namely, congestive heart failure secondary to coronary artery disease; congestive failure resulting from rheumatic heart disease; nephrosis; pulmonary heart disease; and cirrhosis of the liver. He found that all types of fluid retention appeared to respond to chlorothiazide.

Wilkins et al. (1958) reported that orally administered chlorothiazide alone or added to other antihypertensive regimens consistently lowered the blood pressure of patients whose hypertension had not responded to standard treatments. The drug was well-tolerated and was free of serious side effects. The blood pressure of normal control subjects was not significantly altered by the drug.

Freis et al. (1958) administered chlorothiazide to 90 hypertensive patients who were being treated with antihypertensives such as ganglionic blocking agents, veratrum alkaloids, and reserpine. Chlorothiazide, in addition to potentiating the hypotensive effect of the other drugs, was a hypotensive agent in its own right.

Hundreds of preclinical and clinical reports have been published that supported these initial findings with chlorothiazide and extended them to related agents. Many reviews and chapters have also been published (*see*, for example, Taggart, 1958; Beyer and Baer, 1961; Baer and Beyer, 1972; Modell et al., 1976; Gifford, 1976; Allen, 1983; Weiner and Mudge, 1985).

II. The Scientific Departure
Leading to Chlorothiazide: Sulfanilamide

Southworth (1937) noted that two of 50 patients being treated for beta hemolytic streptococcal infections with the antibacterial agent sulfanilamide (Fig. 1) had developed signs of clinical acidosis. As a followup, the author gave sulfanilamide to 15 consecutive patients and monitored the CO_2 combining power of their blood plasmas. All patients showed variable drops in this measurement. Subsequently, Strauss and Southworth (1938) found, in three normal human subjects, that sulfanilamide produced a decrease in the CO_2 combining capacity of the plasma, a definite diuresis, and an increase in the renal excretions of sodium and potassium. These authors made no comment regarding the possible clinical use of sulfanilamide as a diuretic. Marshall et al. (1938), as part of a toxicity study, demonstrated that dogs given sulfanilamide developed very alkaline urines with a coincident large loss of bicarbonate and base (i.e., largely Na^+). Marshall et al. (1938) suggested "...that this may be due to lack of reabsorption of bicarbonate and base from the glomerular filtrate...."

The observations of Southworth (1937) and of Marshall et al. (1938) suggested to Mann and Keilin (1940) the possibility that sulfanilamide and other sulfonamides might be inhibiting the en-

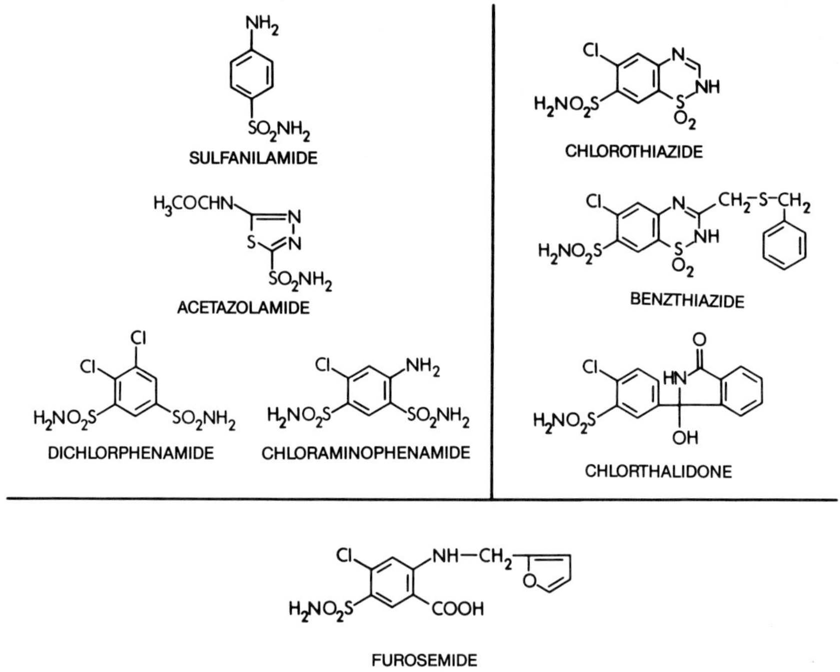

Fig. 1. The structures of chlorothiazide and chemically and/or pharmacologically related substances.

zyme carbonic anhydrase. This enzyme was known to catalyze the reversible reaction

$$CO_2 + H_2O \underset{\text{anhydrase}}{\overset{\text{carbonic}}{\rightleftharpoons}} H_2CO_3 \rightleftharpoons H^+ + HCO_3^-$$

in red blood cells and in gastric mucosa. They found sulfanilamide to be an effective inhibitor. The amino group was necessary for antibacterial action, but was not necessary for carbonic anhydrase inhibition. The unsubstituted sulfonamide group ($-SO_2NH_2$), however, was a strict requirement for enzyme inhibition. Sulfonamide compounds were highly specific in inhibiting carbonic anhydrase: they showed little activity against other enzymes. Locke et al. (1941) confirmed the work of Mann and Keilin (1940).

Davenport and Wilhelmi (1941) reported carbonic anhydrase to be present in significant concentrations in the renal cortex of cats, dogs, and rats. It was suggested that the role of carbonic anhydrase in the kidney could be explored, because it was known that sulfanilamide affected the kidney and was also a powerful inhibitor of carbonic anhydrase.

Sulfanilamide and related agents with unsubstituted sulfonamide groups produced a reversible alkalinization of perfusion fluid as they passed through isolated frog kidneys (Höber, 1942). This investigator surmised that the alkalinization resulted from inhibition of carbonic anhydrase by the sulfanilamide and related compounds, and that this enzyme was involved in catalyzing the reabsorption of bicarbonate by the kidney.

Pitts and Alexander (1945) demonstrated in dogs that a renal mechanism was available for adding acid to the glomerular filtrate as it passed through the renal tubules. It was suggested "...that this addition of acid is effected by the direct exchange of H^+ ions formed within the renal tubular cells for Na^+ ions present in the tubular urine.... The intracellular source of H^+ ions is carbonic acid formed by the hydration of carbon dioxide produced metabolically within the renal cells.... The Na^+ ions which enter the renal tubular cells in exchange for H^+ ions are absorbed into the peritubular blood as sodium bicarbonate." These authors found that administration of sulfanilamide reduced the observed titratable acid of the urine.

Schwartz (1949) noted the concepts of Pitts and Alexander (1945) and theorized from these that sulfanilamide, by inhibiting carbonic anhydrase, should limit the supply of H^+ and thereby lead to a loss of Na^+ and obligatory water. In a study of three patients with congestive heart failure, Schwartz (1949) found that all three showed an increase in Na^+ and K^+ excretion within 24 h after sulfanilamide administration. In the two patients who could tolerate the drug for a week, a weight loss occurred that matched the increase in Na^+ output. The CO_2 combining power of serum decreased sharply, and urine pH increased. It was concluded that the changes could best be explained by an inhibition of carbonic anhydrase in the renal parenchyma, with retention of H^+ and reduction of Na^+ reabsorption. The edemetous condition of two of the three patients was improved. All three patients experienced side effects ranging from slight confusion to nausea, methemoglobinemia, chills, and fever.

Background Contributions Preceding the Discovery of the Carbonic Anhydrase-Inhibiting Action of Sulfanilamide

Meldrum and Roughton (1933) described the preparation and properties of carbonic anhydrase. In summary they stated, "Carbonic anhydrase is an enzyme present in red blood corpuscles (but not in the blood plasma) which catalyzes both phases of the reversible reaction $H_2 CO_3 \leftrightarrows CO_2 + H_2O$. It is thus of prime physiological importance in the formation of CO_2 from bicarbonate in the lung. Without it, CO_2 could not be excreted nearly fast enough for the needs of the body."

Prontosil, a molecule incorporating sulfanilamide in its structure, was synthesized as an azo dye in Germany in 1932. Prontosil was discovered to have chemotherapeutic activities in mice (Domagk, 1935) and sulfanilamide was found to be the active metabolite of prontosil (Tréfouël et al., 1935). Subsequently, Colebrook and Kenny (1936) and Buttle et al. (1936) reported successful results with prontosil and sulfanilamide against puerperal sepsis and meningococcal infections in mice. Colebrook and Kenny (1936) further demonstrated a positive effect of prontosil in a series of 38 puerperal fever cases in humans. Sulfanilamide and related agents were the mainstay of antiinfective therapy until the discovery of penicillin and other antibiotics.

Significant Events Following Sulfanilamide

Schwartz (1949) felt that sulfanilamide was clearly too toxic for prolonged or routine use as a diuretic agent. He emphasized that the structural requirements for sulfonamides viewed as antiinfective agents differed sharply from requirements for sulfonamides viewed as carbonic anhydrase inhibitors. He noted that analogs of sulfanilamide were being studied in an attempt to find one that was as effective as sulfanilamide as a carbonic anhydrase inhibitor but less toxic. A series of heterocyclic sulfonamides was synthesized by Roblin and Clapp (1950), and its activity against carbonic anhydrase was reported by Roblin and associates (Miller et al., 1950). Miller et al. (1950) explicitly expressed their indebtedness to Schwartz for calling their attention to his results (Schwartz, 1949): these results led Miller et al. (1950) to carry out their chemical/pharmacological program. One of their compounds was 330 times more potent than sulfanilamide. This compound, 2-acetylamino-1,3, 4,-thiadiazole-5-sulfonamide (Fig.1), was later given the generic name acetazolamide. The authors also prepared several aromatic sulfonamides, but these had low potency as carbonic anhydrase inhibitors when compared to the best of the heterocyclic compounds.

Acetazolamide was given by Friedberg et al. (1953) to 26 patients with congestive heart failure of diverse origin. The secretion of an acid urine was prevented and the excretion of Na^+ and K^+ increased. Eighteen patients showed diuresis, weight loss, and clinical improvement. Acidosis was evident but mild. With continued thrice-daily administration, the effects of acetazolamide waned: after two to three days, the drug lost its activity completely or partially. Extensive clinical experience has subsequently confirmed the findings of Friedberg et al. (1953). In addition to its limited use in edema, acetazolamide is effective in some forms of epilepsy and glaucoma (Modell et al., 1976).

In the search for better carbonic anhydrase inhibitors, aromatic sulfonamide compounds were given detailed attention in several laboratories. Dichlorphenamide and chloraminophenamide (Fig. 1) resulted from this search. These *meta*-disulfonamide compounds had unexpectedly good activity as carbonic anhydrase inhibitors (Sprague, 1958). Dichlorphenamide is still commercially available for that purpose (Weiner and Mudge, 1985). These compounds were effective diuretics by the oral route and appeared to promote a greater elimination of Cl⁻ than did acetazolamide. In the course of this work, Sprague (1958) discovered that when an acylamino group, instead of an unsubstituted amino group, occupied the benzene ring *ortho* to one of the two sulfonamide groups in a molecule such as chloraminophenamide, a ring closure readily occurred, yielding benzothiadiazine–1, 1-dioxides. These benzothiadiazines were reported to exhibit an order of inhibition of carbonic anhydrase previously seen only among the heterocyclic sulfonamides, such as acetazolamide. As an outgrowth of these chemical findings, the benzothiadiazine compound chlorothiazide (Fig. 1) was eventually synthesized (Novello and Sprague, 1957).

In dogs, chlorothiazide proved to be an effective diuretic agent when given by the oral route (Beyer et al., 1957). Beyer et al. (1957) noted that chlorothiazide was 30 times more potent, in vitro, as a carbonic anhydrase inhibitor than was acetazolamide; yet, unlike acetazolamide, it induced a large and nearly equimolar excretion of Na$^+$ and Cl$^-$ in dogs, without producing acidosis or alkalosis. At doses of 1–3 mg/kg iv and 5 mg/kg orally in dogs, the effect on K$^+$ excretion was slight, and urinary pH was not necessarily increased. Beyer (1958) gave a detailed exposition of the pharmacology of chlorothiazide. He pointed out that, although chlorothiazide resembled a potent organomercurial in its primary effect of increasing Na$^+$, Cl$^-$, and water excretion, and resembled acetazolamide in inhibiting carbonic anhydrase, its spectrum of renotropic effects was unique. Subsequently, the in vitro potency of chlorothiazide against carbonic anhydrase was accurately determined to be only one-twentieth that of acetazolamide (Beyer and Baer, 1961).

Table 1 defines the critical scientific ideas and experiments leading to chlorothiazide and categorizes their origin.

III. Comments on Events Leading to Chlorothiazide

According to Weiner and Mudge (1985), "Acetazolamide is the prototype of a class of agents that have had limited usefulness as diuretics but have played a major role in the development of fundamental renal physiology and pharmacology."

Allen (1983) was of the opinion that

[t]he development of the *meta*-disulfonamides [e.g., dichlorphenamide and related agents] marked the beginning of modern sulfonamide saluretic agents. Like most true progress in drug research, this beginning was characterized by a certain measure of serendipity, as well as close cooperation among medicinal chemists, pharmacologists and clinicians.

Table 1

Profile of Observations and Ideas Crucial to the Development of Chlorothiazide[a]

Sequence: Departure compound[*] to innovative drug[**]	Orient-ation	Nature of study	Research institution	National origin	Nature of discovery	Screening involved	Crucial ideas or observations
Sulfanilamide[*]							
South-worth (1937)	Clinical	Pharma-cology	Uni-versity	USA	Seren-dipitous	No	The antibacterial sulfanilamide produces acidosis (reduces CO_2 combining power of blood in humans).
Mann and Keilin (1940)	Pre-clinical	Pharma-cology	Uni-versity	UK	Orderly	No	Sulfanilamide inhibits carbonic anhydrase.
Davenport and Wil-helmi (1941)	Pre-clinical	Biochem-istry	Uni-versity	USA	Orderly	No	The kidney contains carbonic anhydrase.
Pitts and Alexander (1945)	Pre-clinical	Physi-ology	Uni-versity	USA	Orderly	No	The intracellular hydration of CO_2 supplies the H^+ for the exchange with Na^+ in tubular urine.
Schwartz (1949)	Clinical	Pharma-cology	Uni-versity	USA	Orderly	No	Sulfanilamide causes Na^+ excretion, weight loss, and reduced edema in patients with congestive heart failure, presumably via inhibition of carbonic anhydrase.
Chlorothiazide[**]							
Novello and Sprague (1957)	Pre-clinical	Chem-istry/ pharma-cology	Indus-try	USA	Orderly	Targeted	Chlorothiazide syn-thesized as a carbon-ic anhydrase inhibi-tor; potent diuretic effect not typical of carbonic anhydrase inhibitors; active by oral route.

[a]Taken from Section II. Entries are those contributions without which the discovery of the agent (or additionally, in some cases, a relevant clinical application) would not have taken place or would have been materially delayed.

Baer (1984) reminisced that

> J. M. Sprague...had successfully developed several sulfonamide anti-
> bacterial agents during World War II. K. H. Beyer...had investigated
> the renal transport of sulfonamides and of penicillin...[and] discov-
> ered the penicillin-sparing action of analogs of the sulfonamide type
> [e.g., probenecid]....Based on the competitive inhibition of organic
> acids for renal transport (for which no enzymic mechanism was or is
> evident), we [i.e., Beyer and Baer] presumed that inhibition of inor-
> ganic ion transport might be modulated by organic compounds.

Beyer (1958) noted that his earlier work with a weak carbonic anhydrase inhibitor, *p*-carboxybenzenesulfonamide (Beyer, 1954), suggested that a carbonic anhydrase inhibitor that distributed selectively to the kidney would be preferable to one that distributed more generally. Since measurements of carbonic anhydrase inhibition, in vitro, could make no statements regarding selective distribution of compounds, Beyer decided that, in the renal electrolyte research leading to chlorothiazide, primary emphasis would be placed on in vivo activity rather than on in vitro potency. Presumably, this decision permitted the detection of the unusual properties of chlorothiazide when it was synthesized in the wake of dichlorphenamide (Novello and Sprague, 1957; Sprague, 1958).

Beyer, Sprague, Baer, and Novello received the Albert Lasker Special Award in 1975 for their research work with thiazide diuretics (*see* Beyer, 1977). Weiner and Mudge (1985) considered that the development of chlorothiazide (and related compounds) "...provides an instructive example of the manner in which newly synthesized agents may be endowed with unanticipated efficacious properties."

IV. Developments
Subsequent to Chlorothiazide

The appearance of chlorothiazide stimulated medicinal chemists to synthesize a veritable flood of benzothiadiazine derivatives, all of which contain the sulfonamide group. Hydrochlorothiazide, which was considerably more potent with improved saluretic efficacy, appeared within a year (DeStevens et al., 1958). Hydroflumethiazide, bendroflumethiazide, benzthiazide (Fig. 1), trichlormethiazide, methyclothiazide, and polythiazide followed (Gifford, 1976). In addition, other sulfonamide agents have appeared in which the heterocyclic ring differs substantially from that of chlorothiazide, e.g., chlorthalidone (Fig. 1), quinethazone, metolazone, and indapamide. However, according to Weiner and Mudge (1985) and Gifford (1976), if potency differences are put aside, the pharmacological actions of the whole group appear to be similar, as do their therapeutic actions.

As pointed out by Cragoe (1983), perhaps even more important than the production of benzothiadiazine analogs was the continued exploration of the chemical lead presented by the sulfonamide diuretics. This eventually led to a totally novel subclass of these drugs, exemplified by furosemide (Fig. 1), a very safe, orally effective agent with the high efficacy of the mercurials.

References

Allen, R. C.: Sulfonamide diuretics, in *Diuretics—Chemistry, Pharmacology, and Medicine*, E. J., Cragoe, Jr., ed., pp. 49–200, Wiley, New York, 1983.

Baer, J. E.: Discovery of chlorothiazide, in *Diuretics: Chemistry, Pharmacology, and Clinical Applications*, J. B. Puschett and A. Greenberg, eds., pp. 1–3, Elsevier, New York, 1984.

Baer, J. E. and Beyer K. H.: Subcellular pharmacology of natriuretic and potassium-sparing drugs. *Prog. Biochem. Pharmacol.* 7: 59–93, 1972.

Beyer, K. H.: Factors basic to the development of useful inhibitors of renal transport mechanisms. *Arch. Int. Pharmacodyn.* 98: 97–117, 1954.

Beyer, K. H.: The mechanism of action of chlorothiazide. *Ann. NY Acad. Sci.* 71: 363–379, 1958.

Beyer, K. H., Jr.: Discovery of the thiazides: Where biology and chemistry meet. *Perspect. Biol. Med.* 20: 410–420, 1977.

Beyer, K. H. and Baer, J. E.: Physiological basis for the action of newer diuretic agents. *Pharmacol. Rev.* 13: 517–562, 1961.

Beyer, K. H., Baer, J. E., Russo, H. F., and Haimbach, A. S.: Chlorothiazide (6-chloro-7-sulfamyl-1,2,4-benzothiadiazine–1,1-dioxide): The enhancement of sodium chloride excretion. *Fed. Proc.* 16: 282, 1957.

Buttle, G. A. H., Gray, W. H., and Stephenson, D.: Protection of mice against streptococcal and other infections by p-aminobenzenesulphonamide and related substances. *Lancet* 1: 1286–1290, 1936.

Colebrook, L. and Kenny, M.: Treatment of human puerperal infections, and of experimental infections in mice, with Prontosil. *Lancet* 1: 1279–1286, 1936.

Cragoe, Jr., E. J.: Introduction, in *Diuretics—Chemistry, Pharmacology, and Medicine*, pp. 1–15, Wiley, New York, 1983.

Davenport, H. W. and Wilhelmi, A. E.: Renal carbonic anhydrase. *Proc. Soc. Exp. Biol. Med.* **48:** 53–56, 1941.

DeStevens, G., Werner, L. H., Halamandaris, A., and Ricca, Jr. S.: Dihydrobenzothiadiazine dioxides with potent diuretic effect. *Experientia* **14:** 463, 1958.

Domagk, G.: Ein Beitrag zur Chemotherapie der bakteriellen Infektionen. *Dtsch. Med. Wochenschr.* **61:** 250–253, 1935.

Ford, R. V., Moyer, J. H., and Spurr, C. L.: Clinical and laboratory observations on chlorothiazide (Diuril), an orally effective nonmercurial diuretic agent. *AMA Arch. Intern Med.* **100:** 582–596, 1957.

Friedberg, C. K., Taymor, R., Minor, J. B., and Halpern, M.: The use of diamox, a carbonic anhydrase inhibitor, as an oral diuretic in patients with congestive heart failure. *N. Engl. J. Med.* **248:** 883–889, 1953.

Fries, E. D., Wanko, A., Wilson, I. M., and Parrish, A. E.: Chlorothiazide in hypertensive and normotensive patients. *Ann. NY Acad. Sci.* **71:** 450–455, 1958.

Gifford, Jr., R. W.: A guide to the practical use of diuretics. *J. Am. Med. Assoc.* **235:** 1890–1893, 1976.

Höber, R.: Effect of some sulfonamides on renal secretion. *Proc. Soc. Exp. Biol. Med.* **49:** 87–90, 1942.

Laragh, J. H.: Some effects of chlorothiazide on electrolyte metabolism and its use in edematous states. *Ann. NY Acad. Sci.* **71:** 409–419, 1958.

Locke, A., Main, E. R., and Mellon, R. R.: Carbonic anhydrase inactivation as the source of sulfanilamide "acidosis." *Science* **93:** 66, 67, 1941.

Mann, T. and Keilin, D.: Sulphanilamide as a specific inhibitor of carbonic anhydrase. *Nature* **146:** 164, 165, 1940.

Marshall, E. K., Jr., Cutting, W. C. , and Emerson, K.: The toxicity of sulfanilamide. *J. Am. Med. Assoc.* **110:** 252–257, 1938.

Meldrum, N. U. and Roughton, F. J. W.: Carbonic anhydrase; its preparation and properties. *J. Physiol.* **80:** 113–142, 1933.

Miller, W. H., Dessert, A. M., and Roblin, Jr., R. O.: Heterocyclic sulfonamides as carbonic anhydrase inhibitors. *J. Am. Chem. Soc.* **72:** 4893–4896, 1950.

Modell, W., Schild, H. O., and Wilson, A.: *Applied Pharmacology*, W. B. Saunders, Philadelphia, 1976.

Novello, F. C. and Sprague, J. M.: Benzothiadiazine dioxides as novel diuretics. *J. Am. Chem. Soc.* **79:** 2028, 2029, 1957.

Pitts, R. F. and Alexander, R. S.: The nature of the renal tubular mechanism for acidifying the urine. *Am. J. Physiol.* **144:** 239–254, 1945.

Roblin, Jr. , R. O. and Clapp, J. W.: The preparation of heterocyclic sulfonamides. *J. Am. Chem. Soc.* **72:** 4890–4892, 1950.

Schwartz, W. B.: The effect of sulfanilamide on salt and water excretion in congestive heart failure. *N. Engl. J. Med.* **240:** 173–177, 1949.

Southworth, H.: Acidosis associated with the administration of para-amino-benzene-sulfonamide (Prontylin). *Proc. Soc. Exp. Biol.* **36:** 58–61, 1937.

Sprague, J. M.: The chemistry of diuretics. *Ann. NY Acad. Sci.* **71:** 328–343, 1958.

Stedman's Medical Dictionary, 24th Ed., Williams & Wilkins, Baltimore, 1982.

Strauss, M. B. and Southworth, H.: Urinary changes as a result of sulfanilamide administration. *Bull. J. Hopkins Hosp.* **63:** 41–45, 1938.

Taggart, J. V., consult. ed. *Chlorothiazide and Other Diuretic Agents, Ann. NY Acad. Sci.* **71:** 321–478, 1958.

Tréfouël, J., Tréfouël, J., (Mme.) Nitti, F., and Bovet, D.: Activité du p-aminophénylsulfamide sur les infections streptococciques expérimentales de la souris et du lapin. *Compt. Rend. Soc. Biol.* **120:** 756–758, 1935.

Weiner, I. M. and Mudge, G. H.: Diuretics and other agents employed in the mobilization of edema fluid, in *The Pharmacological Basis of Therapeutics,* 7th Ed., A. G. Gilman, L. S. Goodman, T. W. Rall, and F. Murad, eds., pp. 887–907, Macmillan, New York, 1985.

Wilkins, R. W., Hollander, W., and Chobanian, A. V.: Chlorothiazide in hypertension: Studies on its mode of action. *Ann. NY Acad. Sci.* **71:** 465–472, 1958.

Furosemide

I. Furosemide as an Innovative Therapeutic Agent

Furosemide and ethacrynic acid arrived on the clinical scene in the 1960s. They quickly became known as "loop diuretics" and "high-ceiling diuretics." The former appellation refers loosely to the site of action of these agents within the nephron—the loop of Henle—and the latter to the fact that the maximum diuresis achieved with these drugs far exceeded that obtained with the thiazide diuretics.

Before the loop diuretics, the thiazide and organic mercurial diuretics had been used to good effect as agents for mobilizing edema fluid in congestive heart failure, cirrhosis, and nephrosis. Furosemide and ethacrynic acid were found to be particularly effective in cases that were refractory to the thiazides and mercurials. They were also very effective as emergency intravenous treatments for pulmonary and cerebral edemas and in barbiturate poisoning: diuresis occurred within 15 min, whereas 1–3 h were required for thiazide and mercurial agents to take effect (Stason et al., 1966; Kirkendall and Stein, 1968; Cannon and Kilcoyne, 1969; Modell et al., 1976; Weiner and Mudge, 1985). Unlike the mercurial diuretics, furosemide and ethacrynic acid continued to be effective even when electrolyte and acid–base disturbances were present.

Furosemide has come to be prescribed much more frequently than ethacrynic acid, because of a considerably lower incidence of gastrointestinal side effects and a less steep dose–response curve (Weiner and Mudge, 1985). Loop diuretics, if not carefully administered, may be given in overdose and produce orthostatic hypotension, shock, and prerenal azotemia as a result of excessive diuresis, electrolyte imbalance, or acid–base disturbances. The less steep dose–response curve of furosemide allowed for a more predictable and controllable response in patients than could be obtained with ethacrynic acid. In addition, the relatively brief diuretic action of furosemide allowed for a response in patients that could be quickly and easily controlled by adjustment of dose and by the frequency of administration (Stason et al., 1966).

Hutcheon and Martinez (1986) drew the following conclusions regarding furosemide (and structurally related agents):

1. It was highly effective in producing both natriuresis and lowering of blood pressure in patients with renal failure and edema secondary to renal disease.
2. It represented a major advance in the management of liver disease with ascites.
3. It was especially effective as an adjunct antihypertensive agent in patients with cardiovascular or renal complications, because it lowered renal vascular resistance and thereby maintained renal blood flow and filtration rate despite a hypotension-induced fall in renal artery perfusion pressure.

Hutcheon and Martinez (1986) further noted that furosemide had been well tolerated and was relatively free of untoward reactions when used in recommended therapeutic doses.

Furosemide is an exceptionally efficacious agent. Thus, whereas the peak diuresis from mercurial diuretics, under optimal conditions, amounts to 15–20% of the glomerular filtrate and the maximum effect from thiazide diuretics is approximately half that amount, furosemide has a peak effect as great as 30% or more (Berliner, 1966; Robson et al., 1964; Suki et al., 1965). This was subsequently found to result from the fact that furosemide, in distinction to the thiazides (and mercurials), acts over the entire length of the thick ascending limb of the loop of Henle—both medullary and cortical segments—to inhibit the active transport of Cl^- and the linked, passive reabsorption of Na^+. The thick ascending limb reabsorbs a larger percentage of filtered NaCl than do other parts of the nephron (Stein et al., 1968; Puschett and Goldberg, 1968). Because of its site of action, furosemide inhibits the capacity of the kidneys to both dilute and concentrate the urine. Unlike the thiazides, which produce a hypertonic urine, furosemide promotes an isotonic diuresis and thereby causes considerably greater amounts of water loss than do the thiazides (Jacobson and Kokko, 1976; Allen, 1983). Furosemide is relatively nontoxic. It is 98% bound to plasma proteins, and therefore the amount filtered by the glomerulus is very small. It has a diuretic action because it is actively secreted, in unbound, active form, into the urine of the tubules by the organic acid (anion) transport mechanism (Burg, 1976; Odlind and Beerman, 1980).

Hutcheon et al. (1965) expressed the opinion, "The discovery of furosemide... represents a distinct pharmacological advance over the benzothiadiazine diuretics." According to Allen (1983),

> The introduction of furosemide...into medical practice represented a significant advance in clinical diuretic therapy. Addition of furosemide to the physician's armamentarium presented him with a relatively safe and orally efficacious replacement for the more toxic mercurials, and an alternative to the thiazide-like compounds.

Early Clinical Research History

Kleinfelder (1963) found that furosemide produced a prompt diuretic action in 51 patients with edema of various origins. This author considered furosemide clearly superior to hydrochlorothiazide in edematous patients, since fluid output was 200% greater, and Na^+ output 167% greater, than those obtained with this thiazide.

Furosemide was very effective over a period of 20 months in 80 patients, most of whom were suffering from congestive heart failure. This group included four patients with ascites and edema from hepatic cirrhosis (Stokes and Nunn, 1964). Resistant edemas that did not respond to mercurial and thiazide diuretics were successfully treated with furosemide. Prompt diuresis with intravenous furosemide was of great value in treating acute pulmonary edema.

In 14 patients being treated for heart failure (secondary to rheumatic heart disease in 12 of the 14 cases), furosemide was more effective than the other oral diuretics that were studied, namely, hydrochlorthiazide, chlorthalidone, triamterene, and cyclopenthiazide (Verel et al., 1964). Furosemide compared well with the mercurial mersalyl given intramuscularly. Judging from the pattern of

electrolyte excretion, the authors surmised that furosemide differed
from the oral diuretics in its action on the kidney, but had an action
similar to mersalyl.

Hutcheon et al. (1965) found that furosemide caused a prompt
increase in Na+, K+, Cl−, and water excretion in six normal males and
in 12 patients with edema secondary to congestive heart failure.
These authors also found that the plasma and urinary electrolyte
patterns seen with furosemide, as well as the formation of an acid
urine, resembled those seen with mercurial diuretics.

Stason et al. (1966) treated 39 patients exhibiting abnormal fluid
and Na+ retention, and seven normal people. Most of the patients
were refractory to meralluride, thiazides, acetazolamide, and spiro-
nolactone. Furosemide exhibited a broad dose–response curve in
these patients. At higher doses it was significantly more effective
than the thiazide diuretics. Furosemide, like ethacrynic acid and
unlike thiazide diuretics, interfered both with urinary concentration
during antidiuresis and with urinary dilution during waterloading.
The authors were the first to suggest "...that furosemide acts to block
sodium chloride reabsorption in the ascending limb of Henle's loop
and in more cortical distal diluting segments."

Many reviews and chapters have been devoted to discussion of
the animal and clinical studies with furosemide (*see,* for example,
Suki et al., 1965; Berliner, 1966; Kirkendall and Stein, 1968; Cannon
and Kilcoyne, 1969; Lant and Wilson, 1973; Frazier and Yager,
1973a,b; Suki et al., 1973; Beyer and Baer, 1975; Jacobson and Kokko,
1976; Burg, 1976; Seely and Dirks, 1977; Feit, 1981; Brater, 1983;
Allen, 1983).

II. The Scientific Work
Leading to Furosemide

Muschaweck and Hajdú (1964) commented that, as the sulfonamide (thiazide) diuretics (Fig. 1) gained broad use in the late
1950s, several important side effects of relatively low incidence became evident, for example, increased K+ excretion, elevated blood
glucose, and elevated serum uric acid levels. Because of this,
Muschaweck and Hajdú (1964) considered that there was room for
improvement in the area of sulfonamide diuretics. Synthetic efforts

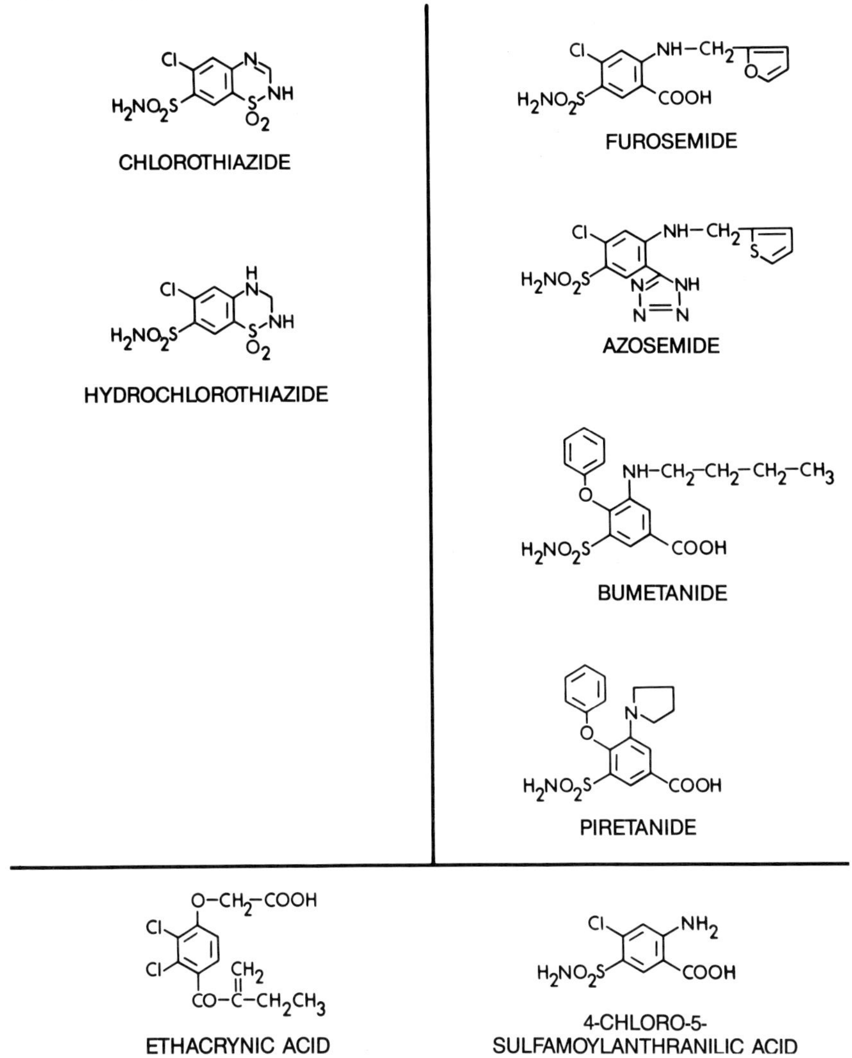

Fig. 1. The structures of furosemide and chemically and/or pharmacologically related substances.

in an aromatic sulfonamide series eventually led to the anthranilic acid derivative furosemide (Fig. 1). In the dog, furosemide effected a considerable and equimolar excretion of Na$^+$ and Cl$^-$, accompanied by a greatly enhanced excretion of water, at doses that did not increase K$^+$ loss. Muschaweck (1963) had already reported earlier, at a symposium, that furosemide had a much higher ceiling for excretion of sodium and chloride ions than did hydrochlorothiazide, and that furosemide increased the diuretic effect when added to the maximum effective dose of hydrochlorothiazide. Furosemide had no influence on blood sugar or uric acid levels, and it was not an inhibitor of carbonic anhydrase. The compound was well tolerated by rats and dogs.

Timmerman et al. (1964) compared the potency (the dose required to produce a standard submaximal diuresis) and efficacy (the maximal diuresis obtainable) of six thiazide diuretics with furosemide in saline-loaded rats. They found that, although the potencies of the thiazides were quite different, their efficacies were similar. On the other hand, furosemide, the least potent of all the compounds, had a natriuretic ceiling (efficacy) that was three times higher than could be obtained with the thiazides and had a considerably steeper dose–reponse curve. Similar results were obtained by these authors in a comparison of hydrochlorothiazide with furosemide in 15 healthy male subjects. Both the maximum Na^+ output and the urine volume obtained with furosemide were considerably in excess of the maximal obtainable with hydrochlorothiazide. Compared to hydrochlorothiazide, furosemide produced an intense action of short duration. Timmerman et al. (1964) concluded, "The unique effect of furosemide suggests that different or, at least, additional modes or sites of action in the nephron might be involved as compared to the action of the thiazides."

Table 1 defines the critical scientific ideas and experiments leading to furosemide and categorizes their origin.

Background Contributions Preceding Furosemide

The sulfonamide antibacterial agent sulfanilamide was shown to inhibit the enzyme carbonic anhydrase (Mann and Keilin, 1940) and to act as a diuretic in humans (Schwartz, 1949). These observations initiated the development of several somewhat more useful diuretics that were very potent inhibitors of this enzyme, for example, a heterocyclic sulfonamide, acetazolamide (Miller, et al., 1950), and an aromatic sulfonamide, dichlorphenamide (Sprague, 1958). Continued molecular modification in the aromatic series eventually led to the synthesis of a heterocyclic benzothiadiazine, chlorothiazide—a vastly superior orally effective sulfonamide diuretic, which

Table 1
Profile of Observations and Ideas Crucial to the Development of Furosemide[*]

Sequence: Route to innovative drug[**]	Orient- ation	Nature of study	Research institution	National origin	Nature of discovery	Screening involved	Crucial ideas or observations
Furosemide[**]							
Muscha- weck and Hajdú (1964)	Pre- clinical	Chem- istry/ pharma- cology	Industry	West Germany	Orderly	Targeted	Furosemide elicits a marked, equimolar excretion of Na and Cl⁻; only trivial increase in K⁺ excretion; no effect on carbohydrate and uric acid metabolism.

[*]Taken from section II. Entries are those contributions without which the discovery of the agent (or additionally, in some cases, a relevant clinical application) would not have taken place or would have been materially delayed.

relied only slightly on inhibition of carbonic anhydrase for its effectiveness (Novello and Sprague, 1957; Beyer, 1958). For greater detail regarding sulfanilamide, carbonic anhydrase inhibition and inhibitors, and thiazide diuretics, *see* section II of the chapter on chlorothiazide.

III. Comments on Events Leading to Furosemide

According to Siedel et al. (1967), Siedel and Sturm of Farbwerke Hoechst AG had been synthesizing heterocyclic carbonic anhydrase inhibitors. They succeeded in 1957 in developing a thiophene disulfonamide that was five times more potent than acetazolamide. This compound did not find therapeutic use because the introduction of the thiazides in 1957 rendered it obsolete. Muschaweck (1984) recollected that it was then that the belief that carbonic anhydrase inhibition alone would produce a diuretic or saluretic effect was abandoned at Hoechst, and it was assumed that genuine diuretics should be saluretic. Muschaweck and Hajdú (1964) noted that in 1959 and 1960 the Hoechst chemists were granted patents on the novel series of aralkylated derivatives of 4-chloro-5-sulfamoylanthranilic acid (Fig. 1) that included furosemide. Allen (1983) commented that the rather weakly active aromatic sulfonamide, 4-chloro-5-sulfamoylanthranilic acid,

> ...provided the bridge from low-ceiling, thiazide-like diuretics to the hitherto unknown class of high-ceiling sulfonamide diuretics. To those working in the diuretic field at the time, such a dramatic change could not have been foreseen...Therefore, it was quite surprising when the Hoechst group, led by Sturm and Muschaweck, reported that substitution of the amino group of this compound with a furfuryl moiety provided a compound (furosemide, frusemide) with markedly increased potency and efficacy.

This unexpected event was seen by Allen as analogous to the unexpected transition from the aromatic carbonic anhydrase inhibitors dichlorphenamide and chloroaminophenamide to the thiazide diuretic chlorothiazide. Furosemide was selected from a group of approximately 300 systematically studied compounds (Muschaweck, 1984).

IV. Developments
Subsequent to Furosemide

In the wake of the discovery of furosemide, related structures were synthesized and studied. Azosemide (Fig. 1), an analog of furosemide in which the acidic tetrazole group replaced the carboxyl group, was equipotent with furosemide and longer lasting by the oral route (Krück et al., 1978). Other structural variants, somewhat more distantly related (bumetanide and piretanide), were developed following the observation that positional isomers related to furosemide, in which the amino group was not ortho to the carboxyl group but meta, had reasonable activities (Feit et al., 1970). Bumetanide (Fig. 1) is a high-ceiling diuretic that is analogous to furosemide but 40–50 times more potent (on a weight basis) in humans. Piretanide (Fig. 1), also a high-ceiling diuretic, has intermediate potency (Allen, 1983).

Muschaweck (1984) pointed out that "...the development of modern diuretics has led to considerable advance in the field of experimental and clinical nephrology....Furosemide became the standard and a necessary tool in experimental nephrology." According to Goldberg et al. (1973),

The development of the orally effective diuretics, the benzothiadiazines, ethacrynic acid and frusemide [furosemide], has not only provided potent methods for treating edema, but also has led to new insights into the physiology of the regulation of sodium excretion.

In the same vein, Seely and Dirks (1977) expressed the opinion that "[d]iuretic drugs continue to attract the interest of renal physiologists not only for their intrinsic tubular effects but equally importantly for the insight that such studies provide into normal and abnormal mechanisms of renal function." In addition, Feit (1981) pointed out, "Due to the complexity of the biochemical processes involved in renal function, the precise mode of action of these diuretics is known only for the carbonic anhydrase inhibitors." Burg (1976), however, noted,

> There was considerable progress in developing better diuretics [in the 1950s and 60s], but this was empirical, based on the synthesis and testing of chemical analogues of known diuretics, and was not guided to an important extent by principles deduced from investigation of the mechanism of drug action.

It is interesting that these comments indicate that the development of sophisticated, nearly perfect diuretics ran parallel to, and was not secondary to, the development of basic knowledge in renal physiology and pharmacology. Indeed, as just cited, these agents have been credited by some authors with having been of significant help in developing such knowledge.

References

Allen, R. C.: Sulfonamide diuretics, in *Diuretics: Chemistry, Pharmacology, and Medicine*, E. J. Cragoe, Jr., ed., pp. 49–200, Wiley, New York, 1983.

Berliner, R. W.: Use of modern diuretics. *Circulation* **33**: 802–809, 1966.

Beyer, K. H.: The mechanism of action of chlorothiazide. *Ann. NY Acad. Sci.* **71**: 363–379, 1958.

Beyer, K. H. and Baer, J. E.: The site and mode of action of some sulfonamide-derived diuretics. *Med. Clin. North Am.* **59**: 735–750, 1975.

Brater, D. C.: Pharmacodynamic considerations in the use of diuretics. *Annu. Rev. Pharmacol. Toxicol.* **23**: 45–62, 1983.

Burg, M. B.: Tubular chloride transport and the mode of action of some diuretics. *Kidney Int.* **9**: 189–197, 1976.

Cannon, P. J. and Kilcoyne, M. M.: Ethacrynic acid and furosemide: Renal pharmacology and clinical use. *Prog. Cardiovasc. Dis.* **12**: 99–118, 1969.

Feit, P. W.: Bumetanide—the way to its chemical structure. *J. Clin. Pharmacol.* **21**: 531–536, 1981.

Feit, P. W., Bruun, H., and Nielsen, C. K.: Aminobenzoic acid diuretics. 1. 4-halogeno-5-sulfamylmetanilic acid derivatives. *J. Med. Chem.* **13**: 1071–1075, 1970.

Frazier, H. S. and Yager, H.: The clinical use of diuretics, part 1. *N. Engl. J. Med.* **288**: 246–249, 1973a.

Frazier, H. S. and Yager, H.: The clinical use of diuretics, part 2. *N. Engl. J. Med.* **288**: 455–457, 1973b.

Goldberg, M., Beck, L. H., Puschett, J. B., and Schubert, J. J.: Sites of action of benzothiadiazines, frusemide and ethacrynic acid, in *Modern Diuretic Therapy, in the Treatment of Cardiovascular and Renal Disease*, A. F. Lant and G. M. Wilson, eds., pp. 135–144, Excerpta Medica, Amsterdam, 1973.

Hutcheon, D. E. and Martinez, J. C.: A decade of developments in diuretic drug therapy. *J. Clin. Pharmacol.* **26**: 567–579, 1986.

Hutcheon, D. E., Mehta, D., and Romano, A.: Diuretic action of furosemide. *Arch. Intern. Med.* **115**: 542–546, 1965.

Jacobson, H. R. and Kokko, J. P.: Diuretics: Sites and mechanisms of action. *Annu. Rev. Pharmacol. Toxicol.* **16**: 201–214, 1976.

Kirkendall, W. M. and Stein, J. H.: Clinical pharmacology of furosemide and ethacrynic acid. *Am. J. Cardiol.* **22**: 162–167, 1968.

Kleinfelder, H.: Experimental investigations and clinical trials of fursemide, a new diuretic. *German med. Mth.* **8**: 459–465, 1963 (a translation of the article in *Dtsch. Med. Wochenschr.* **88**: 1695–1702, 1963).

Krück, F., Bablok, W., Besenfelder, E., Betzien, G., and Kaufmann, B.: Clinical and pharmacological investigations of the new saluretic azosemid. *Eur. J. Clin. Pharmacol.* **14**: 153–161, 1978.

Lant, A. F. and Wilson, G. M., eds.: *Modern Diuretic Therapy in the Treatment of Cardiovascular and Renal Disease*, Excerpta Medica, Amsterdam, 1973.

Mann, T. and Keilin, D.: Sulphanilamide as a specific inhibitor of carbonic anhydrase. *Nature* **146**: 164, 165, 1940.

Miller, W. H., Dessert, A. M., and Roblin, R. O., Jr.: Heterocyclic sulfonamides as carbonic anhydrase inhibitors. *J. Am. Chem. Soc.* **72**: 4893–4896 (letter to the editor), 1950.

Modell, W., Schild, H. O., and Wilson, A.: *Applied Pharmacology*, American Ed., Saunders, Philadelphia, 1976.

Muschaweck, R.: Untitled. *Atti Academia Med. Lombarda* **18**: (Suppl.) 1289–1297, 1963.

Muschaweck, R.: Discovery and development of furosemide: Historical remarks, in *Diuretics: Chemistry, Pharmacology, and Clinical Applications,* J. B. Puschett and A. Greenberg, eds., pp. 4–11, Elsevier, New York, 1984.

Muschaweck, R. and Hajdú, P.: Die salidiuretische Wirksamkeit der Chlor-
N-(2-furylmethyl)-5-sulfamyl-anthranilsäure. *Arzneimittelforsch.* **14**: 44–
47, 1964.

Novello, F. C. and Sprague, J. M.: Benzothiadiazine dioxides as novel diuretics. *J. Am. Chem. Soc.* **79**: 2028, 2029, 1957.

Odlind, B. and Beermann, B.: Renal tubular secretion and effects of furosemide. *Clin. Pharmacol. Ther.* **27**: 784–790, 1980.

Puschett, J. B. and Goldberg, M.: The acute effects of furosemide on acid and
electrolyte excretion in man. *J. Lab. Clin. Med.* **71**: 666–677, 1968.

Robson, A. O., Kerr, D. N. S., Ashcroft, R., and Teasdale, G.: The diuretic
response to frusemide. *Lancet* **2**: 1085–1088, 1964.

Schwartz, W. B.: The effect of sulfanilamide on salt and water excretion in
congestive heart failure. *N. Engl. J. Med.* **240**: 173–177, 1949.

Seely, J. F. and Dirks, J. H.: Site of action of diuretic drugs. *Kidney Int.* **11**:
1–8, 1977.

Siedel, W., Sturm, K., and Muschaweck, R.: L'acide 4-chloro-N-furfuryl-
5-sulfamoylanthranilique (furosémide). *Prod. Prob. Pharm.* **22**: 867–874,
1967.

Sprague, J. M.: The chemistry of diuretics. *Ann. NY Acad. Sci.* **71**: 328–343,
1958.

Stason, W. B., Cannon, P. J., Heinemann, H. O., and Laragh, J. H.: Furosemide: A clinical evaluation of its diuretic action. *Circulation* **34**:
910–920, 1966.

Stein, J. H., Wilson, C. B., and Kirkendall, W. M.: Differences in the acute
effects of furosemide and ethacrynic acid in man. *J. Lab. Clin. Med.* **71**:
654–665, 1968.

Stokes, W. and Nunn, L. C. A.: A new effective diuretic—Lasix. *Br. Med. J.*
2: 910–914, 1964.

Suki, W. N., Eknoyan, G., and Martinez-Maldonado, M.: Tubular sites and
mechanisms of diuretic action. *Annu. Rev. Pharmacol.* **13**: 91–106, 1973.

Suki, W., Rector, Jr., F. C., and Seldin, D. W.: The site of action of furosemide
and other sulfonamide diuretics in the dog. *J. Clin. Invest.* **44**: 1458–1469,
1965.

Timmerman, R. J., Springman, F. R., and Thoms, R. K.: Evaluation of fursemide, a new diuretic agent. *Curr. Ther. Res.* **6**: 88–94, 1964.

Verel, D., Stentiford, N. H., Rahman, F., and Saynor, R.: A clinical trial of
frusemide. *Lancet* **2**: 1088, 1089, 1964.

Weiner, I. M. and Mudge, G. H.: Diuretics and other agents employed in the
mobilization of edema fluid, in *The Pharmacological Basis of Therapeutics*,
7th Ed., A. G. Gilman, L. S. Goodman, T. W. Rall, and F. Murad, eds., pp.
887–907, Macmillan, New York, 1985.

Azathioprine

I. Azathioprine as an Innovative Therapeutic Agent

The replacement of diseased human organs with healthy ones from donors, cadavers, or animals has been a challenge, and an enigma, to surgeons throughout much of the history of medicine. Even in relatively recent times, experiments with homografts* of skin and other organs, such as kidney, indicated that there was virtually no chance for success: the host's immune system rejected and destroyed the donated organ (Medawar, 1944,1945; Dempster, 1953; Hume et al., 1955). Hume et al. (1955) concluded, "Renal homotransplantation has no place in the therapy of human patients at this time."

Before the appearance of azathioprine, attempts were made to suppress the immune response of the human host with total-body irradiation. This method, although known to suppress the immune system of animals (*see* Dempster et al., 1950 for refs.), led to only minimal success in humans (Murray et al., 1960). Irradiation resulted in agranulocytosis and bone marrow depression. Because of severe generalized immunosuppression, patients usually suffered from overwhelming infection, and extensive isolation procedures were often required. The great risks and highly unpredictable effectiveness of the procedure made the undertaking impractical (Starzl, 1978). Nitrogen mustards and cortisone were also used to combat rejection, but were quite toxic.

---

*Homograft (allograft)—a tissue or an organ transplanted from one individual to another of the same species, not identical twins (Stedman, 1982).

With the advent of azathioprine, the situation changed drastically: Homotransplantation of kidneys became feasible. This agent is a cell-cycle-specific, cytotoxic (cytostatic), antimetabolitic, antiproliferative agent. It acts via its dominant metabolite, 6-mercaptopurine, to inhibit cell division, including that of immunologically important lymphocytes, during the phase of the cell cycle when DNA synthesis is maximal (the S phase). In optimal doses, in combination with other immunosuppressing agents, such as corticosteroids, azathioprine prevents rejection of renal homografts in nearly 50% of cases (Schulak and Corry, 1987) without the very serious complications commonly seen with irradiation. In addition, patients retain some capacity to fight environmental antigens (Starzl, 1964). Immunosuppression became clinically practical when it was discovered that azathioprine and prednisone could be used together advantageously (Starzl, 1978). Prednisolone has replaced prednisone in many centers (d'Apice, 1984).

Azathioprine in reasonable doses is relatively free of side effects. In high doses it can cause marrow aplasia, macrocytic anemia, depilation, and hepatic damage. In addition, the immunosuppressant effect of azathioprine is not entirely specific to the transplant; hence the patient, because of general suppression of the immune system, is at some increased risk of developing bacterial, viral, and fungal infections, and certain malignancies.

The combined use of azathioprine and corticosteroids, in addition to advanced techniques in organ preservation, tissue typing, and manipulation of immune responses, has made renal transplantation the therapy of choice in severe renal disease. It is an effective alternative to maintaining patients with end-stage renal disease on chronic dialysis. Renal transplantation may be considered for patients with kidney disease of almost any etiology (Schulak and Corry, 1987).

Currently, in addition to being used in preventing rejection of renal transplants, azathioprine is approved for the treatment of severe rheumatoid arthritis. Azathioprine is also used as an investigational drug for the treatment of systemic lupus erythematosus, Crohn's disease, and other systemic inflammatory states (Calabresi and Parks, 1985).

Early Clinical Research History

Renal Transplantation

Murray et al. (1962) were the first to use azathioprine in human organ-transplant surgery. Six patients undergoing kidney transplants were treated with drugs, rather than with total-body irradiation, as a measure to prevent organ rejection: two with 6-mercaptopurine, a compound known to have immunosuppressant properties in animals (*see* section II); one with azathioprine, a derivative of 6-mercaptopurine; and three with a combination of azathioprine and actinomycin C. Five patients exhibited significant renal function for various lengths of time following the transplant (3–35 d). One patient on the azathioprine and actinomycin C regimen had a functioning kidney 120 d after the operation and was still living when the results were published. The authors concluded that, "Chemical suppression of the immune response...in the human seems promising."

Murray et al. (1963) treated seven additional renal transplant patients with azathioprine. One received only azathioprine; six received a combination of azathioprine and azaserine. There were four survivors, three of whom were alive at the time of the publication (40–110 d after the homografts). Murray and his associates concluded that azathioprine was the single most important drug in the regimen. Azaserine or actinomycin C seemed to increase the ability of azathioprine to prevent rejection. These authors considered the use of drugs to have clear advantages as a mechanism for producing immunosuppression:

1. Continuous inhibition of the immune response;
2. The ability to titrate dose according to the sensitivity and need of the patient; and
3. The ability to start therapy after the transplant operation.

Another advantage was that the host did not become an "immunological cripple"; elaborate precautionary measures to prevent infection were unnecessary.

Numerous clinical trials followed, and have supported and extended these early findings (e.g., Woodruff et al., 1963; Hume et al., 1966; Najarian et al., 1966). Reviews and books on renal transplantation and the role of azathioprine are available (*see*, for example, Starzl, 1964,1978; Calne, 1967; Elion and Hitchings, 1975; Morris, 1984; Schulak and Corry, 1987).

Rheumatoid Arthritis

The introduction of azathioprine into arthritis therapy was based on the fact that there was good evidence that immunological mechanisms played at least a part in the pathogenesis of the disease (Christian and Kunkel, 1963). Furthermore, Jimenez Diaz et al. (1951) and Gubner et al. (1951) had earlier reported that other antimetabolitic or alkylating antiproliferative drugs (aminopterin and nitrogen mustard) had beneficial effects in rheumatoid arthritis in humans (*see* chapters on methotrexate and cyclophosphamide for details). Moens and Brocteur (1965) found in an open study that combined treatment with azathioprine and actinomycin C caused a reduction in inflammatory index in eight of 12 rheumatoid patients who had failed to respond to salicylates, gold salts, antimalarials, and steroids. The regimen did not influence antibody titers, suggesting that, rather than immunosuppression, an antiinflammatory action accounted for the activity.

In an open study, Lorenzen and Videbaeck (1965) found that eight of 11 gravely ill, chronic rheumatoid arthritis patients had their symptoms decreased by a regimen of 6-mercaptopurine followed by azathioprine. These investigators remarked that the treatment, although effective, required careful supervision of patients because of the potential for pancytopenia and sepsis.

Controlled clinical trials followed these early studies and generally confirmed that under careful supervision azathioprine was an effective, reasonably safe drug for patients with rheumatoid arthritis who were not responsive to conventional therapy (Mason et al., 1969; Levy et al., 1972; Urowitz et al., 1973). For additional references *see* Nashel (1985) and Pugh and Pugh (1987).

II. The Scientific Departure
Leading to Azathioprine: 6-Mercaptopurine

Systematic synthesis and screening of purine and pyrimidine analogs in *Lactobacillus casei* by Hitchings and his group (Hitchings et al., 1945; 1948a,b,c; 1950) ultimately led to the synthesis and study

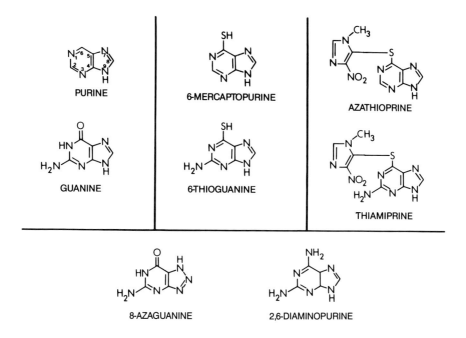

Fig. 1. The structures of azathioprine and chemically and/or pharmacologically related substances.

of the purine antimetabolitic, antiproliferative agent 6-mercaptopurine (Fig.1) (Elion et al., 1951). This compound served as an intermediate for the synthesis of other 6-substituted purines (Elion et al., 1952). Clarke et al. (1953), in association with Hitchings and Elion, found that 6-mercaptopurine prolonged the survival time of mice bearing Sarcoma 180 and induced complete recovery in some animals. Burchenal et al. (1953), in a collaboration with Hitchings and associates, treated patients who had various neoplastic diseases with 6-mercaptopurine. Remissions were seen in 15 of 45 children who were suffering from acute leukemia; a few adults with acute leukemia also experienced temporary remission. The anticancer effects of 6-mercaptopurine were covered in detail the next year (Miner, 1954). 6-Mercaptopurine is still in use for treating some forms of leukemia.

Schwartz et al. (1958) theorized that, since 6-mercaptopurine was considered to prevent cell proliferation by interfering with the utilization of purines for nucleic acid synthesis, and since antibody-producing tissue might be in a "hypermetabolic state," 6-mercapto-purine could be expected to abolish the antibody response to antigen. In further clarification, Schwartz et al. (1959) noted that the formation of antibody was closely linked to nucleic acid production: following administration of an antigen, antibody-producing tissue underwent hypertrophy, cellular proliferation, and an increase in the content of nitrogen, RNA, and DNA (the DNA increase being largely associated with cell multiplication). These authors (Schwartz et al., 1958) found that 6-mercaptopurine, administered to rabbits simultaneously with purified bovine serum albumin, abolished the immune response to this antigen: it sharply suppressed the formation of humoral antibody.

In a followup study, Schwartz and Dameshek (1959) reported that 6-mercaptopurine could bring about a state of "drug-induced immunological tolerance" in rabbits. This state was induced by simultaneous treatment with antigen and 6-mercaptopurine, and sustained by repeated administration of antigen without additional 6-mercaptopurine. The tolerance was specific for the antigen that was given with the 6-mercaptopurine.

Meeker et al. (1959) demonstrated that skin homografts in host rabbits treated with 6-mercaptopurine survived significantly longer than those in untreated host animals. They observed that the toxicity of 6-mercaptopurine limited its use. Schwartz and Dameshek (1960) also showed that untreated rabbits rejected skin homografts three times faster than 6-mercaptopurine-treated rabbits. They felt that the toxicity of 6-mercaptopurine would preclude its use in human transplantation, but that 6-mercaptopurine pointed the way for further studies.

Calne (1960), as a result of the findings of Schwartz and Dameshek (1959), used 6-mercaptopurine in an attempt to modify rejection of renal homografts in dogs. He reported that in some cases 6-mercaptopurine delayed the rejection of grafted kidneys by the host dogs. However, 6-mercaptopurine was effective only at potentially toxic doses, producing leukopenia and causing the death of some of the experimental animals. Calne (1961a) cited the obvious disadvantage of the toxicity of 6-mercaptopurine; however, he indicated that 6-mercaptopurine might offer an approach to renal homografts in humans, especially in chronic uremia, wherein homograft rejection was already depressed.

In an independent study prompted by the report of Schwartz et al. (1959), Zukoski et al. (1960,1961) also demonstrated that, at proper doses, 6-mercaptopurine prolonged the functional survival of renal homografts in dogs.

Background Contributions Preceding the Development of 6-Mercaptopurine as an Antiproliferative Agent

The discovery of 6-mercaptopurine was rooted in the "antimetabolite revolution" that occurred in the late 1930s and early 1940s. According to Wooley (1960), "An antimetabolite is a chemical compound which is closely related in chemical structure to one of the essential compounds functioning in a living organism, and which is able to bring about in a living creature the specific signs of deficiency of that essential compound." The antimetabolite concept is generally considered to have had its start with the ideas of Woods (1940) and Fildes (1940). Woods (1940) demonstrated that the antibacterial action of sulfanilamide was antagonized by para-aminobenzoic acid (PABA), a substance that is essential for the growth of many bacteria. Woods (1940) suggested "...that the enzyme reaction involved in the further utilization of *p*-aminobenzoic acid is subject to competitive inhibition by sulphanilamide, and that this inhibition is due to a structural relationship between sulphanilamide and *p*-aminobenzoic acid...."

8-Azaguanine (guanazolo) (Fig. 1), an antimetabolite of guanine in *Escherichia coli* (Roblin et al., 1945), was the first agent shown to arrest the growth of malignant cells in mice without being severely toxic to the host (Kidder et al., 1949). It was later shown by Malmgren et al. (1952) to reduce antibody titers in the mouse and surmised to be acting at some stage in the process of antibody formation. These observations were not followed up.

Hitchings et al. (1948c) showed that 2,6-diaminopurine (Fig. 1) was an antimetabolite to adenine in *Lactobacillus casei*. Subsequently, with their collaborators they found that this compound increased the survival time in mice with transplanted leukemia (Burchenal et al., 1949). However, it was not very successful against leukemia in humans (Burchenal et al., 1951). The next phase of this group's work led to 6-mercaptopurine, as already described.

Significant Events
Following 6-Mercaptopurine

Hitchings and his colleagues continued their systematic search through many analogs for better anticancer drugs related to 6-mercaptopurine. The 1-methyl-4-nitro-5-imidazolyl derivative of 6-mercaptopurine (BW 57-322, later named azathioprine) (Fig.1) and the identical derivative of 6-thioguanine (BW 57-323, later named thiamiprine) (Fig. 1) showed good activity against Adenocarcinoma 755 (Hitchings and Elion, 1959). Thiamiprine was the more active of the two agents. Numerous reports concerning the antineoplastic activities of thiamiprine appeared (Cancer Chemotherapy Reports, 1960). Elion et al. (1961) summarized azathioprine's positive activity against a variety of transplantable rodent tumors, and Rundles et al. (1961) found it to be comparable to 6-mercaptopurine when used against leukemias in humans. It was noted by Elion et al. (1961) that these heterocyclic-substituted 6-mercaptopurines were made in order to present the thiopurines in a masked form, to reduce metabolic degradation, and to improve tissue distribution.

Because of the reports concerning the immunosuppressant effects of 6-mercaptopurine, Hitchings' group also undertook to study their compounds for effects on the immune response. They acknowledged that a suggestion from Schwartz led them to develop a simple screening program, based on the mouse agglutinin response to administered sheep cells, that was sensitive to 6-mercaptopurine and other antimetabolites (Nathan et al., 1961). Azathioprine and thiamiprine had activities comparable to those of the parent thiopurines in this test; however, azathioprine was active over a wider dose range and at lower fractions of the maximum tolerated dose than were the other agents.

Calne (1961b), Calne and Murray (1961), Calne et al. (1962), and Alexandre and Murray (1962) reported that azathiopine was at least as effective as 6-mercaptopurine in inhibiting rejection of renal homografts in dogs. A combination of azathioprine with either actinomycin C or azaserine produced the best prolongation of the functional survival of the renal transplant. Thiamiprine did not prevent renal homograft rejection, even in toxic doses.

Table 1 defines the critical scientific ideas and experiments leading to azathioprine and categorizes their origins.

III. Comments on Events Leading to Azathioprine

Calne (1976) commented,

In organ grafting the gulf between clinical transplantation and immunologic experimentation and theory has been wide. It has been difficult to provide satisfactory models for organ grafting in man, and fact and fancy have been confused....Biologic principles may be applicable in a wide sense, but the practical value can be completely overshadowed by other factors that were not considered in the experimental model from which the principle was derived.

In a related vein, Schwartz (1976) pointed out,

The development of modern immunosuppressive chemicals occurred during a time when relatively little was known about the fundamentals of immunology. ...And it is difficult to imagine from today's perspective the progress that was achieved in the field of clinical immunology in the face of extraordinary ignorance of fundamental mechanisms.

Schwartz (1976) also stressed that the early history of the development of immunosuppressive therapy was laced with good fortune.

According to Starzl (1978), "The transplantation explosion which eventually occurred from 1962 onwards was dependent upon the use of drugs." Calabresi and Parks (1985) expressed the opinion, "The introduction of mercaptopurine by Elion and coworkers represented a landmark in the history of antineoplastic and immunosuppressant therapy. Today this antipurine and its derivative, azathioprine, are among the most important and clinically useful drugs of the class."

Elion (1989) has recently reviewed the broad aspects of the purine research and the drug discoveries for which she and Hitchings shared in the 1988 Nobel Prize in Medicine.

Table 1
Profile of Observations and Ideas Crucial to the Development of Azathioprine[a]

Sequence: Departure compound* to innovative drug**	Orient-ation	Nature of study	Research institution	National origin	Nature of discovery	Screening involved	Crucial ideas or observations
6-Mercaptopurine*							
Elion et al. (1951)	Pre-clinical	Chem-istry/pharma-cology	Industry	USA	Orderly	Targeted	6-Mercaptopurine, a purine antimetabo-litic, cytotoxic, anti-proliferative agent synthesized.
Schwartz et al. (1958)	Pre-clinical	Pharma-cology	Uni-versity	USA	Orderly	No	In rabbits, 6-mercaptopurine suppresses formation of humoral antibody to bovine albumin.
Schwartz and Dameshek (1959)	Pre-clinical	Pharma-cology	Uni-versity	USA	Orderly	No	6-Mercaptopurine elicits "immunol-ogical tolerance" to a single purified protein antigen.
Calne (1960)	Pre-clinical	Pharma-cology	Uni-versity	UK	Orderly	No	6-Mercaptopurine inhibits rejection of renal homotrans-plants in dogs; poor therapeutic ratio.

(continued)

[a]Taken from Section II. Entries are those contributions without which the discovery of the agent (or additionally, in some cases, a relevant clinical application) would not have taken place or would have been materially delayed.

IV. Developments Subsequent to Azathioprine

Starzl (1978) thought that immunosuppression remained the main problem in organ transplantation. Calne (1976) remarked that, when azathioprine was first used to treat patients undergoing kidney transplants, he considered it a good drug with obvious limi-tations: "I was quite convinced at that time that shortly another agent would be available with a far better therapeutic index. Fifteen

Table 1 (continued)

Sequence: Departure compound* to innovative drug**	Orient- ation	Nature of study	Research institution	National origin	Nature of discovery	Screening involved	Crucial ideas or observations
Azathioprine**							
Hitchings and Elion (1959)	Pre- clinical	Chem- istry/ pharma- cology	Industry	USA	Orderly	Targeted	Azathioprine, a heterocyclic analog of 6-mercaptopurine, synthesized; shown to have anticancer activity.
Nathan et al. (1961)	Pre- clinical	Chem- istry/ pharma- cology	Industry	USA	Orderly	Targeted	Azathioprine inhibits the for- mation of hemag- glutinins to sheep red-blood cells in mice.
Calne (1961b)	Pre- clinical	Pharma- cology	Uni- versity	USA	Orderly	No	Azathioprine as effective as 6- mercaptopurine in inhibiting rejection of renal homotrans- plants in dogs; less toxic than 6-mer- captopurine.

years later azathioprine remains sheet anchor of immunosuppressive therapy together with the corticosteroid drugs..."

Recent research has been aimed at finding a less toxic compound (or regimen) having immunosuppresant activity that is more
selective for the graft—a compound that can suppress the immune
system enough to permit acceptance of a very high percentage of
homografts, without overpowering the entire system and having
the sequela of patient vulnerability to opportunistic infections. The
discovery of cyclosporine seems to be a clear step in this direction.

References

Alexandre, G. P. J. and Murray, J. E.: Further studies of renal homotransplantation in dogs treated by combined Imuran therapy. *Surg. Forum* **13**:
64–66, 1962.

Burchenal, J. H., Bendick, A., Brown, G. B., Elion, G. B., Hitchings, G. H., Rhoads, C. P., and Stock, C. C.: Preliminary studies on the effect of 2,6-diaminopurine on transplanted mouse leukemia. *Cancer* 2: 119, 120, 1949.

Burchenal, J. H., Karnofsky, D. A., Kingsley-Pillers, E. M., Southam, C. M., Myers, W. P. L., Escher, G. C., Craver, L. F., Dargeon, H. W., and Rhoads, C. P.: The effects of the folic acid antagonists and 2,6-diaminopurine on neoplastic disease. *Cancer* 4: 549–569, 1951.

Burchenal, J. H., Murphy, M. L., Ellison, R. R., Skyes, M. P., Tan, T. C., Leone, L. A., Karnofsky, D. A., Craver, L. F., Dargeon, H. W., and Rhoads, C. P.: Clinical evaluation of a new antimetabolite, 6-mercaptopurine, in the treatment of leukemia and allied diseases. *Blood* 8: 965–999, 1953.

Calabresi, P. and Parks, R. E.: Antiproliferative agents and drugs used for immunosuppression, in *The Pharmacological Basis of Therapeutics*, 7th Ed., A. G. Gilman, L. S. Goodman, T. W. Rall, and F. Murad, eds., pp. 1247–1306, Macmillan, New York, 1985.

Calne, R. Y.: Rejection of renal homografts: Inhibition in dogs by 6-mercaptopurine. *Lancet* 1: 417, 418, 1960.

Calne, R. Y.: Observations on renal homotransplantation. *Br. J. Surg.* 48: 384–391, 1961a.

Calne, R. Y.: Inhibition of the rejection of renal homografts in dogs by purine analogs. *Plast. Reconstr. Surg.* 28: 445–461, 1961b.

Calne, R. Y.: *Renal Transplantation*, Edward Arnold, London, 1967.

Calne, R. Y.: Approaches to immunosuppression for organ grafts, in *Design and Achievements in Chemotherapy: A Symposium in Honor of George H. Hitchings*, pp. 42–51, Science and Medicine Publishing, New York, 1976.

Calne, R. Y. and Murray, J. E.: Inhibition of the rejection of renal homografts in dogs by B.W. 57–322. *Surg. Forum* 12: 118–120, 1961.

Calne, R. Y., Alexandre, G. P. J., and Murray, J. E.: Study of effects of drugs in prolonging survival of homologous renal transplants in dogs. *Ann. New York Acad. Sci.* 99: 743–761, 1962.

Cancer Chemother. Reports 8: 36–76, 1960.

Christian, C. L. and Kunkel, H. G., chmn.: Conference on the immunologic aspects of rheumatoid arthritis and systemic lupus erythermatosus. *Arthritis Rheum.* 6: 401–489, 1963.

Clarke, D. A., Philips, F. S., Sternberg, S. S., Stock, C. C., Elion, G. B., and Hitchings, G. H.: 6-Mercaptopurine: Effects in mouse Sarcoma 180 and in normal animals. *Cancer Res.* 13: 594–604, 1953.

d'Apice, A. J. F.: Non-specific immunosuppression: Azathioprine and steroids, in *Kidney Transplantation: Principles and Practice.*, P. J. Morris, ed., Grune and Stratton, London, 1984.

Dempster, W. J.: Kidney homotransplantation. *Br. J. Surg.* 40:447–465, 1953.

Dempster, W. J., Lennox, B., and Boag, J. W.: Prolongation of survival of skin homotransplants in the rabbit by irradiation of the host. *Br. J. Exp. Pathol.* 31: 670–679, 1950.

Elion, G. B.: The purine path to chemotherapy. *Science* 244: 41–47, 1989.

Elion, G. B. and Hitchings, G. H.: Azathioprine, in *Handbuch der experimentellen Pharmakologie*, New Series, vol. 38/2, A. C. Sartorelli and D. G. Johns, eds., pp. 404–425, Springer-Verlag, Berlin, 1975.

Elion, G. B., Burgi, E., and Hitchings, G. H.: Studies on condensed pyrimidine systems. IX. The synthesis of some 6-substituted purines. *J. Am. Chem. Soc.* 14: 411–414, 1952.

Elion, G. B., Hitchings, G. H., and VanderWerff, H.: Antagonists of nucleic acid derivatives. VI. Purines. *J. Biol. Chem.* 192: 505–518, 1951.

Elion, G. B., Callahan, S., Bieber, S., Hitchings, G. H., and Rundles, R. W.: A summary of investigations with 6-[(1-methyl-4-nitro-5-imidazolyl)thio]-purine (B.W. 57-322). *Cancer Chemother. Reports* 14: 93–98, 1961.

Fildes, P.: A rational approach to research in chemotherapy. *Lancet* 1: 955–957, 1940.

Gubner, R., August, S., and Ginsberg, V.: Therapeutic suppression of tissue reactivity. II. Effect of aminopterin in rheumatoid arthritis and psoriasis. *Am. J. Med. Sci.* 221: 176–182, 1951.

Hitchings, G. H. and Elion, G. B.: Activity of heterocyclic derivatives of 6-mercaptopurine and 6-thioguanine in *Adenocarcinoma* 755. (abs.) *Proc. Am. Assoc. Cancer Res.* 3: 27, 1959.

Hitchings, G. H., Elion, G. B., and VanderWerff, H.: The limitations of inhibition analysis. *J. Biol. Chem.* 174: 1037, 1038, 1948a.

Hitchings, G. H., Elion, G. B., and VanderWerff, H.: 2-Aminopurine as a purine antagonist. *Fed. Proc.* 7: 160, 1948b.

Hitchings, G. H., Falco, E. A. and Sherwood, M.B.: The effects of pyrimidines on the growth of *Lactobacillus casei*. *Science* 102: 251, 252, 1945.

Hitchings, G. H., Elion, G. B., VanderWerff, H., and Falco, E. A.: Pyrimidine derivatives as antagonists of pteroylglutamic acid. *J. Biol. Chem.* 174: 765, 766, 1948c.

Hitchings, G. H., Elion, G. B., Falco, E., Russell, P. B., and VanderWerff, H.: Studies on analogs of purines and pyrimidines. *Ann. NY Acad. Sci.* 52: 1318–1335, 1950.

Hume, D., Merrill, J. P., Miller, B., and Thorn, G.: Experiences with renal homotransplantation in the human: Report of nine cases. *J. Clin. Invest.* 34: 327–382, 1955.

Hume, D. M., Lee, H. M., Williams, G. M., White, H. J. O., Ferre, J., Wolf, J. S., Prout, G. R., Jr., Slapak, M., O'Brien, J., Kilpatrick, S. J., Kauffman,

H. M., Jr., and Cleveland, R. J.: Comparative results of cadaver and related donor renal homografts in man and immunologic implications of the outcome of second and paired transplants. *Ann. Surg.* **164:** 352–399, 1966.

Jimenez Diaz, C., Lopez Garcia, E., Merchante, A., and Perianes, J.: Treatment of rheumatoid arthritis with nitrogen mustard. Preliminary report. *J. Am. Med. Assoc.* **147:** 1418, 1419, 1951.

Kidder, G. W., Dewey, V. C., Parks, R. E., Jr., and Woodside, G. L.: Purine metabolism in *Tetrahymena* and its relation to malignant cells in mice. *Science* **109:** 511–514, 1949.

Levy, J., Paulus, H. E., Barnett, E. V., Sokoloff, M., Bangert, R., and Pearson, C. M.: A double-blind controlled evaluation of azathioprine treatment in rheumatoid arthritis and psoriatic arthritis. *Arthritis Rheum.* **15:** 116, 117, 1972.

Lorenzen, I. and Videbaeck, A.: Treatment of collagen diseases with cytostatics. *Lancet* **1:** 558–561, 1965.

Malmgren, R. A., Bennison, B. E., and McKinley, T. W.: The effect of guanazolo on antibody formation. *J. Natl. Cancer Inst.* **12:** 807–818, 1952.

Mason, M., Currey, H. L. F., Barnes, C. G., Dunne, J. F., Hazleman, B. L., and Strickland, I. D.: Azathioprine in rheumatoid arthritis. *Br. Med. J.* **1:** 420–422, 1969.

Medawar, P. B.: The behaviour and fate of skin autografts and skin homografts in rabbits. *J. Anat.* **78:** 176–196, 1944.

Medawar, P. B.: A second study of the behaviour and fate of skin homografts in rabbits. *J. Anat.* **79:** 157–174, 1945.

Meeker, W., Condie, R., Weiner, D., Varco, R., and Good, R.: Prolongation of skin homograft survival in rabbits by 6-mercaptopurine. *Proc. Soc. Exp. Biol. Med.* **102:** 459–461, 1959.

Miner, R. W., ed.: Symposium: 6-Mercaptopurine. *Ann. NY Acad. Sci.* **60:** 183–508, 1954.

Moens, C. and Brocteur, J.: Treatment of rheumatoid arthritis with immunosuppressive drugs. *Acta Rheum. Scand.* **11:** 212–220, 1965.

Morris, P. J., ed.: *Kidney Transplantation, Principles and Practice,* Grune and Stratton, London, 1984.

Murray, J. E., Merrill, J. P., and Harrison, J. H.: Kidney transplantation between seven pairs of identical twins. *Ann. Surg.* **148:** 343–359, 1958.

Murray, J. E., Merrill, J. P., and Harrison, J. H.: Prolonged survival of human-kidney homografts by immunosuppressive drug therapy. *N. Engl. J. Med.* **268:** 1315–1323, 1963.

Murray, J. E., Merrill, J. P., Dammin, G. J., Dealy, J. B., Alexandre, G. W., and Harrison, H. J.: Kidney transplantation in modified recipients. *Ann. Surg.* **156:** 337–355, 1962.

Murray, J. E., Merrill, J. P., Dammin, G. J., Dealy, J. B., Walter, C. W., Brooke, M. S., and Wilson, R. E.: Study on transplantation immunity after total body irradiation: Clinical and experimental investigation. *Surgery* 48: 272–284, 1960.

Najarian, J. S., Gulyassy, P. P., Stoney, R. J., Duffy, G., and Braunstein, P.: Protection of the donor kidney during homotransplantation. *Ann. Surg.* 164: 398–417, 1966.

Nashel, D. J.: Mechanisms of action and clinical application of cytotoxic drugs in rheumatic disorders. *Med. Clin. North Am.* 69: 817–840, 1985.

Nathan, H. C., Bieber, S., Elion, G. B., and Hitchings, G. H.: Detection of agents which interfere with the immune response. *Proc. Soc. Exp. Biol.* 107: 796–799, 1961.

Pugh, M. C. and Pugh, C. B.: Current concepts in clinical therapeutics: Disease-modifying drugs for rheumatoid arthritis. *Clin. Pharm.* 6: 475–491, 1987.

Roblin, R. O., Jr., Lampen, J. O., English, J. P., Cole, Q. P., and Vaughan, J. R., Jr.: Studies in chemotherapy. VIII. Methionine and purine antagonists and their relation to sulfonamides. *J. Am. Chem. Soc.* 67: 290–294, 1945.

Rundles, R. W., Lazlo, J., Itoga, T., Hobson, J. B., and Garrison, F. E., Jr.: Clinical and hematologic study of 6-[(l-methyl-4-nitro-5 imidazolyl) thio] purine (B.W. 57-322) and related compounds. *Cancer Chemother. Reports* 14: 99–115, 1961.

Schulak, J. A. and Corry, R. J.: Transplantation, in *Principles of Basic Surgical Practice,* E. C. James, R. J. Corry, and J. F. Perry, eds., pp. 120–130, Hauley & Belfus, Philadelphia, 1987.

Schwartz, R.: Perspectives on immunosuppression, in *Design and Achievements in Chemotherapy: A Symposium in Honor of George Hitchings,* pp. 39–41, Science and Medicine Publishing, 1976.

Schwartz, R. and Dameshek, W.: Drug-induced immunological tolerance. *Nature* 183: 1682, 1683, 1959.

Schwartz, R. and Dameshek, W.: The effects of 6-mercaptopurine on homograft reactions. *J. Clin. Invest.* 39: 952–958, 1960.

Schwartz, R., Eisner, A., and Dameshek, W. L.: The effect of 6-mercaptopurine on primary and secondary immune responses. *J. Clin. Invest.* 38: 1394–1403, 1959.

Schwartz, R., Stack, J., and Dameshek, W. L.: Effect of 6-mercaptopurine on antibody production. *Proc. Soc. Exp. Biol.* 99: 164–167, 1958.

Starzl, T. E.: *Experience in Renal Transplantation,* W. B. Saunders, Philadelphia, 1964.

Starzl, T. E.: Personal reflections in transplantation. *Surg. Clin. North Am.* 58: 879–893, 1978.

Stedman's Medical Dictionary, 24th Ed., Williams & Wilkins, Baltimore, 1982.

Urowitz, M. D., Gordon, D. A., Smythe, H. A., Pruzanski, W., and Ogryzlo, M. A.: Azathioprine in rheumatoid arthritis. *Arthritis Rheum.* 16:411–418, 1973.

Woods, D. D.: The relation of *p*-aminobenzoic acid to the mechanism of the action of sulphanilamide. *Br. J. Exp. Pathol.* 21: 74–90, 1940.

Woodruff, M. F. A., Robson, J. S., Nolan, B., Lambie, A. T., Wilson, T. I., and Clark, J. G.: Homotransplantation of kidney in patients treated by preoperative local radiation and postoperative administration of an antimetabolite (Imuran). *Lancet* 2: 675–682, 1963.

Wooley, D. W.: The antimetabolite revolution. *Clin. Pharmacol. Ther.* 1: 556–569, 1960.

Zukoski, C. F., Lee, H. M., and Hume, D. M.: Prolongation of functional survival of canine renal homografts by 6-mercaptopurine. *Surg. Forum* 11: 470–472, 1960.

Zukoski, C. F., Lee, H. M., and Hume, D. M.: The effect of 6-mercaptopurine on renal homograft survival in the dog. *Surg. Gynecol. Obstet.* 112: 707–714, 1961.

Cyclosporine

I. Cyclosporine as an Innovative Therapeutic Agent

Prior to the discovery of cyclosporine, azathioprine was the mainstay of immunosuppressant therapy. According to White (1982a), the discovery of azathioprine in 1959 and its subsequent combination with steroids established kidney transplantation as a viable therapy for renal failure. However, although this regimen represented a major step forward, only 50% of the allografts (homografts) achieved with it were functional, and these were accompanied by a 15% mortality rate from secondary infection. Half of the transplanted kidneys were lost within 12 months as a result of rejection (Kahan, 1983; White, 1982b). In only two situations was azathioprine plus corticosteroids consistently effective in renal transplantation: (1) where donors were living, reasonably immune-compatible relatives, or (2) where cadaver organs were given to recipients who tested as weak immune responders. Unfortunately, in the USA, the majority of the young, vigorous population requiring transplants test as strong immune responders (Kahan, 1981).

Azathioprine, via its metabolites, acts as an antimetabolite of adenine and guanine by inhibiting the synthesis of these purines and thus their incorporation into DNA—an effect that renders azathioprine cytotoxic (cytostatic). Azathioprine not only inhibits the replication of immunocompetent lymphocytes, but also tends to inhibit all actively replicating tissues and so, inherently, has a low therapeutic index. With this agent the suppression of myeloid (bone marrow) cells, in particular—with the dual consequence of toxicity and increased susceptibility to infection—lies close to the useful immunosuppression.

The introduction of cyclosporine (formerly called cyclosporin A) in 1978 was a major advance in immunosuppressive therapy. In the case of renal transplantation, in which it has been most extensively used, 90% of cadaveric-kidney recipients escape even a single rejection episode of allografts, and at least 80% of patients have functioning grafts at the end of a year. Moreover, cyclosporine has made renal transplants possible for strong immune responders, older patients, and diabetics (Kahan, 1983). Cyclosporine acts selectively and reversibly on lymphocytes and, unlike cytotoxic immunosuppressant drugs, does not affect myeloid cells, thus sparing considerable immune response for fighting infection.

The response to the antigenic provocation of an organ transplant is a complex host-vs-graft reaction in which the dominant mechanism of rejection is the acute lymphocyte-mediated immune reaction (Berkow, 1982). An activation of selected lymphocytes occurs; this entails several humoral factors (the lymphokines: interleukin-1 and interleukin-2) that are released from cells following appropriate presentation of an antigen (Cohen et al., 1984). By inhibiting the production of interleukin-2 by T-helper lymphocytes, cyclosporine sharply reduces the proliferation and maturation of cytolytic T lymphocytes (the effector cells in the rejection of transplants) and of additional T-helper cells (Morris, 1984, Cohen et al., 1984, Hess et al., 1986, and Lampe, 1986). In contrast to these actions, cyclosporine allows a relative sparing of the generation and activation of suppressor T lymphocytes (a normal dampening control mechanism of the rejection process), which then helps to maintain an unresponsive state to the transplanted graft and to inhibit delayed hypersensitivity responses (Kupiec-Weglinkski et al., 1984). The formation of antibodies against graft antigens is also inhibited as a secondary consequence of cyclosporine-induced inhibition of T-helper lymphocyte function.

According to White (1982b), because of this selective, unique mechanism of action, patients are able to fight infections, few of which are seen with cyclosporine therapy in transplant patients. The lack of myelotoxicity makes cyclosporine an especially valuable immunosuppressant agent for bone marrow transplants that are necessary in treating certain anemias, leukemias, and immunodeficiency diseases in children. Cyclosporine, especially in conjunction with methotrexate, appears to be of some effectiveness in the treatment of acute graft-vs-host disease—a disorder caused by immunologically competent donor cells being given to a heavily suppressed host (Cohen, et al., 1984; Kahan, 1985; Storb et al., 1987). This disease is a very frequent sequela to bone marrow transplantation and is characterized by fever, exfoliative dermatitis, hepatitis, diarrhea, abdominal pain, vomiting, and weight loss, and causes many deaths (Berkow, 1982).

Cyclosporine has proven to be effective in supporting grafts of heart and liver in addition to kidney and bone marrow (Cooley et al., 1983; Starzl et al., 1983, Cohen et al., 1984; Kahan, 1985). Starzl (1983) was of the opinion that cyclosporine made it "...possible to transplant some of the solid organs with a success not previously possible and to carry out other kinds of solid organ transplantation that were previously beyond our grasp." The major obstacle to almost uniform success in transplants of all kinds is the frequent occurrence (25–38%) of cyclosporine-induced nephrotoxicity in humans (Kahan, 1985; Lampe, 1986). This nephrotoxicity is not readily produced in animals. Williams et al. (1986) cautioned that, although cyclosporine is a giant advance in the field of transplantation, its nephrotoxicity can sometimes negate its beneficial effects. Nephrotoxicity may appear as acute or chronic renal insufficiency; hyperkalemia and hypertension may also be observed. In renal transplants it is difficult to differentiate nephrotoxicity from acute rejection. According to Wood et al. (1983), a brief course of cyclosporine in the critical early stage of transplantation may prevent rejection, after which time the drug regimen can be converted to azathioprine and steroids to prevent possible nephrotoxicity.

Other potential uses for cyclosporine are in the treatment of autoimmune diseases, such as rheumatoid arthritis, and in the treatment of insulin-dependent diabetes mellitus (Herold and Rubenstein, 1989).

Early Clinical Research History

Calne et al. (1978b) noted that corticosteroids were essential in preventing organ-graft rejection, however, their many toxic side effects made a safer replacement desirable. Based on promising results with cyclosporine in animals, seven renal-failure patients received transplants from mismatched cadaver donors and were given cyclosporine for immunosuppression. Cyclosporine had a profound immunosuppressive effect and prevented rejection, but nephrotoxicity and transient hepatotoxicity were in evidence. Cyclophosphamide and prednisone were added to the regimen in some cases. Five patients left the hospital with functioning grafts; two had received no steroids. No evidence of bone marrow toxicity was observed.

Calne et al. (1979) extended their studies to 34 recipients of cadaveric kidneys, pancreases, and livers. At the time of publication, 26 of the 32 kidneys had been supporting life for extended periods, three for more than a year. The pancreases and livers were also functioning. Nephrotoxicity, seen in a previous study (Calne et al., 1978b), was ameliorated by perioperative hydration and mannitol infusion. Twenty of the patients were not receiving steroids, and cyclosporine was the sole immunosuppressant used. The authors concluded, "Cyclosporin A is effective on its own and is a very potent immunosuppressive drug." Addition of other immunosuppressive agents to cyclosporine was to be avoided because of a high incidence of infection and because of the two lymphomas that occurred with combined therapy.

Powles et al. (1978) treated five cases of graft-vs-host disease with cyclosporine. Skin lesions were cleared within two days. However, four of the five patients died. Powles et al. (1980) tried cyclosporine as a prophylactic treatment for this disease. Only one out of 20 patients on cyclosporine developed acute graft-vs-host disease and died.

Starzl et al. (1980), reporting on 22 cadaveric kidney transplants, suggested that a combination of cyclosporine and steroids was the appropriate therapy for transplant patients. In a majority of the 22 patients treated with cyclosporine alone, rejection began to develop, but in most instances the process was readily controlled with small doses of prednisone. These workers reported that all but two of their 22 patients had been "liberated from dialysis" and that this high rate of success resulted from a combination of cyclosporine and steroid therapy. Starzl et al. (1980) suggested that with cyclosporine only a small fraction of the steroid therapy necessary in the past was required, and consequently, the risks associated with steroids were greatly minimized. Starzl et al. (1981) felt that the same regimen, cyclosporine and steroids, benefited liver transplants and that cyclosporine had "revitalized" the field of liver transplantation.

Many clinical trials followed that have expanded on these early findings and established cyclosporine in therapy. Some are described by Kahan (1983); also, *see* Sutherland et al. (1984) and the Canadian Multicentre Transplant Study Group (1986). Many reviews and books on cyclosporine have appeared. *See,* for example, White et al. (1979); Tutschka (1979); Borel (1981); Morris (1981, 1984); White (1982a,b); Kupiec-Weglinski et al. (1984); and Williams et al. (1986).

II. The Scientific Work Leading to Cyclosporine

Four publications from the Sandoz research laboratories—Borel et al. (1976), Dreyfuss et al. (1976), Rüegger et al. (1976), Petcher et al. (1976)—established the potential medical significance, microbiological activity, chemical structure, and conformation, respectively, of a new peptide, cyclosporine. As stated by Borel et al. (1976) and Dreyfuss et al. (1976), a screening program for new metabolites from microorganisms led to the isolation of the antibiotics cyclosporin A and C from soil samples. These molecules were isolated from the fermentation broth of two species of fungi, the most important of which was *Trichoderma polysporum* (Link ex Pers.) Rifai.* As antibiotics, the cyclosporins exhibited only a narrow spectrum of activity against fungi and, in addition, only a few species of yeast were sensitive; no inhibition of bacteria was observed (Dreyfuss et al, 1976).

Borel et al. (1976), however, reported interesting immunosuppressant activity. They indicated that cyclosporine (i.e., cyclosporin A) suppressed the appearance of both direct (IgM antibody response) and indirect (IgG antibody response) plaque-forming cells in mice. Unlike the cytotoxic agents cyclosphosphamide and azathioprine, cyclosporine had to be given immediately before or within the

---

*Later corrected to *Tolypocladium inflatum* Gams.

first 24 hours following immunization. Cyclosporine also exhibited an array of other immunosuppressant activities: suppression of hemagglutinin formation in mice in response to sheep erythrocytes, delay of skin graft rejection in mice, delay of the appearance of graft-vs-host disease in mice and rats, and protection of rats from the paralysis of experimental allergic encephalomyelitis and from the induction of Freund's adjuvant arthritis. Unlike cyclosphosphamide and azathioprine, cyclosporine had low myelotoxicity, was not cytotoxic, and was not lympholytic. Given equipotent doses, cyclosporine did not reduce leukocyte counts, whereas azathioprine produced a clear leukopenia. These authors concluded that, because cyclosporine seemed almost devoid of other pharmacological activity and, more important, because of its low myelotoxicity, it should eventually be investigated in human organ transplantation and autoimmune diseases.

Rüegger et al. (1976) and Petcher et al. (1976) elucidated the structure of cyclosporine by chemical degradation and X-ray crystallographic methods (Fig. 1). It was a neutral, hydrophobic, cyclic peptide composed of 11 amino acid residues, seven of which were N-methylated. It also contained a unique unsaturated nine-carbon amino acid in position 1. The four unmethylated nitrogen atoms formed internal hydrogen bonds with carbonyl groups. Borel et al. (1976) suggested that the N-methylation of the amino groups was responsible for the fact that cyclosporine, unlike most peptides, was effective by the oral route: it was rendered unsusceptible to digestive enzymes and to low pH.

Borel et al. (1977) extended their previous studies and showed that cyclosporine depressed both primary and secondary responses of IgM and $IgG2_a$ plaque-forming cells and oxazolone-induced skin reactions in humans. Moreover, cyclosporine did not prevent the formation of IgM antibodies when normal and "nude" mice were immunized with lipopolysaccharide, and since in this immunological model predominantly B lymphocytes are involved, it appeared that cyclosporine did not affect B-cell functions. The authors emphasized that their in vitro results supported the notion that cyclosporine acted at the early stages of lymphoid cell transformation and that it had to be administered during the sensitization phase in order to elicit immunosuppression. In addition, cyclosporine, even at ex-

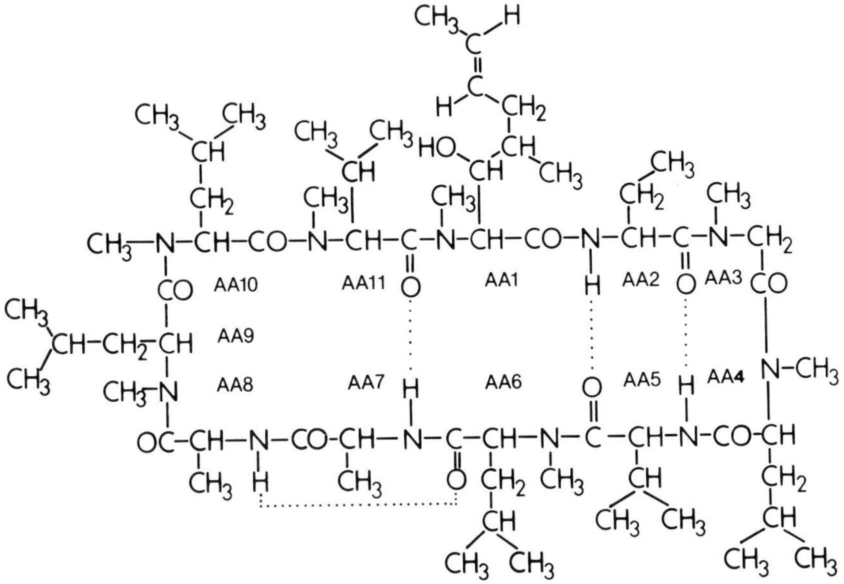

Fig. 1. The structure of cyclosporine.

tremely high doses, produced very little reduction in the number of cells in bone marrow, whereas stem cell proliferation was either not changed or enhanced. Azathioprine, on the other hand, severely affected the number and function of stem cells and caused a transient but severe depletion of bone marrow cells (Borel et al., 1977).

Kostakis et al. (1977) found that rats receiving heart allografts, when treated with cyclosporine dissolved in olive oil at a proper dose, survived an average of 42 d; untreated rats rejected the transplanted hearts at an average of 9 d.

Calne and White (1977) reported that the median survival for 10 dogs given kidney allografts and azathioprine was 27.5 d. Of nine animals treated with cyclosporine, four died, but four were alive more than 20 d after the transplant and still surviving at the time of publication, and one had been alive for 62 d. These investigators concluded that cyclosporine had a "...profound immunosuppressive effect on rejection of dog kidney allografts." and that, in the past, this model proved reliable in predicting the clinical immunosuppressive effect of the drugs tested.

Calne et al. (1978a) subsequently found that cyclosporine was "...more effective in suppressing rejection than any other drug that we have used in pigs with orthotopic cardiac allografts." The median survival in 20 control pigs was 6 d. In contrast, depending on the dose and dosing schedules, pigs treated with cyclosporine survived from 22 to over 68 d, and four animals were alive at the time of publication. Azathioprine plus prednisolone produced a median survival of only 6 d. These authors concluded that cyclosporine was "...sufficiently nontoxic and powerful as an immunosuppressant to make it an attractive candidate for clinical investigation in patients receiving organ grafts."

Table 1 defines the critical scientific ideas and experiments leading to cyclosporine and categorizes their origin.

Background Contributions Preceding Cyclosporine

"Antibiotics are chemical substances produced by various species of microorganisms (bacteria, fungi, actinomycetes) that suppress the growth of other microorganisms and may eventually destroy them" (Sande and Mandell, 1985). The phenomenon of antibiosis is continually ongoing in nature, occurring in soil, sewage, water, and any other habitat of microorganisms. With the coming of the modern age of the organized discovery, production, and medical usage of antibiotics, which started with penicillin in 1941, it has become common practice to sample these habitats in the search for new agents. Samples are brought into the laboratory in order to make extracts, establish activity, isolate the active principle(s) if warranted, characterize and then study the active principle(s) in detail in animals and, eventually, in humans. The discovery of cyclosporine as an immunosuppressant was an outgrowth of such an antibiotic program.

As mentioned earlier, the combined use of azathioprine plus corticosteroids, although a great advance from the vacuum existing prior to their introduction, was only a partial and toxic answer to the rejection problem in renal and bone marrow grafting, and it did little for the grafting of other organs, e.g., heart and liver. It was clear to immunologists, as well as to surgeons, that there was room for improvement in immunosuppressant therapy.

Table 1

Profile of Observations and Ideas Crucial to the Development of Cyclosporine[a]

Sequence: Route to innovative drug[**]	Orient-ation	Nature of study	Research institution	National origin	Nature of discovery	Screening involved	Crucial ideas or observations
Cyclosporine[**]							
Borel et al. (1976)	Pre-clinical	Pharma-cology/ chem-istry	Indus-try	Switzer-land	Orderly	Untargeted	The "failed" anti-biotic cyclosporine (cyclosporin A) has unusual immuno-suppressant activity; unlike cytotoxic agents; no myelo-toxicity; significance for organ transplan-tation in humans recognized.

[a]Taken from section II. Entries are those contributions without which the discovery of the agent (or additionally, in some cases, a relevant clinical application) would not have taken place or would have been materially delayed.

III. Comments on Events Leading to Cyclosporine

Borel (1982) pointed out,

My colleagues who were then involved in isolating metabolites of microbial origin primarily for screening as antibiotics, had learned from experience that these compounds often showed cytostatic or other pharmacological activities greater than the antimicrobial activity for which they had been selected....The chemical structure of these metabolites may also be unusual and thus be valuable for finding new chemical leads and we had, therefore, agreed to include also agents of this type, even the water insolubles ones, in our pharmacological screen.

In the opinion of White (1982b), we owed the development of cyclosporine to Borel, who was convinced by the results of a range of in vitro and in vivo assays that this agent was a specific immuno-suppressant that might have advantages over the cytotoxic im-munosuppressants then in use.

In summarizing reports presented at the first International Cyclosporine Congress in Houston, Starzl (1983) remarked that the transplantation community owed a unique debt to the fathers of cyclosporine, J. Borel, D. White, and R. Calne, as well as to the people at Sandoz who permitted and encouraged a look at the blemishes as well as the perfection of cyclosporine. Borel (1982) noted that "...management [at Sandoz] was flexible enough to recognize firstly the strong and reproducible immunosuppressive activity, and secondly the remarkable lack of side effects of this compound...."

IV. Developments Subsequent to Cyclosporine

The consensus attitude of the organ-transplant community that the nephrotoxicity of cyclosporine placed a limit on its clinical applications (*see* Cohen et al., 1984; Morris, 1984; Kahan, 1985) encouraged the search for a less nephrotoxic analog. Wenger (1983) reported that several of the amino acids in cyclosporine could be replaced with different amino acids and that the products still retained moderate to good immunosuppressant activity in animal models. Some of these compounds may prove to be suitable for clinical trial. Unfortunately, reliable animal models of cyclosporine-induced human nephrotoxicity are not available. The major goal for future work is the development of selective, specific, safe suppressants of the immune system.

It should be noted that cyclosporine has had a large impact not only on clinical practice, but also on the basic immunology of graft rejection (Borel, 1982, 1983; Kahan, 1983). Hess et al. (1986) noted that

> ...the studies to date suggest that CsA [cyclosporine] is not only a unique effective immunosuppressive agent offering great potential for the control of transplant rejection, but is also a valuable tool in which to probe mechanisms of tolerance induction and suppressor, helper, and cytotoxic T-cell activation.

References

Berkow, R., ed.: Immunology; allergic-disorders, in *The Merck Manual*, 14th Ed., pp. 265–347, Merck Sharp & Dohme Research Laboratories, Rahway, NJ, 1982.

Borel, J. F.: Cyclosporin-A, Present experimental status. *Transplant. Proc.* **13**: 344–348, 1981.

Borel, J. F.: The history of cyclosporin A and its significance, in *Cyclosporin A*, D. J. G. White, ed., pp. 5–17, Elsevier, Amsterdam, 1982.

Borel, J. F.: Cyclosporine: Historical perspectives. *Transplant. Proc.* **15** (Suppl. 1): 2219–2229, 1983.

Borel, J. F., Feurer, C., Gubler, H. U., and Stähelin, H.: Biological effects of cyclosporin A: A new anti-lymphocytic agent. *Agents Actions* **6**: 468–475, 1976.

Borel, J. F., Feurer, C., Magneé, C., and Stähelin, H.: Effects of the new anti-lymphocytic peptide cyclosporin A in animals. *Immunology* **32**: 1017–1025, 1977.

Calne, R. Y. and White, D. J. G.: Cyclosporin A—A powerful immunosuppressant in dogs with renal allografts. *IRCS Med. Sci.* **5**: 595, 1977.

Calne, R. Y., White, D. J. G., Rolles, K., Smith, D. P., and Herbertson, B. M.: Prolonged survival of pig orthotopic heart grafts treated with cyclosporin A. *Lancet* **1**: 1183–1185, 1978a.

Calne, R. Y., White, D. J. G., Thiru, S., Evans, D. B., McMaster, P., Dunn, D. C., Craddock, G. N., Pentlow, B. D., and Rolles, K.: Cyclosporin A in patients receiving renal allografts from cadaver donors. *Lancet* **2**: 1323–1327, 1978b.

Calne, R. Y., Rolles, K., White, D. J. G., Thiru, S., Evans, D. B., McMaster, P., Dunn, D. C., Craddock, G. N., Henderson, R. G., Aziz, S., and Lewis, P.: Cyclosporin A initially as the only immunosuppressant in 34 recipients of cadaveric organs: 32 kidneys, 2 pancreases and 2 livers. *Lancet* **2**: 1033–1036, 1979.

The Canadian Multicentre Transplant Study Group: A randomized clinical trial of cyclosporine in cadaveric renal transplantation: Analysis at three years. *N. Engl. J. Med.* **314**: 1219–1225, 1986.

Cohen, D. J., Loertscher, R., Rubin, M. F., Tilney, N. L., Carpenter, C. B., and Strom, T. B.: Cyclosporine: A new immunosuppressive agent for organ transplantation. *Ann. Intern. Med.* **101**: 667–682, 1984.

Cooley, D. A., Frazier, O. H., Painvin, G. A., Boldt, L., and Kahan, B. D.:

Cardiac and cardiopulmonary transplantation using cyclosporine for immunosuppression: Recent Texas Heart Institute experience. *Transplant. Proc.* **15** (Suppl. 1): 2567–2572, 1983.

Dreyfuss, M., Harri, E., Hofmann, H., Kobel, H., Pache, W., and Tscherter, H.: Cyclosporin A and C. New metabolites from *Trichoderma polysporum* (link ex pers) rifai. *Eur. J. Applied Microbiol.* **3**: 125–133, 1976.

Herold, K. C. and Rubenstein, A. H.: Immunosuppression for insulin-dependent diabetes. *N. Engl. J. Med.* **318**: 701, 702, 1989.

Hess, A. D., Colombani, P. M. and Esa, A.: Cyclosporine: Immunologic aspects in transplantation, in *Kidney Transplant Rejection: Diagnosis and Treatment*, G. M. Williams, J. F. Burdick, and K. Solez, eds., pp. 353–382, Marcel Dekker, New York, 1986.

Kahan, B. D.: Cosmas and Damian in the 20th century? *N. Engl. J. Med.* **305**: 280, 281, 1981.

Kahan, B. D.: Cosmas and Damian revisited. *Transplant. Proc.* **15** (Suppl. 1): 2211–2216, 1983.

Kahan, B. D.: Cyclosporine: The agent and its actions. *Transplant. Proc.* **17** (Suppl. 1): 5–18, 1985.

Kahan, B. D., ed.: Symposium. First international congress on cyclosporine. *Transplant. Proc.* **15** (Suppls. 1,2): 2207–3188, 1983.

Kostakis, A. J., White, D. J. B., and Calne, R. Y.: Prolongation of rat heart allograft survival by cyclosporin A. *IRCS Med. Sci.* **5**: 280, 1977.

Kupiec-Weglinski, J. W., Filho, M. A., Strom, T. B. ,and Tilney, N. L.: Sparing of suppressor cells: A critical action of cyclosporine. *Transplantation* **38**: 97–101, 1984.

Lampe, K. F., ed.: Immunomodulators, in *Drug Evaluations*, 6th Ed., pp. 1147–1165, American Medical Association, Chicago, 1986.

Morris, P. J.: Cyclosporin A. *Transplantation* **32**: 349–354, 1981.

Morris, P. J.: Cyclosporine, in *Kidney Transplantation: Principles and Practice*, P. J. Morris, ed., pp. 261–279, Grune and Stratton, London, 1984.

Petcher, T. J., Weber, H. P., and Rüegger, A.: Crystal and molecular structure of an iodo-derivative of the cyclic undecapeptide cyclosporin A. *Helv. Chim. Acta* **59**: 1480–1488, 1976.

Powles, R. L., Barrett, A. J., Clink, H., Kay, H. E. M., Sloane, J., and McElwain, T. J.: Cyclosporin A for the treatment of graft-versus-host disease in man. *Lancet* **2**: 1327–1331, 1978.

Powles, R. L., Clink, H. M., Spence, D., Morgenstern, G., Watson, J. G., Selby, P. J., Woods, M., Barrett, A., Jameson, B., Sloane, J., Lawler, S. D., Kay, H. E. M., Lawson, D., McElwain, T. J., and Alexander, P.: Cyclosporin A to prevent graft-versus-host disease in man after allogeneic bone-marrow transplantation. *Lancet* **1:** 327–329, 1980.

Rüegger, A., Kuhn, M., Lichti, H., Loosli, H. R., Huguenin, R., Quiquerez, C., and von Wartburg, A.: Cyclosporin A, a peptide metabolite from *Trichoderma polysporum Rifai* with a remarkable immunosuppressive activity. *Helv. Chim. Acta* **59:** 1075–1092, 1976.

Sande, M. A. and Mandell, G. L.: Antimicrobial agents. General considerations, in *The Pharmacological Basis of Therapeutics*, 7th Ed., A. G. Gilman, L. S. Goodman, T. W. Rall, and F. Murad, eds., pp. 1066–1094, Macmillan, New York, 1985.

Starzl, T. E.: Clinical aspects of cyclosporine therapy: A summation. *Transplant. Proc.* **15** (Suppl. 1): 3103–3107, 1983.

Starzl, T. E., Hakala, T. R., Rosenthal, J. T., Iwatsuki, S., and Shaw, B. W., Jr.: The Colorado-Pittsburgh cadaveric renal transplantation study with cyclosporine. *Transplant. Proc.* **15** (Suppl. 1): 2459–2462, 1983.

Starzl, T. E., Iwatsuki, S., Klintmalm, S., Schröter, G. P. J., Weil, R. III, Koep, L. J., and Porter, K. A.: Liver transplantation, 1980, with particular reference to cyclosporin-A. *Transplant. Proc.* **13** (No . 1): 281–285, 1981.

Starzl, T. E., Weil, R. III, Iwatsuki, S., Klintmalm, G., Schröter, G. P. J., Koep, L. J., Iwaki, Y., Terasaki, P. I., and Porter, K. A.: The use of cyclosporin A and prednisone in cadaver kidney transplantation. *Surg. Gynecol. Obstet.* **151:** 17–26, 1980.

Storb, R., Deeg, H. J., Whitehead, J., Farewell, V., Appelbaum, F. R., Beatty, P., Bensinger, W., Buckner, C. D., Clift, R. A., Doney, K., Hansen, J. A., Hill, R., Lum, L. G., Martin, P., McGuffin, R., Sanders, J. E., Singer, J., Stewart, P., Sullivan, K. M., Witherspoon, R. P., and Thomas, E. D.: Marrow transplantation for leukemia and aplastic anemia: Two controlled trials of a combination of methotrexate and cyclosporine v cyclosporine alone or methotrexate alone for prophylaxis of acute graft-v-host disease. *Transplant. Proc.* **19:** 2608–2613, 1987.

Sutherland, D. E. R., Goetz, F. C., and Najarian, J. S.: Pancreas transplants from related donors. *Transplantation* **38:** 625–633, 1984.

Tutschka, P. J.: Cyclosporin A—A new outlook for immunosuppression in clinical transplantation. *Blut* **39:** 81–87, 1979.

Wenger, R.: Synthesis of cyclosporine and analogues. Structure activity relationships of new cyclosporine derivatives. *Transplant. Proc.* **15** (Suppl. 1): 2230–2241, 1983.

White, D. J. G.: Foreword to *Cyclosporin A*, D. J. G. White, ed., p. v, Elsevier Biomedical, Amsterdam, 1982a.

White, D. J. G.: Cyclosporin A. Clinical pharmacology and therapeutic potential. *Drugs* **24**: 322–334, 1982b.

White, D. J. G., Plumb, A. M., Pawelec, G., and Brons, G.: Cyclosporin A: An immunosuppressive agent preferentially active against proliferating T cells. *Transplantation* **27**: 55–58, 1979.

Williams, G. M., Burdick, J. F., and Solez, K.: Preface, in *Kidney Transplant Rejection: Diagnosis and Treatment*, G. M. Williams, J. F. Burdick, and K. Solez, eds., pp. v,vi, Marcel Dekker, New York, 1986.

Wood, R. F. M., Thompson, J. F., Allen, N. H., Ting, A., and Morris, P. J.: The consequences of conversion from cyclosporine to azathioprine and prednisolone in renal allograft recipients. *Transplant. Proc.* **15** (Suppl. 1): 2862–2868, 1983.

Psychiatry Group

Chlorpromazine
Haloperidol
Imipramine
Iproniazid
Lithium
Chlordiazepoxide
Diazepam

Chlorpromazine

I. Chlorpromazine as an Innovative Therapeutic Agent

Schizophrenia is a mysterious, crippling illness characterized by disordered thinking, delusions, hallucinations, and withdrawal from the external world. Until the early 1950s it was treated with electroconvulsive shock or hypoglycemic shock induced with insulin, often resulting in memory dysfunction, amnesia, and subtle impairment of cognitive function (Taylor, 1982; Squire, 1982). In addition, drugs (barbiturates, morphine, and other sedatives) were used to calm (control) the agitated patient. Sleep therapy was in vogue. Unfortunately, paranoia, delusions, hallucinations, and disturbed thought processes were not affected by either shock or sleep therapies. As pointed out by Hollister (1972), pneumonia and cardiovascular collapse were often associated with the aggressive use of sedatives. These "therapies" prevented the creation of rapport with the patient and the initiation of psychotherapy. Chlorpromazine completely removed this impasse: it calmed highly agitated patients and dramatically improved other symptoms of psychosis. It was evident that the efficacy of chlorpromazine transcended its sedative actions. Chlorpromazine could be used regardless of age or sex, in the hospital or on an outpatient basis, and was effective at any stage of the illness.

Chlorpromazine revolutionized the specialty of psychiatry. It brought legitimacy to the concept of biological psychiatry by demonstrating that a drug could influence the course of a major psychosis. Once chlorpromazine was available, psychiatrists began to design complex studies to evaluate its effects and those of other neuroleptics. According to Sherman and Rothstein (1966), chlorpromazine and other psychoactive drugs created scientists out of clinicians and methodologists out of practitioners. Psychiatric rating scales were developed, allowing clinical data to be standardized. Controlled clinical trials were performed with large homogeneous samples of patients; recording became objective, and statistical analyses were employed (Hollister, 1972).

Chlorpromazine became the treatment of choice for schizophrenia. Its most important contribution was that the resident population of mental hospitals was reduced by 80% (Hollister, 1983). Today chlorpromazine and related compounds are used as calmative agents no matter what the cause of agitation: acute or chronic brain syndrome, manic depression, or severe anxiety. Chlorpromazine is still widely used for the management of acutely disturbed patients (Burrows and Davies, 1985). Chlorpromazine has also been used to control extreme nausea and to potentiate analgesia in intractable pain.

Because of its tricyclic-propylamine structure, chlorpromazine displays significant antiadrenergic and anticholingeric actions and exerts adverse effects secondary to these actions: orthostatic hypotension, dry mouth, blurred vision, constipation, and urinary retention. Sedation is common. With high doses extrapyramidal reactions may occur, and with prolonged use tardive dyskinesia may develop. This latter movement disorder is frequently slow to reverse or may be irreversible.

Early Clinical Research History

In the case of chlorpromazine the early clinical history permeates the scientific work leading to its discovery and is, therefore, covered in section II.

II. The Scientific Departure Leading to Chlorpromazine: Promethazine

Laborit (1949), a naval surgeon, was concerned with problems relating to surgical shock, volatile anesthetics, and postsurgical phlebitis. He theorized that histamine, released by surgical intervention, elicited capillary hyperpermeability, which in turn led to the arousal of defense mechanisms (e.g., vasoconstriction) and, inappropriately, to shock. He proposed the use of a combination of pharmacological agents (eventually termed a "lytic cocktail") to dampen the arousal of these mechanisms, with synthetic antihistamines being used to combat capillary hyperpermeability. He recognized in his studies that promethazine—Rhone-Poulenc (RP) compound number 3277 (Fig. 1)—produced useful analgesia and drowsiness. With promethazine in the mixture, there was no need for postsurgical morphine: patients were calm, relaxed, peaceful, and drowsy. Sigwald et al. (1949), in a large study of neurological patients, noted that diethazine and promethazine produced drowsiness. Promethazine was useful in controlling pain and in inducing sleep; patients lost their apprehensiveness for an anticipated painful injection. It was suggested by Sigwald et al. (1949) that some of these properties of promethazine be exploited. Laborit and Leger (1950) stated, "The antihistamine properties of Phenergan [promethazine] are intense, but are also present in other antihistamines. Its side effects are unique to this substance." They stated that the centrally mediated side effects of promethazine were of "indisputable" advantage.

Guiraud and David (1950) suggested that the drowsiness that was produced by antihistamines might be of interest to psychiatry. Promethazine calmed 24 anxious, excited patients; abolished or shortened manic attacks; and brought some patients under control for long periods of time. These investigators did not continue their work with promethazine.

Background Contributions Preceding the Discovery of the CNS Usefulness of Promethazine

A series of phenolic ethers that displayed selective sympatholytic activity had been synthesized by Fourneau (Fourneau and Bovet, 1933). Later, Bovet and his graduate student, Staub (Staub, 1939), tested the series of phenolic ethers against histamine. With thymoxydiethylamine (929F) and, subsequently, the aniline derivative 1571F, they found clear experimental support for Bovet's theoretical concept of selective antihistamine activity. The first therapeutically useful antihistamine, Antergan (RP 2339) (also an aniline derivative), was reported by Halpern (1942).

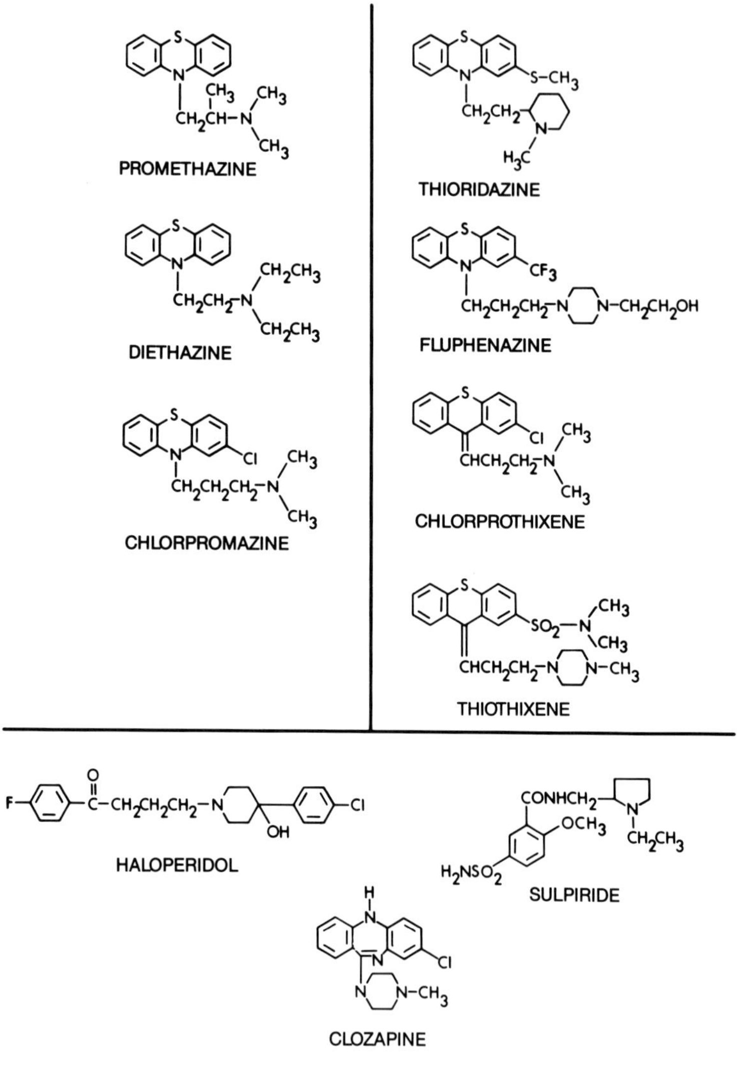

Fig. 1. The structures of chlorpromazine and chemically and/or pharmacologically related substances.

Knowledge of the phenothiazine nucleus had come from the synthetic dye industry, where analyses of the structures of Lauth's violet and methylene blue led to its description. Phenothiazines became known for their antihelminthic action, and it was known that amine chains were associated with antimalarial activity in other molecules. These two pieces of knowledge were fused when Charpentier (1947) reported synthesizing alkyl amine derivatives of phenothiazines as possible antiparasite compounds in 1944. However, they were without significant antimalarial, antihelminthic, or trypanocidal activity. Halpern (1947) discovered the antihistaminic activities of these phenothiazine derivatives and drew attention to the high potency of promethazine.

Significant Events Following Promethazine

Charpentier et al. (1952) reported that they had condensed 1-chloro phenothiazine, 3-chloro phenothiazine, and 3-methoxy phenothiazine with 3-chloro-1-dimethyl amino propane and obtained 11 new compounds with propylamine sidechains. They indicated that all the compounds had specific pharmacological properties that would be presented elsewhere. The 3-chloro derivative (RP 4560) (Fig. l) had the generic name of chlorpromazine proposed for it.

Laborit and Huguenard (1951) had been troubled by the fact that the pharmacological aspect of the surgical technique they had developed was too complex. They reported preliminary work with chlorpromazine, which they judged to be very effective in conjunction with promethazine and diethazine. They felt that chlorpromazine probably had both peripheral and central actions that would simplify their procedures. Laborit et al. (1952) stated that chlorpromazine had "interesting properties" in potentiating general anesthesia. It was not an antihistamine, but had properties in common with promethazine and diethazine. When used alone

> ...the product does not cause any loss of consciousness, no alteration of the psychic state, but merely a certain tendency to sleep and especially "disinterest" on the part of the patient in his environment...The facts suggest certain indications of the product in psychiatry, whereby its potentiating action can be used as a sleep agent with a positive reduction of the use of barbiturates.

Hamon et al. (1952), influenced by Laborit, treated a patient who had a long history of manic outbursts—not controlled by either electroshock or insulin shock—with a combination of chlorpromazine, barbiturates and analgesics. The patient immediately became calm and, after some period of therapy, was released. Hamon et al. (1952) suggested that chlorpromazine was a sedative that could be useful in sleep disorders and neurotic conditions, and a pharmacological product that could enrich psychiatric therapy.

Delay et al. (1952a) stated, "Although this product is generally used as a potentiator of anesthetics, analgesics and hypnotics, it seemed to us more rational to use it by itself." Delay et al. (1952a) alluded to work done in rats. Conditioned rats under the influence of chlorpromazine became indifferent to stimuli. This indifference ceased once chlorpromazine administration was stopped. The indifference could not be obtained with barbiturates. The experimental work devoted to RP 4560 "...indicate a predominantly central action, which led us to use the medication in psychiatry." Delay et al. (1952 a,b) treated a variety of mental disorders including agitation, confusion, anxiety, depression, and schizophrenia. Patients who before the drug had to be put in restraint became calm and smiling. They appeared normal but indifferent to exterior stimuli, "...separated from their environment as if by an invisible wall." The remissions exhibited by the patients were better than would have been expected with insulin shock or electroshock. Delay and his colleagues suggested that chlorpromazine could be of considerable interest to psychiatry and that its central actions could be used to bring about a state resembling artificial hibernation.

Courvoisier et al. (1953), colleagues of Charpentier et al. (1952), published the pharmacology of chlorpromazine. Of note was its effect on conditioned avoidance in rats. They utilized the method that Winter (1948) and Winter and Flataker (1951) had devised to study what was considered the unwanted side effect of antihistamines—sedation. Rats were conditioned to climb a rope at the sound of a bell. Under the influence of chlorpromazine, rats ignored the sound of the bell, and were uncoordinated and disoriented. Courvoisier and associates concluded that the central actions of chlorpromazine, which had negligible antihistamine activity, were manifested by its effect on conditioned reflexes as well as by the capacity to potentiate general anesthetics, hypnotics, and analgesics.

Table 1 defines the critical scientific ideas and experiments leading to chlorpromazine and categorizes their origin.

Table 1
Profile of Observations and Ideas Crucial to the Development of Chlorpromazine[a]

Sequence: Departure compound* to innovative drug**	Orient- ation	Nature of study	Research institution	National origin	Nature of discovery	Screening involved	Crucial ideas or observations
Promethazine*							
Laborit (1949)	Clinical	Surgery	Hospital	Tunisia[b]	Seren- dipitous	No	The antihistamine promethazine has CNS side effects useful in anesthesiol- ogy and surgery.
Laborit and Leger (1950)	Clinical	Surgery	Hospital	France	Orderly	No	Promethazine has uniquely useful CNS side effects.
Chlorpromazine**							
Charpentier et al. (1952)	Pre- clinical	Chem- istry/ pharma- cology	Indus- try	France	Orderly	Targeted	Chlorpromazine and other analogs of promethazine synthe- sized and screened.
Delay et al. (1952a, b)	Clinical	Psy- chiatry	Uni- versity	France	Orderly	No	Chlorpromazine, by itself, is useful in psychiatric disorders.

[a]Taken from section II. Entries are those contributions without which the discovery of the agent (or additionally, in some cases, a relevant clinical application) would not have taken place or would have been materially delayed.
[b]In a French naval hospital.

III. Comments on Events Leading to Chlorpromazine

Acceptance of chlorpromazine was swift in Europe. Between the report of its first use in psychiatric patients (in 1952) and 1954, according to Viaud (1954), 500 publications appeared, mainly in the European literature, on the clinical uses of chlorpromazine. Accep- tance of chlorpromazine into psychiatric practice was slower in other parts of the world. Lehmann and Hanrahan (1954), in Canada, reported that 71 psychiatric patients in agitated states became emotionally indifferent with wooden facial expressions, did not dis- play interfering behavior, and yet were easily accessible to talk to and exhibited no clouding of consciousness. Their general appearance resembled that of Parkinsonism. Chartan (1954), in England, found chlorpromazine to be the drug of choice for acute excitement, especially because it facilitated psychotherapeutic contact. Goldman (1955), in the USA stated that since chlorpromazine had created a sense of optimism rarely seen with any other technique in the treatment of psychotic states, it was time to put timidity and fearfulness aside and push the drug to the limits of its possibilities.

Subsequently, a vast clinical literature has developed regarding the place of chlorpromazine in psychiatry. Chlorpromazine has been the subject of books and reviews both as an entity in itself and in the context of the science of psychotherapeutics (*see,* for example, Caldwell, 1970,1973; Swazey, 1974; Hollister, 1972, 1983; Bernstein, 1984; Burrows and Davies, 1985).

Some strong feelings concerning the distribution of credit for the development and use of chlorpromazine have been expressed in the literature. A fervid account of the discovery of chlorpromazine was presented by Caldwell (1970). She felt that without Laborit the use of chlorpromazine in psychiatry would never have occurred. Caldwell (1970,1973) states that Laborit clearly understood the intrinsic similarity between postoperative disease and mental illness and that it was a natural step for a surgeon who is familiar with the reactions of anxiety and depression to introduce chlorpromazine into psychiatry.

Swazey (1974), in the epilogue to her exhaustive, dispassionate treatise on the development of chlorpromazine (CPZ) has the following comments:

> The most complex and controversial issues in the history of CPZ's development and entrance into psychiatry turn around Henri Laborit's role.
> ...published and unpublished documents from the early 1950s generally cited the nature and import of Laborit's work as it bore on CPZ's synthesis and first uses in psychiatry. From the mid-1950s on, discussions of CPZ's "history," with few exceptions, neglected or minimized his contributions.
> Although CPZ did not enter French psychiatry through an organized program of clinical trials, its use and dissemination in France and other countries was facilitated by Delay's imprimatur.

IV. Developments Subsequent to Chlorpromazine

Once the clinical efficacy of chlorpromazine in psychiatry was established, many pharmacological and behavioral studies followed, thus providing tools for screening for new antipsychotic drugs.

Potent activity was found in the thioxanthene analogs of phenothiazine (if the nitrogen atom in the phenothiazine ring is replaced with a carbon atom, the thioxanthene nucleus is formed) (Fig. 1). In addition to finding activity in both series when the aliphatic amine side chain was present, higher potency was found with phenothiazines that had a piperidine substitution in the side chain, e.g., thioridazine (Fig. 1). Even higher potencies were found with both ring systems when the side chains contained piperazine moieties (Fig. 1). There are numerous phenothiazines available today.

The butyrophenones, especially haloperidol (Fig. 1), were the first neuroleptic agents to represent a clear chemical departure from the phenothiazines (*see* chapter on haloperidol). Other structural classes of neuroleptics have appeared: indoles, dibenzoxazepines, dibenzdiazepines, and benzamides.

Recognition in the late 1950s and 1960s of late-appearing abnormal movement disorders, having insidious onset and frequently being irreversible (tardive dyskinesia), dimmed the luster of chlorpromazine (and, to date, all other neuroleptics as well). Available evidence suggests that the blockade of dopamine receptors in limbic areas of the brain accounts for antipsychotic activity, whereas their blockade in striatal areas accounts for early extrapyramidal motor side effects and, ultimately, for tardive dyskinesia. There are now 20 antipsychotic drugs on the market. They all bind to dopamine receptors with varying potencies (Bernstein, 1984). Clozapine, a dibenzdiazepine, and sulpiride, a benzamide (Fig. 1), in addition to the phenothiazine derivative, thioridazine, appear to have less propensity to produce extrapyramidal side effects than do other available neuroleptics. The ultimate goal is to discover drugs with highly specific antipsychotic actions, lacking extrapyramidal activity.

The availability of chlorpromazine and related agents permitted the basic pharmacologic studies of their interactions with brain dopamine to be carried out in animals. This work, in turn, eventually led to the construction of the dopamine hypothesis of schizophrenia (Carlsson and Lindquist, 1963; Carlsson, 1975,1978).

References

Bernstein, J. G.: Rational use of antipsychotic drugs, in *Clinical Psychopharmacology*, J. G. Bernstein, ed., pp. 145–165, John Wright PSG, Boston, 1984.

Burrows, G. D. and Davies, B. M.: An introduction to the use of antipsychotic drugs, in *Antipsychotic Drugs in Psychiatry*, vol. 3, G. D. Burrows, T. R. Norman, and B. Davies, eds., pp. 3–8, Elsevier, Amsterdam, 1985.

Caldwell, A. E.: *Origins of Psychopharmacology*, Charles C. Thomas, Springfield, IL, 1970.

Caldwell, A. E.: History of psychopharmacology, in *Principles of Psychopharmacology*. W. E. Clark and J. del Guidice, eds., pp. 9–30, Academic, New York, 1973.

Carlsson, A.: Antipsychotic drugs and catecholamine synapses, in *Catecholamines and Schizophrenia*, S. W. Matthysse and S. S. Kety, eds., pp. 57–64, Pergamon, NewYork, 1975.

Carlsson, A.: Antipsychotic drugs, neurotransmitters, and schizophrenia. *Am. J. Psychiatry* **135:** 164–173, 1978.

Carlsson, A. and Lindquist, M.: Effect of chlorpromazine and haloperidol on formation of 3-methoxytyramine and normetanephrine in mouse brain. *Acta Pharmacol. Toxicol.* **20:** 140–144, 1963.

Charpentier, P.: Sur la constitution d'une dimethylamino-propyl-N-phenothiazine. *Comptes Rendus* **225:** 306–308, 1947.

Charpentier, P., Gailliot, P., Jacob, R., Gaudechon, J., Buisson, P., and Delepine, M.: Chimie organique—Recherches sur les dimethylamino-propyl-N phenothiazines substituee. *Comptes Rendus* **235:** 59,60, 1952.

Chartan F. B. E.: An evaluation of chlorpromazine ("Largactil") in psychiatry. *J. Ment. Sci.* **100:** 882–893, 1954.

Courvoisier, S., Fournel, J., Ducrot, R., Kolsky, M., and Koetschet, P.: Proprietes pharmacodynamiques du chlorohydrate de chloro-3(dimethylamino-3'propyl)-10 phenothiazine (4560 R.P.). *Arch. Int. Pharmacodyn.* **92:** 305–361, 1953.

Delay, J. Deniker, P., and Harl, J. M.: Utilisation en therapeutique psychiatrique d'une phenothiazine d'action centrale elective (4560 R.P.). *Ann. Méd.-Psychol.* (Paris) **110:** 112–117, 1952a.

Delay, J., Deniker, P., and Harl, J. M.: Traitement des etats d'excitation et

d'agitation par une methode medicamenteuse derivee de l'hiberno-
therapie. *Ann. Méd.-Psychol.* (Paris) **110**: 267–273, 1952b.

Fourneau, E. and Bovet, D.: Recherches sur l'action sympathicolytique
d'un nouveau dérivé du dioxane. *Arch. Int. Pharm. Ther.* **46**: 178–191,
1933.

Goldman, D.: Treatment of psychotic states with chlorpromazine. *JAMA*
157: 1274–1278, 1955.

Guiraud, M. P., and David, C.: Traitement de l'agitation motrice par un antihistaminique (3277 R.P.). *C. R. Cong. Alien. Neurol. France* **48**: 599–602,
1950.

Halpern, B. N.: Les antihistaminiques de synthese. Essais de chimio-
therapie des états allergiques. *Arch. Int. Pharm. Ther.* **68**: 339–408, 1942.

Halpern, B. N.: Experimental research on a series of new chemical substances with powerful antihistaminic activity: The thiodiphenylamine
derivatives. *Allergy* **18**: 263–272, 1947.

Hamon, Paraire, and Velluz: Remarques sur l'action due 4560 R.P. sur
l'agitation maniaque. *Ann. Med.-Psychol.* (Paris) **110**: 331–335, 1952.

Hollister, L. E.: Clinical use of psychotherapeutic drugs. I: Antipsychotic
and antimanic drugs. *Drugs* **4**: 321–360, 1972.

Hollister, L. E.: *Clinical Pharmacology of Psychotherapeutic Drugs*, 2nd Ed.,
Churchill Livingston, New York, 1983.

Laborit, H.: Sur l'utilization de certains agents pharmacodynamiques a action neuro-vegetative en periode per- et postoperatoire. *Acta Chir. Belg.*
48: 485–492, 1949.

Laborit, H. and Huguenard, P.: Notes de technique chirurgicale. *Presse
Méd.* **59**: 1329, 1951.

Laborit, H. and Leger, L.: Utilisation d'un antihistaminique de synthese
en therapeutique pre, per, et post-operatoire. *Presse Méd.* **58**: 492, 1950.

Laborit, H., Huguenard, P., and Alluaume, R.: Un nouveau stabilisateur
vegetatif (le 4560 R.P.). *Presse Méd.* **60**: 206–208, 1952.

Lehmann, H. E. and Hanrahan, G. E.: Chlorpromazine. New inhibiting
agent for psychomotor excitement and manic states. *AMA Arch. Neurol.
Psych.* **71**: 227–237, 1954.

Sherman, L. J. and Rothstein, E.: Methodological models for the study of
drugs in the treatment of alcoholism. *Psychosom. Med.* **28**: 627–635, 1966.

Sigwald, J. Durel, P., and Pellerat, J.: Emploi de certain derives de la di-
benzoparathiazine dans le maladie de Parkinson et divers syndromes
neurologiques. *ARS Medici* **4**: 74–77, 1949.

Squire, L. R.: Neuropsychological effect of ECT, in *Electroconvulsive Therapy:
Biological Foundation and Clinical Applications*, R. Abrams and W. B.
Essman, eds., pp. 169–186, MTP, New York, 1982.

Staub, A. M.: Recherches sur quelques bases synthétiques antagonistes de l'histamine. *Ann. Inst. Pasteur* **63:** 400–436; 485–524, 1939.

Swazey, J. P.: *Chlorpromazine in Psychiatry,* MIT Press, Cambridge, MA, 1974.

Taylor, M. A.: Indications for electroconvulsive treatment, in *Electroconvulsive Therapy: Biological Foundations and Clinical Applications,* R. Abrams and W. B. Essman, eds., pp. 7–39, MTP, New York, 1982.

Viaud, P.: Les amines derivees de la phenothiazine. *J. Pharm. Pharmacol.* **6:** 361–389, 1954.

Winter, C. A.: Potentiating effect of antihistaminic drugs upon the sedative action of barbiturates. *J. Pharmacol. Exp. Ther.* **94:** 7–11, 1948.

Winter, C. A. and Flataker, L.: The effect of antihistaminic drugs upon the performance of trained rats. *J. Pharmacol. Exp. Ther.* **101:** 156–162, 1951.

Haloperidol

I. Haloperidol as an Innovative Therapeutic Agent

Although chlorpromazine was the first synthetic neuroleptic drug discovered and represented a major innovation in the therapy of psychoses, its use was eroded by later generations of more potent phenothiazine drugs and, in particular, by the nonphenothiazine, haloperidol. In the two decades between 1958 and 1978, haloperidol became one of the most frequently prescribed neuroleptics in the world (Ayd, 1978) and the World Health Organization listed it, along with chlorpromazine and fluphenazine, as an essential psychotherapeutic drug (WHO, 1979).

Haloperidol does not owe its status as an innovative agent to any sharp differences in antipsychotic effectiveness between it and the phenothiazines, but to a combination of properties that makes it very acceptable and safe for a wide spectrum of patients. As a result of its structure, haloperidol exhibits high neuroleptic potency. Because of this high potency, and because it lacks the tricyclicpropylamine structure, haloperidol interacts less than chlorpromazine with autonomic and other receptors. This, in turn, results in less sedation, less anticholinergic and cardiovascular effect, and less lowering of convulsive threshold (Ayd, 1978). Haloperidol undoubtedly owes some of its status as an innovative therapeutic agent to the fact that it is structurally so distinct from the phenothiazines and is not a "spin-off" from chlorpromazine. On the negative side, haloperidol, like most high-potency neuroleptics, has a greater tendency than chlorpromazine to cause extrapyramidal motor effects—akinesia, dyskinesia, akathisia, and Parkinsonism. This greater tendency is expressed in rapidity of appearance and in intensity, but not in frequency of occurrence.

Haloperidol is useful in the treatment of schizophrenia and acute psychoses (Bennett, 1983), being particularly effective in the treatment of symptoms of overactivity, agitation, and mania (Goldstein et al., 1968). According to Ayd (1978), "Excited persons are candidates for haloperidol. Depressed persons generally are not." Thus, haloperidol, like most antipsychotic drugs, is useful in controlling aggressive behavior in mentally subnormal people, in emotionally disturbed children, in epileptics, in organic psychoses, in alcoholic delerium, and in assaultive criminal psychotics (Ban, 1973; Ayd, 1978), but, also like these other agents, it is not very effective in treating the shallow, inappropriate affect and regressive behavior seen in hebephrenic schizophrenics (Ban, 1973). Depression, apathy, and retardation are not very responsive to haloperidol or other antipsychotic drugs (Crane, 1967).

Haloperidol is also used in combination with lithium in the treatment of mania, particularly in early therapy (Ayd, 1978). It has also found use in the treatment of confused, negativistic geriatric patients, in senile psychosis, paranoid reactions, and other psychic and behavioral disorders of the aged (Ban and Pecknold, 1976; Ayd, 1978).

Haloperidol is effective in Gilles de la Tourette's syndrome (a rare disorder characterized by tics of the face, arms, and legs; other involuntary movements; barking sounds; and obscene vocalizations) and in Huntingon's chorea (Ban, 1973; Baldessarini, 1985). In addition, haloperidol is a potent antiemetic (Bennett, 1983).

Early Clinical Research History

Divry et al. (1958) were the first to try haloperidol in humans. In a preliminary study using intravenous administration in psychiatric patients, haloperidol was a potent sedative of psychomotor agitation, with rapid onset, and with 3–5 h duration of effect. This same group (Divry et al., 1959) administered haloperidol by the oral route to 50 psychiatric patients in average doses of 7.5–15 mg. A host of Parkinson-like effects occurred: akinesia, hypertonia, asthenia-abulia. In addition, other extrapyramidal effects were noted, e.g., hyperkinesia, buccal dystonia. The authors commented on the occurence of "...emotional inhibitions of great therapeutical interest." Ultimately, the same group, (Divry et al., 1960), on the basis of experience in 94 patients, considered haloperidol to be the best drug available for treating manic patients, to be highly active in anxious depression, to inhibit impulsive and aggressive behavior in psychopaths, and to constitute a major weapon for treating schizophrenia.

Paquay et al. (1959) found that small oral doses of haloperidol (2–5 mg) given for 2–3 mo to chronic schizophrenics and to patients with agitation or character disturbances gave excellent results without serious side effects. Parkinson-like symptoms were seldom observed.

Delay et al. (1960) clearly categorized haloperidol as a neuroleptic, i.e., very similar in activity to phenothiazines and reserpine. Its range of action in 62 psychotic patients was essentially the same as that of other neuroleptics: haloperidol was very effective in mania, acute schizophrenia, delerious episodes, paranoid delusions, and hallucinations. In low doses, which avoided the pronounced Parkinson-like, neurological side effects, haloperidol was an "...excellent neuroleptic: easy to handle, very well tolerated by the patients even when the course of treatment extends over months, and very effective."

A considerable preclinical and clinical literature regarding haloperidol has been developed and has substantiated these earlier findings (*see*, for references, Crane, 1967; Goldstein, 1967; Goldstein et al., 1968; Janssen, 1970; Ban, 1973; Ban and Pecknold, 1976; Ayd, 1978; Bennett, 1983; Hollister, 1983; Janssen and Tollenaere, 1983).

II. The Scientific Work
Leading to Haloperidol

Janssen et al. (1959a) made note of their earlier chemical and pharmacological work in the field of substituted piperidines related to meperidine (Fig. 1). This program had led to the discovery of a potent propiophenone narcotic analgesic agent, R951 (Fig. 1) (Janssen et al., 1958, 1959b). (*See* section II of chapter on fentanyl for additional information.) Unexpectedly, it also yielded the discovery that 4-(4-hydroxy-4-phenylpiperidino)butyrophenone (Fig. 1) was a potent CNS depressant. On the basis of screening hundreds of basic ketones related to this butyrophenone in simple in vivo pharmacological tests in mice (inhibition of righting reflex, pentobarbital

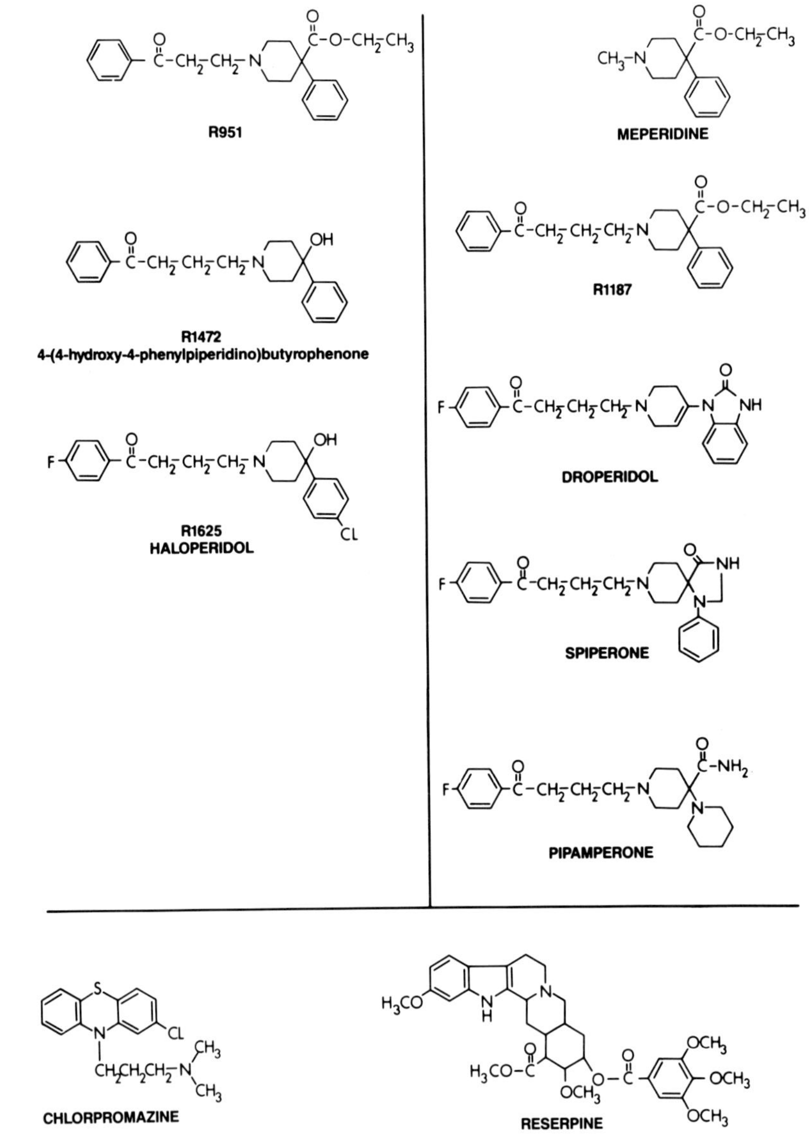

Fig. 1. The structures of haloperidol and chemically and/or pharmacologically related substances.

potentiation, hot plate, mydriactic activity, rotorod test of coordination), eight derivatives bearing halogen, methyl, or no substitutions on the two aromatic rings were judged to be of special interest: they exhibited a CNS depressant profile distinguishable from those of the narcotics, barbiturates, and meprobamate, but not readily distinguishable from those of the phenothiazine, chlorpromazine (Fig. 1), and its active congeners (Janssen et al., 1959a). Like the phenothiazines, these structurally unrelated butyrophenone compounds produced sedation at low dose levels, followed by progressive reduction of spontaneous and induced motor activities, and, ultimately, by the loss of righting reflex as doses were increased. The butyrophenones were more effective potentiators of barbiturate sleep time than were most of the phenothiazines. One of the eight compounds, R1625 (Fig. 1), was given the generic name "haloperidol," and studies were initiated with it in psychiatric patients (Janssen et al., 1959a).

Table 1 defines the critical scientific ideas and experiments leading to haloperidol and categorizes their origin.

Background Contributions Preceding Haloperidol

Meperidine (pethidine) was the first totally synthetic narcotic analgesic and was prepared and studied by Eisleb and Schaumann (1939).

Reserpine (Fig. 1), the active principle of *Rawolfia serpentina* Benth, was isolated by Müller et al. (1952). It was initially used in therapy for its hypotensive properties, but when cardiologists reported that it caused "psychic indifference," study of the drug in psychiatry was instituted.

Chlorpromazine was synthesized by Charpentier et al. (1952), and its propensity for producing psychic indifference in patients was also characterized (Delay et al., 1952a,b).

Not long after their introductions into therapy, both reserpine and chlorpromazine were shown to produce Parkinson-like extrapyramidal syndromes (Steck, 1954).

Delay and Deniker (1957) summarized and emphasized the important therapeutic characteristics that were shared by chlorpromazine and reserpine despite major differences in the chemical

Table 1
Profile of Observations and Ideas Crucial to the Development of Haloperidol[a]

Sequence: Route to innovative drug[**]	Orient- ation	Nature of study	Research institution	National origin	Nature of discovery	Screening involved	Crucial ideas or observations
Haloperidol[**]							
Janssen et al. (1959a)	Pre- clinical	Pharma- cology/ chem- istry	Indus- try	Belgium	Seren- dipitous	Targeted, untargeted	Following unsought-for discovery of chlorpromazine-like activity in a butyro-phenone-substituted hydroxy-phenyl-piperidine, synthesis and screening led to haloperidol.

[a]Taken from section II. Entries are those contributions without which the discovery of the agent (or additionally, in some cases, a relevant clinical application) would not have taken place or would have been materially delayed.

structures of these two agents (Fig. 1). They termed these shared properties "neuroleptic" (i.e., "that which takes the neuron"). The properties are:

1. Strong sedative action: not narcotic, not sleep, but a state of indifference
2. Control of excitation, agitation, aggressiveness, and impulsiveness not controlled by classic sedatives
3. Antipsychotic action
4. Autonomic and extrapyramidal symptoms that accompany the other actions
5. A dominant subcortical site of action

With the entry of reserpine and chlorpromazine into therapy, the modern era of psychopharmacology and psychiatry was launched, and many other drugs followed, including haloperidol.

III. Comments on Events Leading to Haloperidol

Janssen and Tollenaere (1983) recollected that they and their colleagues unknowingly started on the path to haloperidol when they commenced a thorough study of 4-phenylpiperidines related to meperidine in the mid-1950s. Their objective was to increase meperidine's morphine-like properties by replacing the *N*-methyl group with other simple chemical groups. The propiophenone derivative R951 (Fig. 1) turned out to be 100 times more potent than meperidine. When, *inter alia*, they lengthened the alkyl chain of R951 by one carbon, producing a butyrophenone compound (R1187, Fig. 1), the morphine-like potency fell significantly, but was now associated with chlorpromazine-like effects: the animals became progressively calm, sedated, and slightly catatonic. After the synthesis of many additional compounds, 4-(4-hydroxy-4-phenylpiperidino) butyrophenone (R1472, Fig. 1) was prepared. It was devoid of morphine-like activity and indistinguishable from chlorpromazine. Appropriate halogenation of this compound produced haloperidol (R1625, Fig. 1) (Janssen and Tollenaere, 1983).

Janssen and Tollenaere (1983) candidly commented that, "Today we can only guess as to what guided us to pick up that particular combination of molecular fragments [i.e., the 4-OH-4-phenylpiperidine group of R1472 in place of the 4-COOalkyl-4-phenylpiperidine group of R1187] out of many thousands of possible combinations we could have synthesized. A certain insight in the structure–activity relationship, luck and serendipity were definitely important factors on our side.... Hard work, an open mind for the unexpected and serendipity eventually culminated in a structurally novel compound that is called haloperidol."

IV. Developments
Subsequent to Haloperidol

Following the success of haloperidol, there was intense interest in butyrophenone derivatives. Janssen and his colleagues have dominated developments in this area to the present day. Some 25 butyrophenone-type drugs were put into clinical trial by this group (Janssen and Tollenaere, 1983). At present, in addition to haloperidol, there are nine butyrophenone neuroleptics that are in use in human and veterinary medicine in parts of the world: fluanisone, trifluperidol, pipamperone (Fig. 1), moperone, droperidol (Fig. 1), benperidol, azaperone, spiperone (Fig. 1), and bromperidol. Droperidol is a potent, very fast, short-acting, well-tolerated neuroleptic agent used in conjunction with the short-acting narcotic fentanyl in anesthesiology. Fluanisone is a specific tranquilizer for poultry, and azaperone is used to tranquilize pigs and other animals. The other butyrophenones were primarily intended for a variety of human indications: violent psychopathic syndromes, hypersexual tendencies, mood normalization, disturbed sleep patterns, agitation, hallucinations, and resistant chronic schizophrenia (Janssen, 1970; Janssen and Tollenaere, 1983). Hollister (1983) has remarked on the large number of butyrophenones available, and noted that it remains to be seen how many can be successfully introduced into clinical practice in the USA.

Ban (1973) felt that more important than the therapeutic impact of haloperidol was the fact that studies with this butyrophenone contributed to the changes in psychiatry's thinking and understanding of psychopathological syndromes.

References

Ayd, F. J., Jr.: Haloperidol: Twenty years' clinical experience. *J. Clin. Psychiatry* **39:** 807–814, 1978.

Baldessarini, R. J.: Drugs and the treatment of psychiatric disorders, in *The Pharmacological Basis of Therapeutics*, 7th Ed., A. G. Gilman, L. S. Goodman, T. W. Rall, and F. Murad, eds., pp. 387–445, Macmillan, New York, 1985.

Ban, T. A.: Haloperidol and the butyrophenones. *Psychosomatics* **14:** 286–297, 1973.

Ban, T. A. and Pecknold, J. C.: Haloperidol in the therapy of severe behavior disorders. *Curr. Psychiatr. Ther.* **16:** 127–137, 1976.

Bennett, D. R., ed.: Antipsychotic drugs, in *AMA Drug Evaluations*, 5th Ed., pp. 235–237, American Medical Association, Chicago, 1983.

Charpentier, P., Gailliot, P., Jacob, R. M., Gaudechon, J., and Buisson, P.: Recherches sur les dimethylaminopropyl-N-phenothiazines substitutee. *Comptes Rendus Chimie Organique* **235:** 59, 60, 1952.

Crane, G. E.: A review of clinical literature on haloperidol. *Int. J. Neuropsychiatr.* **3:** S110–S123, 1967.

Delay, J. and Deniker, P.: Caractéristiques psycho-physiologiques des médicaments neuroleptiques, in *Psychotropic Drugs*, S. Garattini and V. Ghetti, eds., pp. 486–501, Elsevier, Amsterdam, 1957.

Delay, J., Deniker, P., and Harl, J. M.: Utilization en therapeutique psychiatrique d'une phenothiazine d'action central elective (4560 R.P.) *Ann. Méd.-Psychol.* (Paris) **110:** 112–117, 1952a.

Delay, J. Deniker, P., and Harl, J. M.: Traitment des etats d'excitation et d'agitation par une methode medicamenteuse derivee de l'hiberno-therapie. *Ann. Méd.-Psychol.* (Paris) **110:** 267–273, 1952b.

Delay, J., Pichot, P., Lempériére, T. and Elissalde, B.: Halopéridol et chimio-thérapie des psychoses. *Presse Méd.* **68:** 1353–1355, 1960.

Divry, P., Bobon, J., and Collard, J.: Le "R1625": Nouvelle thérapeutique symptomatique de l'agitation psychomotrice. *Acta Neurol. Psychiatr. Belg.* **58:** 878, 888, 1958.

Divry, P., Bobon, J., and Collard, J.: Rapport sur l'activite neuro-psycho-pharmacologique du halopéridol (R1625). *Acta Neurol. Belg.* **60:** 7–19, 1960.

Divry, P., Bobon, J., Collard, J., Pinchard, A., and Nols, E.: Etude et expéri-mentation cliniques du R1625 on haloperidol, nouveau neuroleptique et "neurodysleptique." *Acta Neurol. Psychiatr. Belg.* **59:** 337–366, 1959.

Eisleb, O. and Schaumann, O.: Dolantin, ein neuartiges Spasmolytikum und Analgetikum. *Dtsch. Med. Wochenschr.* **65:** 967, 968, 1939.

Goldstein, B. J., ed.: Haloperidol. *Int. J. Neuropsychiatr.* **3:** S1–S153, 1967.

Goldstein, B. J., Clyde, D. J., and Caldwell, J. M.: Clinical efficacy of the butyrophenones as antipsychotic drugs, in *Psychopharmacology, A Re-view of Progress, 1957–1967* (Public Health Service Publication No. 1836), D. H. Efron, ed., US Gov't. Printing Office, Washington, DC, 1968.

Hollister, L. E.: *Clinical Pharmacology of Psychotherapeutic Drugs*, 2nd Ed., Churchill Livingstone, New York, 1983.

Janssen, P. A.: The butyrophenone story, in *Discoveries in Biological Psychi-atry*, F. J. Ayd and B. Blackwell, eds., pp. 165–179, J. B. Lippincott, Phila-delphia, 1970.

Janssen, P. A. and Tollenaere, J. P.: The discovery of the butyrophenone-type neuroleptics, in *Discoveries in Pharmacology*, vol. 1, M. J. Parnham and J. Bruinvels, eds., pp. 181–196, Elsevier, Amsterdam, 1983.

Janssen, P. A., Jageneau, A. H., Van Proosdij-Hartzema, E. G., and DeJongh, D. K.: The pharmacology of a new potent analgesic, R951 2 [*N*-(4-car-bethoxy-4-phenyl)-piperidino]-propiophenone HCl. *Acta Physiol. Phar-macol. Neerl.* **7:** 373–402, 1958.

Janssen, P. A., Van de Westeringh, C., Jageneau, A. H., Demoen, P. J. Hermans, B. K., Van Daele, G. H., Schellekens, K. H., Van der Eycken, C. A., and Niemegeers, C. J.: Chemistry and pharmacology of CNS de-pressants related to 4-(4-hydroxy-4-phenylpiperidino)butyrophenone. Part I—Synthesis and screening data in mice. *J. Med. Pharmaceut. Chem.* **1:** 281–297, 1959a.

Janssen, P. A., Jageneau, A. H., Demoen, P. J. Van de Westeringh, C., Raeymaekers, A. H., Wouters, M. S., Sanczuk, S., Hermans, B. K., and Loomans, J. L.: Compounds related to pethidine. I. Mannich bases derived from norpethidine and acetophenones. *J. Med. Pharmaceut. Chem.* **1:** 105–120, 1959b.

Müller, J. M., Schlittler, E., and Bein, H. J.: Reserpin, der sedative Wirkstoff aus *Rauwolfia serpentina*. *Experientia* **8:** 338, 1952.

Paquay, J., Arnould, F., and Burton, P.: Etude clinique de l'action du R1625 á doses modérées en psychiatrie. *Acta Neurol. Belg.* **59:** 882–891, 1959.

Steck, H.: Le syndrome extra-pyramidal et diencéphalique au cours des traitments au Largactil et du Serpasil. *Ann. Méd.-Psychol.* (Paris) **112** (2): 737–743, 1954.

World Health Organization: The selection of essential drugs; Second report of the WHO Expert Committee (Technical Report Series, 641), World Health Organization, Geneva, 1979.

Imipramine

I. Imipramine as an Innovative Therapeutic Agent

Depression has been defined as "a sinking of spirits [affect] so as to constitute a clinically discernible condition" (Stedman, 1982). In earlier times, it was called melancholia. It comprises two major types: (1) severe depression of mood associated with psychomotor retardation or agitation, self-reproach or guilt, as well as other symptoms, all of which occur in the apparent absence of a precipitating cause; (2) severe depression of mood associated directly with an intensely sad external situation, which is relieved by removal of the external situation. The former is referred to as endogenous depression and the latter as reactive depression.

According to Baldessarini (1983), severe disorders of mood are among the most common major psychiatric disorders. Approximately 12% of the general population can expect to experience a medically significant affective disorder during their lifetime. In the decade prior to the development of effective drugs for depression in the 1950s, electroconvulsive treatment (ECT) was the only useful therapy, but its effects were frequently short-lived and coupled with diminished efficacy upon repetition. Prior to ECT, there was no really effective treatment. Lehmann (1983) reminisced about having tried some of the following pre-ECT procedures for treating serious depression: photosensitizing hematoporphyrin, tincture of opium (which in higher doses gave some temporary relief), nitrogen-induced anoxia, X-ray irradiation, nitrous oxide inhalation, dinitrile succinate, methedrine, testosterone, and nicotinic acid. Results were uniformly disappointing.

133

Klein et al. (1980) noted that the psychopharmacological agents, including imipramine and other tricyclic antidepressants, radically altered all phases of treatment of patients with affective disorders. Tricyclic antidepressants elevated mood and alertness, increased physical activity, and represented a major advance in psychiatry. Imipramine was the first tricyclic antidepressant described, and it still remains one of the mainstays in the treatment of endogenous and reactive depressions.

Imipramine, as well as more recently developed tricyclic antidepressants, has been tried experimentally, with some success, for a variety of indications: enuresis, alcoholism, eating disorders (bulimia), panic reactions, obsessive–compulsive disorders, chronic pain, neuralgias, migraine, and peptic ulcer (Hollister, 1978; Baldessarini, 1985).

The common side effects of imipramine, as well as other tricyclic antidepressants, are a result of their capacity to block cholinergic and adrenergic receptors and thus, in some circumstances, to elicit flushing, sweating, dry mouth, constipation, blurred vision, tachycardia, and blood pressure reduction. These effects may be especially troublesome in elderly patients.

Early Clinical Research History

The earliest clinical history of imipramine is intimately involved in its discovery and will be presented in section II.

II. The Scientific Work
Leading to Imipramine

Charpentier et al. (1952) of Rhone-Poulenc reported the synthesis of the phenothiazine compound, chlorpromazine (Fig. 1). Laborit (a surgeon), and his associates found that chlorpromazine was useful in potentiating general anesthesia and that it produced in patients a disinterest in their environment (Laborit et al., 1952). Delay et al. (1952a,b) administered this agent, by itself, to patients who were exhibiting a variety of serious mental disorders, including agitation, confusion, anxiety, depression, and schizophrenia. Form-

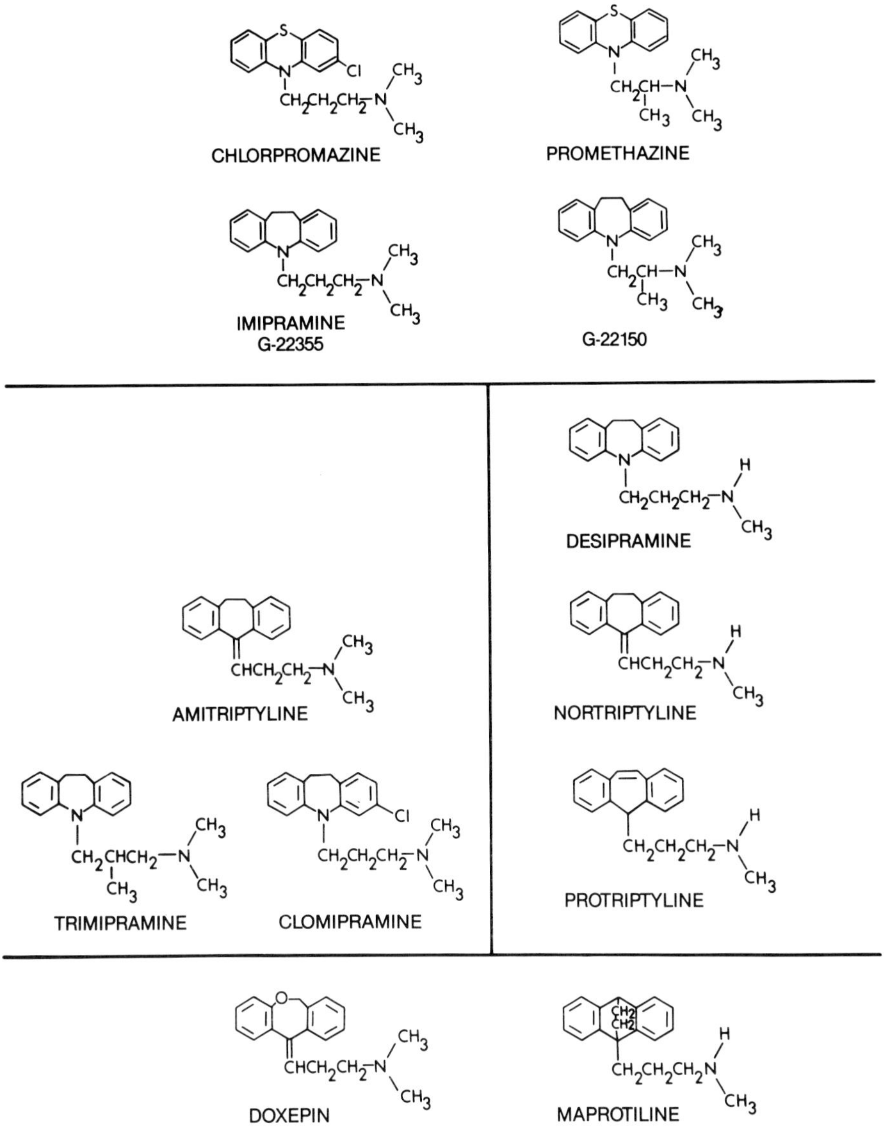

Fig. 1. The structures of imipramine and chemically and/or pharmacologically related substances.

erly uncontrollable patients became calm and smiling. They appeared normal, but were indifferent to external stimuli. Delay et al. (1952a,b) suggested that chlorpromazine would be of considerable interest to psychiatry. Acceptance of chlorpromazine into psychiatric practice for the treatment of schizophrenia was rapid in Europe.

Stimulated by the results with chlorpromazine, the Geigy Co. (Basel) initiated psychiatric evaluations of many iminodibenzyl derivatives in 1954 (Kuhn, 1957). The compounds had been synthesized earlier at Geigy as structural analogs of Rhone-Poulenc's antihistamine and anti-Parkinson phenothiazine compounds (Schindler and Häfliger, 1954)* (discussed more fully in the background section, following). In a three-year period, more than 500 patients were used by Kuhn to screen different compounds from this chemical series for their effectiveness in schizophrenia and in a variety of other mental disorders, including depression. None of the substances tested was as effective as chlorpromazine in ameliorating the symptoms of schizophrenia. One compound, G-22355 (Fig. 1), was the direct structural analog of promazine (promazine being chlorpromazine without Cl). G-22355 was discovered in an open study to have a distinct influence on depressive states (Kuhn, 1957). Later named imipramine, it was especially effective in endogenous depression. Patients became generally more active and more talkative. Crying and complaining ceased, hypochondriacal and neurasthenic complaints receded, relations with other people were reestablished, and moods and behavior became balanced (Kuhn, 1957). Kuhn concluded, "A substance such as G-22355, which influences depressive states, is of great interest theoretically as well as practicically."

Table 1 defines the critical scientific ideas and experiments leading to imipramine and categorizes their origin.

Background Contributions Preceding Imipramine

Charpentier (1947) reported synthesizing, *inter alia*, the phenothiazine derivative promethazine (Fig. 1) as a possible antiparasitic

---

*According to Häfliger (1959), "The iminodibenzyl derivatives gained for us in importance and interest when it was shown by Delay and Deniker that a phenothiazine derivative, chlorpromazine, was of therapeutic value in the treatment of psychiatric disorders."

Table 1
Profile of Observations and Ideas Crucial to the Development of Imipramine[a]

Sequence: Route to innovative drug[**]	Orient- ation	Nature of study	Research institution	National origin	Nature of discovery	Screening involved	Crucial ideas or observations
Imipramine[**]							
Charpentier (1952)	Pre- clinical	Chem- istry/ pharma- cology	Indus- try	France	Orderly	Targeted	The phenothiazine, chlorpromazine, syn- thesized; structurally, it is closely related to the CNS-active pheno- thiazine antihista- mine, promethazine.
Delay et al. (1952a, b)	Clinical	Psy- chiatry	Uni- versity	France	Orderly	No	Chlorpromazine is effective in psychi- atric disorders.
Schindler and Häfliger (1954)	Pre- clinical	Chem- istry/ pharma- cology	Indus- try	Switzer- land	Orderly	Targeted, untargeted	Iminodibenzyl compounds, close structural analogs of promethazine, synthesized and screened in animals as antihistamines (*inter alia*) beginning in late 1940s.
Kuhn (1957)	Clinical	Psy- chiatry	Hospital	Switzer- land	Orderly	Targeted, untargeted	In 1950, the direct iminodibenzyl ana- log of promethazine found by Kuhn to have only little pro- methazine-like CNS effects in humans; in 1954, subsequent to the reports of Delay et al. (1952a, b) on chlorpromazine, additional imino- dibenzyl analogs given to Kuhn to screen for chlor- promazine-like activity; the direct structural analog of promazine, G-22355 (imipramine), is not chlorpromazine- like, but has anti- depressant activity.

[a]Taken from section II. Entries are those contributions without which the discovery of the agent (or additionally, in some cases, a relevant clinical application) would not have taken place or would have been materially delayed.

compound in 1944. However, it was inactive as a parasiticide. Subsequently, Halpern (1947) reported that promethazine was a highly potent antihistamine.

Schindler and Häfliger (1954) of the Geigy company commented that they first became interested in the iminodibenzyl ring system (in 1948) because it was a close structural analog of the phenothiazine ring system from which several clinically useful substances had been developed, including the antihistamine promethazine. They synthesized 42 iminodibenzyl compounds, including the direct structural analog of the antihistamine, promethazine (Geigy compound G-22150) (Fig. 1). These compounds were tested in standard animal preparations for antihistaminic, anticholinergic, and local anesthetic effects, as well as for a spasmolytic action against barium-induced contractions, for analgesic actions, and for iv toxicity in the mouse (Schindler and Häfliger, 1954). No CNS effects were reported.

Laborit (1949), who used promethazine for its antihistaminic properties in his surgical work, recognized that it produced the useful side effects of analgesia and drowsiness: patients were calm, relaxed, peaceful, and drowsy. Laborit and Leger (1950) noted that "...the antihistamine properties of Phenergan [promethazine] are intense, but are also present in other antihistamines. Its side effects are unique to this substance." They stated that the centrally mediated side effects of promethazine were of "indisputable" advantage.

Kuhn (1957) commented that he was asked by the Geigy Co. in 1950 to study G-22150, the iminodibenzyl analog of promethazine, for possible sedative–hypnotic effects in humans. Sedative–hypnotic properties were not pronounced with this compound. Other compounds in this series were not given clinical evaluation by Kuhn at this time.

III. Comments on Events
Leading to Imipramine

Sulser and Mishra (1983) noted that it has often been said that serendipity played a major role in the discovery of the antidepressant effect of imipramine, an activity that clearly could not have been predicted from the pharmacological data available. Kuhn

(1970) commented that, in his screening of iminodibenzyl derivatives, a really important decision was not to pass a verdict until they
had been tried in depressive illness. "Thoroughness was not our
only reason for doing this—there was also our conviction that it
must be possible to find a drug effective in endogenous depressions." Sulser and Mishra credited Kuhn with having a mind that
was "prepared" to accept his unusual findings.

Since the efficacy of imipramine had been defined only by an
open study, medical scientists spent considerable time and effort in
establishing a firmer foundation for it—and subsequent tricyclic
agents as well—because of its theoretical as well as its practical
importance. During the first decade of their use, 77% (50 out of 65)
of controlled studies indicated that tricyclic antidepressants were
superior to a placebo; in no study was a placebo found superior
(Klein et al., 1980). As also pointed out by Klein et al. (1980), "Though
imipramine is clearly superior to a placebo, the quantitative superiority of the drug is not overwhelming (i.e., about 30%)." Therefore,
even well-designed studies required large patient samples to detect
moderate drug–placebo differences. It was not surprising that
imipramine and other tricyclics were not found to be superior to
placebo in all trials. Klerman (1972) was of the opinion that tricyclic
antidepressants were the most effective antidepressant medication
available.

IV. Developments
Subsequent to Imipramine

Synthesis of new tricyclic antidepressants followed quickly on
the discovery of the antidepressant action of imipramine. Desmethylimipramine, the monodemethylated analog of imipramine
(Fig. 1), was found to be effective. More recently, the clomipramine
and trimipramine derivatives of imipramine have been developed
(Fig. 1). Other ring systems, which were structurally analogous to
the iminodibenzyl ring system, were synthesized, and *N,N*-di-
methylpropyl or *N*-methylpropyl side chains identical to those of
imipramine and desmethylimipramine, respectively, were added at
the appropriate positions. By this procedure several clinically effective agents were developed. The dibenzocycloheptadiene ring sys-

tem has yielded amitriptyline and nortriptyline (Fig. 1). The dibenzocycloheptatriene ring system yielded protriptyline (Fig. 1). More recent variants of the tricyclic ring system have yielded doxepin and maprotiline (Fig. 1). Controlled comparisons of the various tricyclic antidepressants have usually concluded that they are essentially equivalent drugs (Hollister, 1978; Klein et al., 1980). Although there are differences in dosages required with the various agents, this should not be confused with differences in therapeutic efficacy. The possibility remains, although it is as yet unproven, that the different tricyclic agents may be useful in different subtypes of depression.

The availability of tricyclic antidepressants, in addition to reserpine, MAO inhibitors, and a few other drugs, permitted the basic pharmacologic studies of their interactions with biogenic amines in the CNS of animals. This work, in turn, allowed for the rationalization of the amine hypothesis of depression (Schildkraut, 1965; Schildkraut and Kety, 1967), and for a subsequent variation on this hypothesis (Sulser et al., 1978).

References

Baldessarini, R. J.: *Biomedical Aspects of Depression and its Treatment*, American Psychiatric Press, Washington, DC, 1983.

Baldessarini, R. J.: Drugs and the treatment of psychiatric disorders, in *The Pharmacologic Basis of Therapeutics*, 7th Ed., A. G. Gilman, L. S. Goodman, T. W. Rall, F. Murad, eds., pp. 387–445, Macmillan, New York, 1985.

Charpentier, P.: Sur la constitution d'une dimethylamino-propyl-N-phénothiazine. *Comptes Rendus* **225**: 306–308, 1947.

Charpentier, P., Gaillot, P., Jacob, R., Gaudechon, J., and Buisson, P.: Chimie organique—Recherches sur les dimethylaminopropyl-N-phenothiazines substitutuee. *Comptes Rendus* **235**, 59, 60, 1952.

Delay, J., Deniker, P., and Harl, J. M.: Utilisation en therapeutique psychiatrique d'une phenothiazine d'action central elective (4560 R.P.) *Ann. Méd.-Psychol.* (Paris) **110**: 112–117, 1952a.

Delay, J., Deniker, P., and Harl, J. M.: Traitement des etats d'excitation et d'agitation par une methode medicamenteuse derivee de l'hibernotherapie. *Ann. Méd.-Psychol.* (Paris) **110**: 267–273, 1952b.

Häfliger, F.: Chemistry of Tofranil. *Can. Psychiatr. Assoc.* **4**: S 69–S 74, 1959.

Halpern, B. N.: Experimental research on a series of new chemical substances with powerful antihistaminic activity: The thiodiphenylamine derivatives. *J. Allergy* **18**: 263–272, 1947.

Hollister, L. E.: Tricyclic antidepressants. *N. Engl. J. Med.* **299:** 1106–1109, 1978.

Klein, D. F., Gittelman, R., Quitkin, F., and Rifkin, A.: *Diagnosis and Drug Treatment of Psychiatric Disorders,* 2nd Ed., Williams & Wilkins, Baltimore, 1980.

Klerman, G. L.: Drug therapy of clinical depressions—current status and implications for research on neuropharmacology of the affective disorders. *J. Psychiatr. Res.* **9:** 253–270, 1972.

Kuhn, R.: Über die Behandlung depressiver Zustände mit einem Iminodibenzyl-derivat (G 22355). *Schweiz. Med. Wochenschr.* **35/36:** 1135–1140, 1957.

Kuhn, R.: The imipramine story, in *Discoveries in Biological Psychiatry*, F. J. Ayd and B. Blackwell, eds., pp. 205–217, Lippincott, Philadelphia, 1970.

Laborit, H.: Sur l'utilisation de certains agents pharmacodynamiques à action neuro-végétative en période per- et postoperatoire. *Acta Chir. Belg.* **48:** 485–492, 1949.

Laborit, H. and Leger, L.: Utilisation d'un antihistaminique de synthèse en thérapeutique pré, per, et post-opératoire. *Presse Méd.* **58:** 492, 1950.

Laborit, H., Huguenard, P., and Alluame, R.: Un nouveau stabilisateur vegetatif (le 4560 R. P.). *Presse Méd.* **60:** 206–208, 1952.

Lehmann, H. E.: Tricyclic antidepressants: Recollections by H. E. Lehmann, in *Discoveries in Pharmacology,* vol. 1, M. J. Parnham and J. Bruinvels, eds., pp. 211–216, Elsevier, Amsterdam, 1983.

Schildkraut, J. J.: The catecholamine hypothesis of affective disorders; a review of supporting evidence. *Am. J. Psychiatry* **122:** 509–522, 1965.

Schildkraut, J. J. and Kety, S. S.: Biogenic amines and emotion. *Science* **156:** 21–30, 1967.

Schindler, W. and Häfliger, F.: Über Derivate des Iminodibenzyls. *Helv. Chim. Acta* **37:** 472–483, 1954.

Stedman's Medical Dictionary, 24th Ed., Williams & Wilkins, Baltimore, 1982.

Sulser, F. and Mishra, R.: The discovery of tricyclic antidepressants and their mode of action, in *Discoveries in Pharmacology,* vol. 1, M. J. Parnham and J. Bruinvels, eds., pp. 233–247, Elsevier, Amsterdam, 1983.

Sulser, F., Vetulani, J., and Mobley, P. L.: Mode of action of antidepressant drugs. *Biochem. Pharmacol.* **27:** 257–261, 1978.

Iproniazid

I. Monoamine Oxidase Inhibitors (MAOIs) as Innovative Therapeutic Agents

Iproniazid, the first clinically effective MAOI, was studied extensively for its psychiatric effects for a year or two following the favorable report on its effects in withdrawn patients by Loomer, Saunders, and Kline (1957). These authors noted that iproniazid was the first useful drug to "energize" rather than sedate depressed patients. They considered this an important distinction when treating diseases that were associated with deep depression of mood and lack of reactivity to the environment. Unfortunately, iproniazid had to be withdrawn from the market in 1961 because of what was considered an unacceptable incidence of hepatitis (Kline 1970; Kline and Cooper 1980; Kauffman 1979). Other MAOIs were subsequently introduced and studied extensively. However, as noted by Kline and Cooper (1980), the use of MAOIs gradually faded for several reasons. Chief among these was the risk of hypertensive attacks being precipitated by consumption of foods rich in the pressor amine tyramine, since this amine was normally prevented from entering the circulation by MAO activity in intestine and liver (the so-called "cheese effect"). Sandler et al. (1979) considered that the cheese effect was almost entirely responsible for limiting the more general application of the MAOIs. As pointed out by Klein et al. (1980) "...clinical lore suggests that a MAOI should be used only in depressed patients refractory to other treatment methods."

Despite this air of negativity, there has been a continuing clinical interest in the MAOIs. Some studies have supported the notion that with adequate dosage they may be particularly useful in neurotic or atypical depressions, whereas tricyclic agents may be particularly useful in endogenous depression (*see* Raskin et al., 1974; Robinson et al., 1973 for refs.).

Neurotic or atypical depression is characterized by phobic anxiety and hysterical symptoms, such as fatigue and somatic complaints, in addition to marked depression of mood. Endogenous depression is characterized by marked depression of mood, psychomotor retardation or agitation, lack of reactivity to the environment, self-reproach, early awakening, feeling worse in the morning and weight loss. Klein et al. (1980) considered that MAOIs have been underutilized and agreed with the British Medical Journal editorial, (Lock, 1976) that a resurgence of interest in MAOIs was timely.

In addition to their use in depression, MAOIs have had use as antihypertensive agents (especially pargyline).

At present the two MAOIs most widely used in depression are the hydrazine derivative phenelzine and the nonhydrazine compound tranylcypromine. Kline and Cooper (1980) pointed out that the FDA had rated phenelzine as the only MAOI effective in the treatment of depression, but this was followed by approval of isocarboxazid and tranylcypromine. Since it is difficult to single out a specific MAOI as having had remarkable clinical success to date, and thus to be categorized as the innovative therapeutic agent, only the history of iproniazid will be presented in section II. The development of phenelzine and tranylcypromine will be emphasized in section IV, which deals with all the MAOIs developed subsequent to iproniazid. Reviews of MAO and MAOIs are available (*see*, for example, Sackler and Sackler, 1958; Pletscher et al., 1966; Kaiser and Zirkle, 1970; Biel et al., 1978; Singer et al., 1979; Zeller, 1983; Benedetti and Dostert, 1987).

Early Clinical Research History

The clinical history of iproniazid is intimately involved in its discovery and will be presented in section II.

II. The Scientific Work Leading to Iproniazid

Isoniazid and iproniazid (Fig. 1), two hydrazine derivatives of isonicotinic acid, were tested as antitubercular agents in a series of 92 "hopeless" tuberculous patients and were reported to be spec-

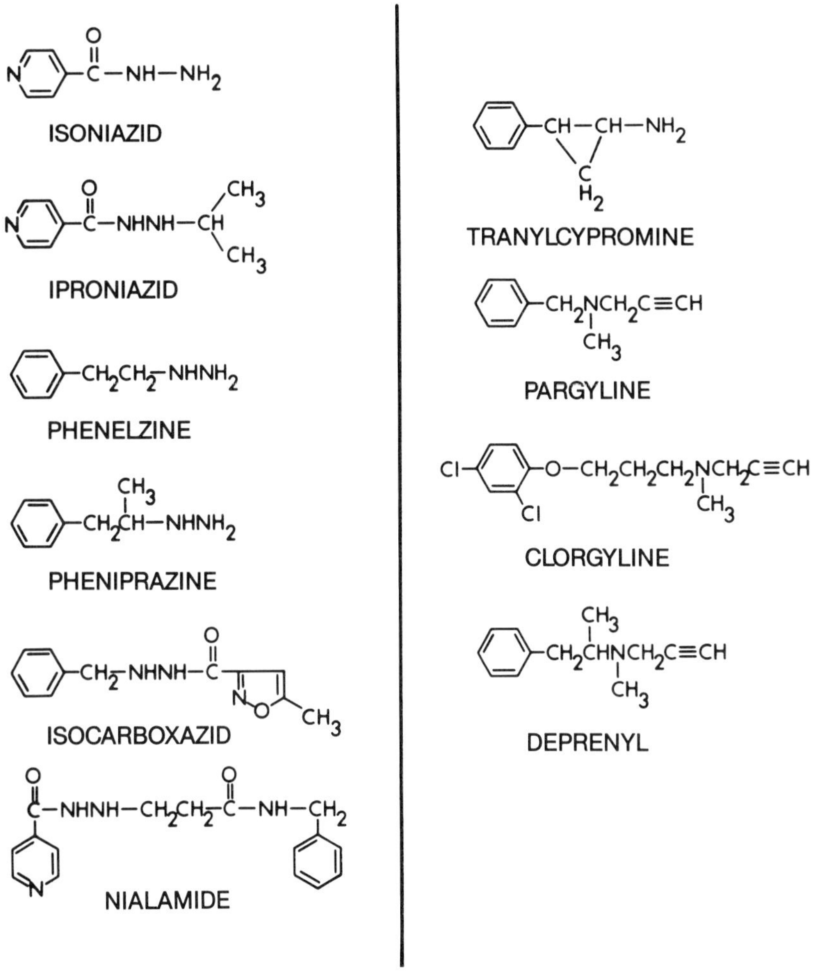

Fig. 1. The structures of iproniazid and chemically and/or pharmacologically related substances.

tacularly effective. Many patients rapidly experienced a great sense of well-being, a return of appetite, and weight gain (Robitzek et al., 1952). The investigators stated, "The mortally ill patients we have studied have obtained therapeutic benefit beyond anything we have ever seen with any of the chemotherapeutics or antibiotic agents previously utilized by us." Robitzek and Selikoff (1952), in a series of 44 caseous-pneumonic tuberculous patients, noted that, in addition to an antitubercular effect, patients usually felt better before any objective measurement of improvement in their disease. The authors noted many side effects with these two agents, including twitching of the extremities, dizziness, ataxia, urinary retention, constipation, hyperreflexia, drowsiness, insomnia, and dryness of the mouth. These were ascribed in part to CNS actions and in part to peripheral sympathetic actions of the drugs. Isoniazid produced fewer reactions per patient than did iproniazid.

Zeller, who had a long-standing interest in hydrazines and other bases as inhibitors of amine oxidases, tested both compounds. He found that, in vitro, iproniazid, but not isoniazid, inhibited monoamine oxidase preparations from liver and brain of several species (Zeller et al., 1952a,b). Likewise, when administered in vivo to rats and guinea pigs, iproniazid, but not isoniazid, blocked monoamine oxidase in mitochondrial preparations from liver and brain (Zeller and Barsky, 1952). The authors stated, "The above results may also offer an explanation for the sympathetic and general mental stimulation observed after administration of isonicotinyl-hydrazides to patients and animals."

O'Connor et al. (1953) pointed out that great improvement in the sense of well-being, ravenous appetite, and marked and rapid weight gain occurred regularly with 27 tuberculous patients taking iproniazid, but far less frequently or impressively with 32 patients on isoniazid treatment. Symptomatic relief with iproniazid was out of proportion to objective improvement as determined by X-ray or bacteriologic studies. When treatment was stopped these "side effects" promptly disappeared. O'Connor et al. (1953) concluded that "...the initial favorable symptomatic response to iproniazid may actually be ...a side effect of the drug." They also reported that three prepsychotic patients developed frank psychoses when given iproniazid.

Smith (1953), prompted by the reports of mental stimulation in tuberculosis patients, treated 11 cases of mental disease with iproniazid. He found no evidence of marked or sustained improvement. Likewise, Kamman et al. (1953) found only small positive effects with iproniazid in a placebo-controlled study of 90 female psychotic patients.

Crane (1956a) carried out a study to evaluate the nature, extent and frequency of the psychiatric side effects of iproniazid in tuberculous patients. Nineteen debilitated patients were included. All patients experienced some psychiatric effect. Subjective feelings of well-being were expressed by 10 patients, manic behavior was seen in six, and overt psychotic action in four. In a followup study, the main purpose of which was to investigate the psychological reactions to iproniazid, Crane (1956b) reported that 12 of 20 tuberculous patients showed the desired psychological response to the drug and gained an average of 20 pounds. However, six patients became behavior problems and two developed mental disorders and their treatments were discontinued. In a third study, in which the emphasis was shifted from treatment of physical debilitation to treatment of psychiatric disturbances, Crane (1957) studied 20 tuberculous patients of which eight were clinical neurotics, four were psychotics, and one had a psychopathic personality. Eleven patients had marked psychological improvement. Crane noted that "...patients with depressions (reactive or psychogenic) responded more favorably than individuals with hysterical or unstable personalities."

Loomer, Saunders, and Kline (1957), in an open study, treated a group of 17 nontuberculous, chronically institutionalized, psychiatric patients. They all fit the criteria of being withdrawn, regressed, deteriorated, colorless, and of flattened affect. Iproniazid at 50 mg three times per day induced a favorable response in 70% of the patients by causing varying degrees of improved general attitude and behavior, better ward adjustment, increased weight, heightened affective mood, and added interest in self and environment. Loomer, Saunders, and Kline (1957) pointed out that dosage had to be individualized in order to optimize the response and to minimize neurological and psychological changes. It was noted that iproniazid had been shown to be an amine oxidase inhibitor by Zeller and Barsky (1952) and that this might explain, in part, its effect on nervous and mental function by altering the metabolic degradation of epinephrine, norepinephrine, and serotonin. These authors stated, "Whatever the mechanism of iproniazid may be, it would appear as though with it a new pharmacological approach is now available for adjunctive therapy in psychiatry."

Table 1 defines the critical scientific ideas and experiments leading to iproniazid and categorizes their origin.

Background Contributions Preceding the Discovery of the Antidepressant Effect of Iproniazid

Blaschko et al. (1937a) described a specific enzyme, obtained from cell-free extracts of liver, kidney, and small intestine, that catalyzed the oxidation of adrenaline (epinephrine). Blaschko et al. (1937b) also demonstrated that this enzyme and two other enzymes, described earlier by other investigators as tyramine oxidase and as aliphatic amine oxidase, were identical. Eventually this enzyme was given the name monoamine oxidase (MAO).

Fox synthesized isoniazid in 1951 while attempting to prepare a pyridine analog of the German antitubercular compound, tibione. Isoniazid was an intermediate in this synthesis. It proved to be very active when screened against murine tuberculosis (Fox, 1960). Fox and Gibas (1953), in a continuing search for tuberculostats, synthesized alkyl, cycloalkyl, and arylalkyl derivatives of isoniazid, one of which was iproniazid.

III. Comments on Events Leading to Iproniazid

Loomer, Saunders, and Kline (1957) stated that their decision to evaluate iproniazid followed upon the observations of Chessin et al. (1956) and Brodie et al. (1956) that animals given iproniazid, and subsequently reserpine, instead of becoming sedated, became excited and overactive. Saunders (1959), however, pointed out that, "...I suggested the application of amine oxidase inhibitors to psychiatry in 1955 on the theoretical basis of their action on amine metabolism in the brain, with the probability that they would alleviate depression."* The clinical work of Selikoff, Robitzek, and coworkers, as well as that of Crane and other authors, was known to these workers (Loomer, Saunders, and Kline, 1957; Kline, 1970; Kline and Cooper, 1980).

*Saunders informed the authors that he won legal actions against Kline over credit for iproniazid's use in depressed patients: "(Appellate Division of the Supreme Court, First Judicial County of New York, Index No. 7770, April 15, 1980; New

Table 1
Profile of Observations and Ideas Crucial to the Development of Iproniazid[a]

Sequence: Route to innovative drug**	Orient- ation	Nature of study	Research institution	National origin	Nature of discovery	Screening involved	Crucial ideas or observations
Iproniazid							
Robitzek and Selikoff (1952)	Clinical	Pul- monary	Hospital	USA	Seren- dipitous	No	Isoniazid and iproniazid give a sense of well-being to tuberculous patients. This occurs before objective measures of improvement of the tuberculosis; some neurologic effects noted.
O'Connor et al. (1953)	Clinical	Pul- monary	Uni- versity	USA	Orderly	No	Iproniazid, not isoniazid, is responsible for improved sense of well-being and also for serious side effects in tuberculous patients.
Loomer, Saunders, and Kline (1957)	Clinical	Psy- chiatry	Hospital	USA	Orderly	No	70% of depressed, withdrawn psychiatric patients respond favorably to iproniazid.

[a]Taken from section II. Entries are those contributions without which the discovery of the agent (or additionally, in some cases, a relevant clinical application) would not have taken place or would have been materially delayed.

Kline (1970) and Kline and Cooper (1980) believed that the withdrawal of iproniazid by the FDA because of hepatotoxicity was not scientifically sound. He estimated that 400,000–600,000 patients were given iproniazid during its first year in psychiatric use. In those patients who developed jaundice, the condition was indistinguishable from infectious hepatitis. It might have been anticipated that at least 100 persons would have developed jaundice in the absence of iproniazid. There were actually 127 cases of iproniazid-associated hepatitis reported. Since there were no controls, iproniazid was implicated as causative. Kline and Cooper (1980) noted that a high incidence of hepatitis had not materialized in association with the use of clinically available MAOIs.

York Court of Appeals, Decision of the Appellate Division of the Supreme Court, Upheld in Saunders vs Kline, No. 141, March 26, 1981)."

IV. Developments
Subsequent to Iproniazid

The demonstration by Zeller and his colleagues (Zeller et al., 1952a,b; Zeller and Barsky, 1952) that iproniazid was a MAOI simultaneously provided a possible mechanism for its central actions and a basis for the targeted development of successor compounds by chemists and pharmacologists.

Within two years of the initial report on iproniazid (Loomer, Saunders, and Kline 1957), a report appeared on the positive antidepressant activities of four hydrazine derivatives from three pharmaceutical companies. These MAOIs included phenelzine and pheniprazine (Bailey et al., 1959) (Fig. 1). Isocarboxazid and nialamide, both hydrazides, were developed soon thereafter (Fig. 1). Pheniprazine was eventually withdrawn because of toxicity—it produced transient red–green color blindness from retrobulbar neuritis. Isocarboxazid, a relatively weak agent, is currently available but not actively marketed, and nialamide is not available for medical use (Klein et al., 1980).

In an attempt to produce less-toxic MAOIs, nonhydrazine derivatives were studied. Pargyline and tranylcypromine (Fig. 1) were the result. Both are available for clinical use today. Pargyline, however, has only been approved by the FDA for use as an antihypertensive agent.

Phenelzine is the MAOI that has been most widely studied as an antidepressant. However, as noted by Klein et al. (1980), there is a dearth of placebo-controlled studies with phenelzine in endogenous depression. In addition, in many studies in the past, doses may have been too low and the study durations too short. In an influential and widely quoted multicenter study conducted by the Medical Research Council (MRC) in the UK (1965), 250 endogenously depressed patients were treated with electroconvulsant therapy (ECT), imipramine, phenelzine, and, for a short time, placebo. ECT and imipramine increased the frequency of recovery above the spontaneous rate seen with placebo. Phenelzine, on the other hand, demonstrated no advantage over, or was worse than, the placebo. Robinson et al. (1978) noted that in the MRC study the patient population that was chosen had a low probability of responding to MAOIs, since available data from less-rigorous studies pointed toward MAOIs having their greatest benefit in nonendogenous (atypical) depressions (e.g., West and Dally, 1959; Sargant, 1961; Sargant and Dally, 1962). Robinson et al. (1973) carried out a double-blind, placebo-controlled, balanced-design study involving 87 out-patients, in which precise, structured, standardized interviews were used to estimate effects, and doses of phenelzine were adjusted to maintain at least 80% inhibition of MAO (as measured in platelets). These investigators showed that phenelzine as compared with placebo was especially effective in improving subscale scores for irritability, hypochondriasis-agitation, and psychomotor change. They concluded that "MAO inhibitors may have a special efficacy in treating depressive illnesses with atypical features such as anxiety, fatigue, phobia, or other somatic complaints."

Regarding tranylcypromine, Klein et al. (1980) noted that, "...although the number of studies contrasting tranylcypromine to a placebo is small, in three of four the drug was found superior." They concluded that available evidence argued for the likelihood that tranylcypromine had antidepressant properties in endogenous and reactive depressions.

Baldessarini (1983) credited a renewal of interest in MAOIs in part to the work of Robinson and his colleagues with phenelzine. In addition, interest in MAOIs continues because there appears to be two forms of MAO, namely, MAO type A and MAO type B (Youdim, 1972). Each form has its relatively selective inhibitors. MAO type A has a greater propensity for oxidizing certain substrates, such as serotonin, than it has for phenethylamine or benzylamine, whereas with MAO type B, the selectivity is reversed. Clorgyline (Fig. 1) is a relatively selective inhibitor of MAO type A and deprenyl (Fig. 1) of MAO type B (Knoll, 1976, 1979). As can be seen in Fig. 1, both clor-gyline and deprenyl are propargylamine compounds. Interesting-ly, so is pargyline, which has a modest preference for MAO type B (Baldessarini, 1983; Maxwell and White, 1978).

Unfortunately, as noted by Baldessarini (1983), although de-prenyl does not potentiate the cardiovascular effects of tyramine (lack of cheese effect) it also appears to be a poor antidepressant agent in man, whereas clorgyline appears to be the better anti-depressant compound in man, but is a strong potentiator of the cardiovascular effects of tyramine. Additional work aimed at pro-ducing an effective, nonhydrazine MAOI antidepressant, free of the cheese effect, is being actively pursued.

Drug Discovery

References

Bailey, S. d'A., Bucci, L., Gosline, E., Kline, N. S., Park, I. H., Rochlin, D., Saunders, J. C., and Vaisberg, M.: Comparison of iproniazid with other amine oxidase inhibitors, including W-1544, JB-516, RO 4-1018 and RO 5-0700. *Ann. NY Acad. Sci.* **80:** 652–668, 1959.

Baldessarini, R. J.: *Biomedical Aspects of Depression.* American Psychiatric Press, Washington, DC, 1983.

Benedetti, M. S. and Dostert, P.: Overview of the present state of MAO inhibitors. *J. Neural Transm.* (Suppl.) **23:** 103–119, 1987.

Biel, J. H., Bopp, B., and Mitchell, B. D.: Chemistry and structure-activity relationships of psychotropic drugs, in *Principles of Psychopharmacology*, 2nd Ed., W. G. Clark and J. Guidice, eds., pp. 9–40, Academic, New York, 1978.

Blaschko, H., Richter, D., and Schlossmann, H.: The inactivation of adrenaline. *J. Physiol.* (London) **90:** 1–17, 1937a.

Blaschko, H., Richter, D., and Schlossmann, H.: CCLXVIII. The oxidation of adrenaline and other amines. *Biochem. J.* **31:** 2187–2196, 1937b.

Brodie, B. B., Pletscher, A., and Shore, P. A.: Possible role of serotonin in brain function and in reserpine action. *J. Pharmacol. Exp. Ther.* **116:** 9, 1956.

Chessin, M., Dubnick, B., Kramer, E. R., and Scott, C. C.: Modifications of pharmacology of reserpine and serotonin by iproniazid. *Fed. Proc.* **15:** 409, 1956.

Crane, G. E.: The psychiatric side-effects of iproniazid. *Am. J. Psychiatry* **112:** 494–501, 1956a.

Crane, G. E.: Further studies on iproniazid phosphate; isonicotinyl-isopropyl-hydrazine phosphate, marsilid. *J. Nerv. Ment. Dis.* **124:** 322–331, 1956b.

Crane, G. E.: Iproniazid (Marsilid) phosphate, a therapeutic agent for mental disorders and debilitating diseases. *Psychiatric Res. Rep.* **8:** 142–152, 1957.

Fox, H. H.: Chemotherapy of acid-fast infections, in *Medicinal Chemistry*, 2nd Ed., A. Burger, ed., pp. 970–996, Interscience, New York, 1960.

Fox, H. H. and Gibas, J. T.: Synthetic tuberculostats. VII. Monoalkyl derivatives of isonicotinylhydrazine. *J. Org. Chem.* **18:** 994–1002, 1953.

Kaiser, C. and Zirkle, C. L.: Antidepressant drugs, in *Medicinal Chemistry*, 2nd Ed., A. Burger, ed., pp. 1470–1497, Wiley, New York, 1970.

Kamman, G. R., Freeman, J. G., and Lucero, R. J.: The effect of 1-isonicotinyl-2-isopropyl hydrazide (IIH) on the behavior of long-term mental patients. *J. Nerv. Ment. Dis.* **118:** 391–407, 1953.

Kauffman, G. B.: The discovery of iproniazid and its role in antidepressant therapy. *J. Chem. Ed.* **56:** 35–36, 1979.

Klein, D. F., Gittelman, R., Quitkin, F., and Rifkin, A.: *Diagnosis and Treatment of Psychiatric Disorders: Adults and Children*, 2nd Ed., Williams & Wilkins, Baltimore, 1980.

Kline, N. S.: Monoamine oxidase inhibitors: An unfinished picaresque tale, in *Discoveries in Biological Psychiatry*, F. J. Ayd and B. Blackwell, eds., pp. 194–204, Lippincott, Philadelphia, 1970.

Kline, N. S. and Cooper, T. B.: Monoamine oxidase inhibitors as antidepressants, in *Psychotropic Agents*, F. Hoffmeister and G. Stille, eds., pp. 369–397, Springer-Verlag, Berlin, 1980.

Knoll, J.: Analysis of the pharmacological effect of selective MAOI, in *Monoamine Oxidase and Its Inhibition, CIBA Foundation Symposium 39*, pp. 135–161, North Holland, Amsterdam, 1976.

Knoll, J.: Structure–activity relationships of the selective inhibitors of MAO-B, in *Monoamine Oxidase: Structure, Function and Altered Functions*, T. P. Singer, R. W. VonKorff, and D. L. Murphy, eds., pp. 431–446, Academic, New York, 1979.

Lock, S., ed.: New look at monoamine oxidase inhibitors. *Br. Med. J.* **2:** 69, 1976.

Loomer, H. P., Saunders, J. C., and Kline, N. S.: A clinical and pharmacodynamic evaluation of iproniazid as a psychic energizer. *Psychiatric Res. Rep.* **8:** 129–141, 1957.

Maxwell, R. A. and White, H. L.: Tricyclic and monoamine oxidase inhibitors antidepressants: Structure–activity relationships, in *Handbook of Psychopharmacology*, vol. 14, L. L. Iversen, S. D. Iversen, and S. H. Snyder eds., pp. 83–155, Plenum, New York, 1978.

Medical Research Council: Clinical trial of the treatment of depressive illness. *Br. Med. J.* **1:** 881–886, 1965.

O'Connor, J. B., Howlett, K. S., Jr., and Wagner, R. R.: Side effects accompanying use of iproniazid. *Am. Rev. Tuberc.* **68:** 270–272, 1953.

Pletscher, A., Gey, K. F., and Burkard, W. P.: Inhibitors of monoamine oxidase and decarboxylase of aromatic amino acids, in *Handbook of Experimental Pharmacology*, vol. 19, O. Eichler and A. Farah eds., pp. 593–735, Springer-Verlag, Berlin, 1966.

Raskin, A., Schulterbrandt, J. G., Reatig, N., Crook, T. H., and Odle, D.: Depression subtypes and response to phenelzine, diazepam, and a placebo. *Arch. Gen. Psychiatry* **30:** 66–75, 1974.

Robinson, D. S., Nies, A., Ravaris, C. L., and Lamborn, K. R.: The monoamine oxidase inhibitor, phenelzine, in the treatment of depressive-anxiety states. *Arch. Gen. Psychiatry* **29:** 407–413, 1973.

Robinson, D. S., Nies, A., Ravaris, C. L., Ives, J. O., and Bartlett, D.: Clinical pharmacology of phenelzine. *Arch. Gen. Psychiatry* **35:** 629–635, 1978.

Robitzek, E. H., and Selikoff, I. J.: Hydrazine derivatives of isonicotinic acid (rimifon, marsilid) in the treatment of active progressive caseous-pneumonic tuberculosis; preliminary report. *Am. Rev. Tuberc.* **65**: 402–428, 1952.

Robitzek, E. H., Selikoff, I. J., and Ornstein, G. G.: Chemotherapy of human tuberculosis with hydrazine derivatives of isonicotinic acid. *Q. Bull. Sea View Hosp.* **13**: 27–51, 1952.

Sackler, A. M. and Sackler, M. D., eds.: Symposium on the biochemical and clinical aspects of Marsilid and other monoamine oxidase inhibitors. *J. Clin. Exp. Psychopathol.* **19**: (Suppl. 1), 1–186, 1958.

Sandler, M., Glover, V., Elsworth, J. D., Lewinsohn, R., Reveley, M. A.: Monoamine oxidase and its inhibition: Some clinical implications, in *Monoamine Oxidase: Structure, Function, and Altered Functions*, T. P. Singer, R. W. VonKorff, and D. L. Murphy, eds., pp. 447–456, Academic, New York, 1979.

Sargant, W.: Drugs in the treatment of depression. *Br. Med. J.* **1**: 225–227, 1961.

Sargant, W. and Dally, P.: Treatment of anxiety states by antidepressant drugs. *Br. Med. J.* **1**: 6–9, 1962.

Saunders, J. C.: Discussion in Amine Oxidase Inhibitors. *Ann. NY Acad. Sci.* **80**: 719–724, 1959.

Singer, T. P., VonKorff, R. W., and Murphy, D. L., eds.: *Monoamine Oxidase: Structure, Function and Altered Functions*, Academic, New York, 1979.

Smith, J. A.: The use of the isopropyl derivative of isonicotinylhydrazine (marsilid) in the treatment of mental disease. *Am. Pract. Digest. Treatment* **4**: 519, 520, 1953.

West, E. D. and Dally, P. J.: Effects of iproniazid in depressive syndromes. *Br. Med. J.* **1**: 1491–1494, 1959.

Youdim, M. B. H.: Multiple forms of monoamine oxidase and their properties, in *Monoamine Oxidases: New Vistas*, vol. 5 of *Advances in Biochemical Psychopharmacology*, E. Costa and M. Sandler, eds., pp. 67–77, Raven, New York, 1972.

Zeller, E. A. and Barsky, J.: *In vivo* inhibition of liver and brain monoamine oxidase by 1-isonicotinyl-2-isopropyl hydrazine. *Proc. Soc. Exp. Biol. Med.* **81**: 459–461, 1952.

Zeller, E. A., Barsky, J., Fouts, J. R., Kirchheimer, W. F., and Van Orden, L. S.: Influence of isonicotinic acid hydrazide (INH) and 1-isonicotinyl-2-isopropyl hydrazide (IIH) on bacterial and mammalian enzymes. *Experientia* **8**: 349, 350, 1952a.

Zeller, E. A., Barsky, J., Berman, E. R., and Fouts, J. R.: Action of isonicotinic acid hydrazide and related compounds on enzymes involved in the autonomic nervous system. *J. Pharmacol. Exp. Ther.* **106**: 427, 428, 1952b.

Lithium

I. Lithium (Li⁺)* as an Innovative Therapeutic Agent

Manic-depressive illness is a major psychosis. The classic picture is the episodic bipolar cycle: euphoria, grandiosity, cyclothymia, retardation, depression. This psychosis loses its intensity after periods of days or months, but, because it is typically a chronic illness, there can be frequent relapses. The mood swings can be subtle, or explosive and disruptive, and do not respond to environmental or interpersonal factors. Exaggerated symptoms of mania, endangering the patient and those nearby, require immediate and vigorous action, usually with drugs.

Before the use of Li, the treatment of choice for manic-depressive illness was a combination of electroshock therapy, barbiturates, and other sedatives. Electroshock therapy produced fast results, but frequently the beneficial results were of short duration. Repeated treatment was often not as effective as the initial treatment and led on occasion to memory impairment. Patients developed fear of the method. Barbiturates, on the other hand, caused patients to feel drugged, drowsy, and mentally dull. With the advent of the phenothiazines, chlorpromazine—and later, other neuroleptics—became the dominant pharmacotherapy for acute mania. These antipsychotic agents effectively suppressed manic attacks (Goodwin and Zis, 1979) but only at doses that sedated and elicited subnormal psychomotor activity.

The advent of Li so changed the situation that Rifkin and Siris (1983) were prompted to say, "Drug treatment of mania is one of the great successes of psychopharmacology." Goodwin (1979) consid-

---

*For convenience lithium ion (administered as a salt) will be abbreviated as Li.

ered Li to be "...the major advance in the treatment of major mental disorders since introduction of the phenothiazines and the tricyclic antidepressants..."

Li has become the treatment of choice for manic-depressive illness. Seventy to eighty percent of patients respond to therapy with major improvement within five to eight days (Lazarus, 1986). It is most effective in patients who experience frequent relapses or are hypomanic. Li is more effective in "normalizing" the mood of patients than are neuroleptics (Schou, 1968). The dose of Li necessary to bring about control of mania does not cause major CNS side effects, as do neuroleptics. Many years of prophylactic treatment with Li has not affected normal functions or restricted the normal emotional range of happiness and sorrow. Li has stabilized the undulating life course of many manic-depressives (Schou, 1968). According to Lazarus (1986), Li represents one of the most significant therapeutic advances in psychiatry in this century.

Li was the first drug to demonstrate clear-cut prophylaxis for both phases of manic-depressive illness (Rosenbaum et al., 1979). In addition, Li has been found to be effective, although perhaps less so, in unipolar depression (Bunney and Garland, 1984). Fieve and Peselow (1983), in reviewing the clinical literature, concluded that many investigators found Li to be as effective as, or superior to, antidepressants as a prophylaxis against unipolar depression. This point is still controversial.

Li can be a very toxic substance, therefore, serum Li levels must be kept within a narrow range in order to achieve therapeutic benefit while avoiding acute adverse reactions (gastrointestinal, cutaneous, CNS, renal, and others) and longer-term intoxication that can lead to renal impairment and, in extreme cases, to death.

The FDA approved the use of Li for acute mania in 1970 and for maintenance therapy in 1974. Subsequent to the demonstration of its effectiveness in mania, Li has been tried, with varied success, in a wide variety of disorders. Youngerman and Canino (1978) reported Li to be effective in the treatment of children and adolescents with manic-depressive illness. Extreme cases of depression, not responsive to standard antidepressants, have been treated with Li (Nelson and Byck, 1982). Li is also used in gastric disorders accompanied by secretory diarrhea, such as pancreatic cholera syndrome

(Pandol et al., 1980). It is used in the therapy of resistant chronic cluster headaches (Ekbom, 1981). Other possible uses of Li are in the treatment of alcoholism and drug abuse.

Early Clinical Research History

In the case of Li, the clinical history is, in essence, the scientific work leading to its discovery and will be covered in section II.

II. The Scientific Work Leading to Lithium as an Antimanic Agent

Cade in the late 1940s commenced investigations to demonstrate whether some excreted toxin could be detected in the urine of manic patients. In connection with this work, he attempted to determine whether uric acid would enhance the toxicity of urea in guinea pigs (Cade, 1949). He elected to use the most soluble salt of uric acid, lithium urate. To determine if the lithium ion *per se* might affect the toxicity of urea, Cade substituted lithium carbonate for lithium urate. Lithium carbonate had a strong protective action against the convulsant death elicited by urea. In running appropriate controls for his experiments, Cade found that when lithium carbonate was given alone (i.e., without urea challenge) "...after a latent period of about two hours, the animals, although fully conscious, became extremely lethargic and unresponsive to stimuli for one to two hours before once again becoming normally active and timid." Cade concluded that, "It appeared worthwhile in view of these results to try lithium salts in ...mania, in view of their sedative effect;..." Cade treated manic patients in his hospital with Li. Case I, a 51-yr-old male, had been manic for 5 yr and confined to a closed chronic ward. After 5 d of Li therapy he was noticeably more settled, after 3 wk he was transferred to a less restrictive ward, and after 2 mo he was released from the hospital to return to work. He was readmitted to the hospital 6 mo later because he had stopped taking the Li. After a month of Li therapy, he was again well enough to leave the hospital. Nine additional patients were treated. All the manic patients given Li improved. One patient, who was manic and also had hallucinations and delusions, became calm, but continued to have hallucinations and delusions. Three depressed patients did not worsen, but after several weeks were not improved. Cade stated,

> There is no doubt that in mania patients' improvement has closely paralleled treatment and that this criterion has been fulfilled in the chronic and subacute cases just as closely as in the cases of more recent onset. The quietening effect on restless non-manic psychotics is additional strong evidence of the efficacy of lithium salts, especially as such restlessness returned on cessation of treatment.

Cade's findings prompted other Australian psychiatrists to try Li in mania. Roberts (1950) and Ashburner (1950) exchanged comments on the efficacy and toxicity of Li. Noack and Trautner (1951) treated 100 patients suffering from a variety of mental disorders with Li; no serious toxicity was observed. Out of 30 manic patients treated, only one did not improve. Glesinger (1954) substituted Li for electroshock therapy, which had not been very effective in chronic patients. He considered Li to be a step toward an ideal treatment, if properly administered, and that Li could be of value in both in-hospital and outpatient use. Gershon (Gershon and Yuwiler, 1960), building on his earlier pharmacokinetic work and that of colleagues (Noack and Trautner, 1951; Trautner et al., 1955; Gershon and Trautner, 1956), pointed out that Li treatment was safe and could be continued indefinitely when regular plasma assays and careful clinical observations were made, but that grave risks were run without these controls.

Corroborative clinical studies were carried out rapidly in France and Denmark and later in England. Schou et al. (1954) conducted the first controlled studies with Li. They considered it "astonishing" that reports of the striking effect of Li aroused little interest among psychiatrists. They attributed this, in part, to the fact that the many pitfalls in the clinical study of drugs—diagnosis errors, suggestibility, poor quantitation, spontaneous remissions—produced skepticism about the reports. They set a goal of minimizing these sources of error. Thirty-eight manic patients, male and female, were housed in special wards to ensure constancy of observation. Li was given in "open" treatment for a certain period and then in a double-blind, placebo-controlled, crossover procedure. Treatment consisted of 2 wk on Li and two on placebo, randomly arranged, and including placebo–placebo and Li–Li groups. Electroshock was not used during this time and the use of other drugs was curtailed. Fourteen patients showed positive effect, 18 a possible effect , and six no effect. The researchers concluded that Li not only had therapeutic usefulness, but also held theoretical interest because it counteracted manic symptoms. It could, therefore, be of use in understanding the pathophysiology of psychosis (Schou et al., 1954).

Cade (1949) and other Australian investigators had alluded to a possible prophylactic effect of Li, as did Schou et al. (1954), Hartigan (1963), Schou (1963), and Baastrup (1964). Baastrup and Schou (1967) provided convincing controlled data that established this prophylactic action, with their study of 88 manic-depressive, or recurrently depressed, females. The patients were observed for more than 6 yr, and prophylactic Li had been administered for 1–5 yr. Calculations were made of the relapse frequency (episode starts/year) and psychosis rate (months/year in a psychotic state) for periods with and without Li treatment. The results were statistically highly significant. Li markedly reduced relapse rate and psychosis rate. Li was also effective against relapses in recurrent depression. These investigators concluded that Li was the first drug to have a clear-cut prophylactic action against these diseases, and its unique feature was that it did not interfere with normal mental processes.

A considerable amount of investigation has evolved concerning the clinical efficacy of Li since these disclosures, and many reviews are available (e.g., Schou, 1968; Gershon, 1970; Kline and Kistner, 1971; Johnson and Cade, 1975; Davis, 1976; Goodwin and Zis, 1979; Fieve and Peselow, 1983; Lazarus, 1986).

Table 1 defines the critical scientific ideas and experiments leading to Li as an antimanic agent and categorizes their origin.

Background Contributions Preceding the Use of Lithium as an Antimanic Agent

There is no modern (twentieth-century) literature that can be considered to support convincingly the antimanic properties of Li, prior to the contribution of Cade (1949). However, Yeragani and Gershon (1986) noted that William Hammond (Bellevue Hospital,

Table 1
Profile of Observations and Ideas Crucial to the Development of Lithium[a]

Sequence: Route to innovative drug[**]	Orientation	Nature of study	Research institution	National origin	Nature of discovery	Screening involved	Crucial ideas or observations
Lithium[**]							
Cade (1949)	Pre-clinical	Pharma-cology	Hospital	Australia	Seren-dipitous	No	Guinea pigs quieted by Li.
Cade (1949)	Clinical	Psy-chiatry	Hospital	Australia	Orderly	No	Manic patients controlled by Li.

[a]Taken from section II. Entries are those contributions without which the discovery of the agent (or additionally, in some cases, a relevant clinical application) would not have taken place or would have been materially delayed.

New York) published *Treatise on Diseases of the Nervous System* in 1871, in which he clearly reported the successful treatment of acute mania with high doses of lithium bromide. Unfortunately, this observation was never followed up and faded into obscurity.

III. Comments on Events Leading to Lithium

As noted by Gershon (1970), Li was introduced to the scientific world in 1949 and, therefore, preceded chlorpromazine and reserpine as the first modern drug in psychopharmacology.

Kline and Kistner (1971) credited Cade with being a good enough clinician to test whether the calming effect of Li on guinea pigs might carry over into manic patients. Cade (1970) conceded that there seemed to be a great distance between lethargy in guinea pigs and excitement in psychotics, but that the association of these two ideas was explicable because he was looking for some toxin in the urine of manic patients when he discovered the sedative qualities of Li. He maintained that his discovery of the antimanic effect of Li was unexpected, but in retrospect was a result of his interest in the etiology of manic-depressive illness. Johnson and Cade (1975) maintained, "[t]hat [although] the therapeutic efficacy of lithium was unsuspected when the experimental work was commenced, [this] in no way made the final outcome entirely the product of chance."

Davis (1976) felt that great credit should go to the early Australian workers who followed up on Cade's discovery and developed the clinical information and tactics for the safe use of Li, and who discovered the prophylactic properties of Li to replace maintenance electroshock treatment. Goodwin (1979) states the view that Cade discovered the therapeutic use of Li, and Schou provided the firm scientific basis for its major clinical use.

Psychiatrists in the USA were reluctant to use Li because in the 1940s lithium chloride had been recommended as a substitute for sodium chloride for patients who had to be on a salt-free diet, and kidney toxicity and a number of fatal intoxications had resulted from its liberal intake. Cade (1970) noted that 1949, the year that Li was found to be active in mania, was the same year that it was reported to be toxic. He felt that 1949 was the least favorable year to try to introduce Li as a therapeutic agent, especially considering that the attempt was being made by an unknown psychiatrist with no research training, and primitive techniques and equipment, who was working in a small hospital. Johnson and Cade (1975) thought, in addition, that the introduction of chlorpromazine at the same time as Li, for the same indications, hindered the acceptance of Li. Chlorpromazine had an "edge over Li" because chlorpromazine had a wide margin of safety and brought highly agitated patients under rapid control. Schou (1959) held that Li being totally different, chemically and pharmacologically, from available drugs used to treat extreme agitation was one reason that physicians were put off from trying it. Baldessarini and Lipinski (1975) also suggested that lack of interest by the pharmaceutical industry in a cheap, unpatentable mineral was one of the reasons why it took Li a long time to be accepted in the USA. Li was eventually approved for use in the USA more than twenty years after Cade's initial report.

IV. Developments
Subsequent to Lithium

Li is an unusual drug in that it has spawned no progeny. Li, an inorganic ion, leaves little, if any, room for manipulation by medicinal chemists. In addition, there are no good animal models of mania, the behavioral pharmacology of Li is not very specific, and the pro-

posed biochemical mechanisms for the antimanic action of Li are
moot. Gershon (1970), Baldessarini and Lipinski (1975), and Jefferson
et al. (1983) all pointed out that, despite considerable work, the
mechanism of the antimanic action of Li was unknown at the time of
their writing. More recently, Bunney and Garland-Bunney (1987)
suggested tentatively that a "serotonergic enhancing activity" of Li
was compatible with an antidepressant activity, as was its capacity
to down-regulate beta receptors. A "muscarinic-cholinergic enhancing action" of Li or its inhibition of "second messenger cyclic-AMP-
mediated processes," as well as other actions, were speculated to be
possible mechanisms for an antimanic activity.

An important outgrowth of Li therapy has been better and
more accurate diagnosis of manic and depressive psychiatric illnesses (Baldessarini and Lipinski, 1975).

References

Ashburner, J. V.: Correspondence: A case of chronic mania treated with
   lithium citrate and terminating fatally. *Med. J. Aust.* **2:** 386, 1950.
Baastrup, P. C.: The use of lithium in manic-depressive psychosis. *Compr.
   Psychiatry* **5:** 396–408, 1964.
Baastrup, P. C. and Schou, M.: Lithium as a prophylactic agent. *Arch. Gen.
   Psychiatry* **16:** 162–172, 1967.
Baldessarini, R. J. and Lipinski, J. F.: Lithium salts 1970–1975. *Ann. Intern.
   Med.* **83:** 527–533, 1975.
Bunney, W. E. and Garland-Bunney, B. L.: Mechanisms of action of lithium
   in affective illness: Basic and clinical implications, in *Psychopharmacology:
   The Third Generation of Progress*, H. Y. Meltzer, ed., pp. 553–565, Raven,
   New York, 1987.
Bunney, W. E. and Garland, B. L.: Lithium and its possible mode of action,
   in *Neurobiology of Mood Disorders*, R. M. Post and J. C. Ballenger, eds., pp.
   731–743, William & Wilkins, Baltimore, 1984.
Cade, J. F. J.: Lithium salts in the treatment of psychotic excitement. *Med.
   J. Aust.* **2:** 349–352, 1949.
Cade, J. F. J.: The story of lithium, in *Discoveries in Biological Psychiatry*,
   F. J. Ayd and B. Blackwell., eds., pp. 218–229, J. B. Lippincott, Philadel-
   phia, 1970.
Davis, J. M.: Overview: Maintenance therapy in psychiatry: II Affective dis-
   orders. *Am. J. Psychiatry* **133:** 1–13, 1976.

Ekbom, K.: Lithium for cluster headache: Review of the literature and preliminary results of long-term treatment. *Headache* **21:** 132–139, 1981.

Fieve, R. R. and Peselow, E. D.: Lithium: Clinical application, in *Drugs in Psychiatry*, vol. 1, G. D. Burrows, T. R. Norman, and B. Davies, eds., pp. 277–321, Elsevier Science, New York, 1983.

Gershon, S.: Lithium in mania. *Clin. Pharm. Ther.* **11:** 168–187, 1970.

Gershon, S. and Trautner, E. M.: The treatment of shock-dependency by pharmacological agents. *Med. J. Aust.* **1:** 783–787, 1956.

Gershon, S. and Yuwiler, A.: Lithium ion: A specific psychopharmacological approach to the treatment of mania. *J. Neuropsychiatry* **1:** 229–241, 1960.

Glesinger, B.: Evaluation of lithium in treatment of psychotic excitement. *Med. J. Aust.* **1:** 277–283, 1954.

Goodwin, F. K.: The lithium ion. Impact on treatment and research. Introduction. *Arch. Gen. Psychiatry* **36:** 833, 834, 1979.

Goodwin, F. K. and Zis, A. P.: Lithium in the treatment of mania. Comparison with neuroleptics. *Arch. Gen. Psychiatry* **36:** 840–844, 1979.

Hartigan, G. P.: The use of lithium salts in affective disorders. *Br. J. Psychiatry* **109:** 810–814, 1963.

Jefferson, J. W., Greist, J. H., and Ackerman, D. L.: *Lithium Encyclopedia for Clinical Practice*, pp. 1–29, American Psychiatric Press, Washington, DC, 1983.

Johnson, F. N. and Cade, J. F. J.: The historical background to lithium research and therapy, in *Lithium Research and Therapy*, F. N. Johnson, ed., pp. 10–22, Academic, London, 1975.

Kline, N. S. and Kistner, G. A.: Lithium: The history of its use in psychiatry, in *Lithium and Psychiatry; Journal Articles*, D. J. Kupfer, ed., pp. 279–295, Medical Examination, New York, 1971.

Lazarus, J. H.: Lithium—history and pharmacology, in *Endocrine and Metabolic Effects of Lithium*, pp. 1–30, Plenum Medical, New York, 1986.

Nelson, J. C. and Byck, R.: Rapid response to lithium in phenelzine nonresponders. *Br. J. Psychiatry* **141:** 85, 86, 1982.

Noack, C. H. and Trautner, E. M.: The lithium treatment of maniacal psychosis. *Med. J. Aust.* **2:** 219–222, 1951.

Pandol, S. J., Korman, L. Y., McCarthy, D. M., and Gardner, J. D.: Beneficial effects of oral lithium carbonate in the treatment of pancreatic cholera syndrome. *N. Engl. J. Med.* **302:** 1403, 1404, 1980.

Rifkin, A. and Siris, G.: Drug treatment of mania, in *Schizophrenia and Affective Disorders*, A. Rifkin, J. Wright, eds., pp. 79–94, PSG, Boston, 1983.

Roberts, E. L.: A case of chronic mania treated with lithium citrate and terminating fatally. *Med. J. Aust.* **2:** 261, 262, 1950.

Rosenbaum, A. H., Maruta, T., and Richelson, E.: Clinical pharmacology: Drugs that alter mood. II Lithium. *Mayo Clin. Proc.* **54:** 401–407, 1979.

Schou, M.: Lithium in psychiatric therapy. *Psychopharmacologia* **1**: 65–78, 1959.

Schou, M.: Normothymotics, "mood-normalizers. " *Br. J. Psychiatry* **109**: 803–809, 1963.

Schou, M.: Lithium in psychiatric therapy and prophylaxis. *J. Psychiatry Res.* **6**: 67–95, 1968.

Schou, M., Juel-Nielsen, N., Stromgren, E., and Voldby, H.: The treatment of manic psychoses by the administration of lithium salts. *J. Neurol. Neurosurg. Psychiatry* **17**: 250–260, 1954.

Trautner, E. M., Morris, R., Noack, C. H., and Gershon, S.: The excretion and retention of ingested lithium and its effects on the ionic balance of man. *Med. J. Aust.* **2**: 280–291, 1955.

Yeragani, V. K. and Gershon, S.: Hammond and lithium: Historical update. *Biol. Psychol.* **21**: 1101, 1102, 1986.

Youngerman, J. and Canino, I. A.: Lithium carbonate use in children and adolescents. *Arch. Gen. Psychiatry* **35**: 216–224, 1978.

Chlordiazepoxide and Diazepam

I. Chlordiazepoxide and Diazepam as Innovative Therapeutic Agents

Anxiety has been most succinctly defined as "...the distressing experience of dread and foreboding [coupled] with an array of autonomic concomitants" (Rosenbaum, 1982). A more extensive definition was given by Rickels (1981b): "Anxiety is perceived as a subjective feeling of heightened tension and diffused uneasiness, defined as the conscious and reportable experience of intense dread and foreboding, conceptualized as internally derived and unrelated to external threat."

Anxiety is a frequent cause for seeking medical attention. The nature and significance of anxiety has been the subject of ruminations by philosophers, psychologists, and theologians, and has been discussed exhaustively by physicians (Lader, 1972; Lewis, 1980; Cassano, 1983). Lader (1972) pointed out, "Anxiety is an ubiquitous phenomenon in everyday life." Because of its common occurrence, some forms of anxiety are labeled as normal. However, in many instances, anxiety can be so profound as to be considered pathological. Anxiety, on occasion, may be related to external threat, but the emotional response it evokes is usually greatly out of proportion to the magnitude of the threat.

Facial expression is one of the most obvious signs of anxiety. Symptoms include tightness in the throat, difficulty in breathing, a sense of constriction in the chest, epigastric discomfort or pain, palpitations, dizziness and weakness, and dryness of the mouth (Lader, 1972). Running in panic, screaming, tremor, sudden mictu-

165

rition or defecation, vomiting, and sweating may also occur. Anxiety has been estimated to occur in 2–5% of the total population and in 7–16% of psychiatric patients (Burrows and Davies, 1984).

Prior to the introduction of chlordiazepoxide, the first benzodiazepine compound, the barbiturates and meprobamate were the agents used to treat serious anxiety conditions. Unfortunately, the barbiturates had a propensity for tolerance to their useful actions to develop. Moreover, physical dependence and potentially lethal reactions upon withdrawal were common occurrences. Meprobamate exerted an unclear separation between its antianxiety effects and heavy sedation. It also caused physical dependence and was quite toxic on acute overdosage (Baldessarini, 1985). Hollister (1984) noted that chlordiazepoxide (as well as diazepam and subsequent congeners) resembled conventional "sedative–hypnotics," and was included in the same pharmacological category as the barbiturates and meprobamate, the effects of all three being characterized by sedation proceeding to hypnosis, and by muscle relaxation and an anticonvulsant action. However, for chlordiazepoxide and other benzodiazepines, the ratio of the sedating dose to the anxiolytic dose, in humans, is relatively large compared to the ratios for the barbiturates and meprobamate (Rickels, 1978; Klein et al., 1980; Greenblatt and Shader, 1981). An antianxiety effect can generally be achieved without clouding of the sensorium.

It was generally agreed that chlordiazepoxide, diazepam, and related benzodiazepines are much safer on acute administration than are the barbiturates and meprobamate, although benzodiazepines have a low propensity to produce a mild tolerance and physical dependence on sustained usage (Rickels, 1978, 1981a; Hollister, 1981a,b; 1984; Rosenbaum, 1982; Greenblatt et al., 1983b). A clear benefit that accrued from the replacement of barbiturates by the benzodiazepines was a reduction in the number of successful suicides from barbiturate overdosage (Hollister, 1981a).

Benzodiazepines do not depress respiration or influence cardiac output. They also do not inhibit or induce hepatic microsomal enzymes and therefore have few, if any, drug interactions.

Chlordiazepoxide, diazepam, and related agents have also found use in the treatment of insomnia, muscle spasticity, repetitive grand mal seizures (status epilepticus), and alcohol withdrawal (Greenblatt et al., 1983b; Hollister, 1984). These agents, particularly diazepam, are also useful for preanesthetic medication and as mild anesthetics inducing sedation for procedures such as endoscopy and cardioversion. Diagnostically, lack of response to these agents may indicate that the anxiety is masking major psychiatric disorders such as depression and schizophrenia.

Greenblatt and Shader (1981) considered that "[t]he availability of benzodiazepines for the treatment of anxiety and insomnia clearly constitutes a therapeutic advance in drug efficacy and safety."

Early Clinical Research History

The initial reports describing the major effects of chlordiazepoxide were presented in a symposium entitled *Newer Antidepressant and Other Psychotherapeutic Drugs*, which was held at the University of Texas Medical Branch in Galveston, Texas in 1959 and published in 1960. Tobin et al. (1960) administered chlordiazepoxide to 79 patients whose predominant symptomatology was anxiety. Eighteen patients were judged to have had excellent relief of their anxiety, 27 a good response, and 19 a fair response—an incidence of success of 81%. Kinross-Wright et al. (1960) found that the action of chlordiazepoxide was limited mainly to reduction of anxiety and tension: it was effective in 77% of neurotic clinic patients who were exhibiting anxiety. At effective doses there was no clouding of consciousness. Bowes (1960) reported chlordiazepoxide to be effective in long-standing anxiety and phobic reactions, and in obsessional states. He remarked that it was not as effective as phenothiazines in schizophrenia. Farb (1960) found that 44 of 45 patients, the majority of which were psychoneurotics, were afforded relief. The ability of the compound to reduce anxiety without interfering with work efficiency and without aggravating depression was noteworthy. Breitner (1960) reported that chlordiazepoxide "...was very useful in combating such hard-to-treat manifestations of tension as obsession, agitation accompanying depression and excessive use of alcohol." Fifty-four of 63 patients exhibited fair to good response.

Many books, reviews, and chapters covering the clinical uses of chlordiazepoxide, diazepam, and congeners have appeared (*see*, for example, Symposium, 1960; Symposium, 1961; Rickels, 1978; Klein et al., 1980; Hollister, 1981a; Costa, 1983; Greenblatt et al., 1983a,b; Randall, 1983; Trimble, 1983; Burrows et al., 1984).

II. The Scientific Work Leading to Chlordiazepoxide and Diazepam

Chlordiazepoxide (first given the generic name methaminodiazepoxide) (Fig. 1) was synthesized by Sternbach and Reeder (1961a). Chlordiazepoxide and related agents were formed when 6-chloro-2-chloromethyl-4-phenylquinazoline 3-oxide was reacted with a series of primary amines. Such reactions were expected to form a series of secondary amino derivatives of quinazoline 3-oxide. Unexpectedly, a ring enlargement occurred, yielding 2-amino derivatives of 7-chloro-5-phenyl-3H-1,4-benzodiazepine 4-oxide in addition to the expected products. When methylamine was the primary amine, this "side" reaction yielded chlordiazepoxide. Sternbach and Reeder (1961a) commented that chlordiazepoxide "...showed, as found by L. O. Randall and coworkers, interesting psychosedative properties."

Randall et al. (1960) reported that chlordiazepoxide had muscle-relaxant and sedative effects in mice and depressed the avoidance responding and spontaneous locomotor activity of normal rats. Furthermore, it had a calming effect on rats made irritable by lesions in the septum. Perhaps even more significantly, in ordinarily vicious monkeys, a loss of aggressive behavior occurred at doses that did not depress general activity or avoidance behavior. Chlordiazepoxide was considered to be in many ways similar to meprobamate as a tranquilizer, but was qualitatively more potent, and had taming effects. Randall (1960) noted, in addition, that chlordiazepoxide had the tranquilizing properties of chlorpromazine and reserpine, but lacked the autonomic blocking effects of these compounds. Chlordiazepoxide also had anticonvulsant properties similar to those of phenobarbital, but did not induce hypnosis.

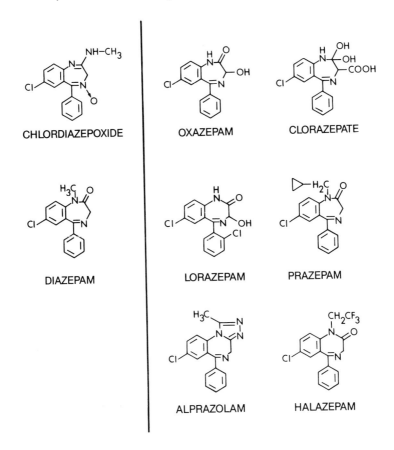

Fig. 1. The structures of chlordiazepoxide, diazepam, and chemically and/or pharmacologically related substances.

Diazepam (Fig. 1), which was five times more potent than chlordiazepoxide, appeared shortly after the latter agent. Pharmacological studies showed that a lactam degradation product formed from chlordiazepoxide in solution was very active, as was the lactam from which the N-oxide oxygen was removed. These observations led to an intense program of synthesis that eventually yielded diazepam (Sternbach and Reeder, 1961b; Randall et al., 1961). Diazepam was the most frequently prescribed drug in the United States for more than 12 years (Ayd, 1980).

Table 1 defines the critical scientific ideas and experiments leading to chlordiazepoxide and diazepam and categorizes their origin.

Background Contributions
Preceding Chlordiazepoxide

The arrival on the clinical scene of chlorpromazine, reserpine, iproniazid, imipramine, meprobamate, and lithium in the early 1950s created a revolution in psychiatry. These drugs established an atmosphere of receptivity in a medical discipline in which drugs, aside from barbiturates, had little impact heretofore. A ferment of research ensued that was aimed at determining the mechanisms of action of these agents and at the development of additional novel treatments for psychiatric illnesses. Chlordiazepoxide and diazepam were two of the results.

III. Comments on Events Leading
to Chlordiazepoxide and Diazepam

According to Sternbach (1978), the Hoffman-LaRoche Co. decided in the mid-1950s to enter the area of tranquilizer research. The "...chemists were asked to produce a novel compound which would have the desired properties, would be patentable and....would be superior to the then existing tranquilizers." Haefely (1983) noted that the medicinal chemists at Hoffman-LaRoche were requested not to make derivatives of barbiturates, mephenesin, or any compounds structurally related to other existing CNS agents, such as reserpine and chlorpromazine. "We planned to look for a completely new type of tranquilizer and to work with a new class of compounds not known to possess any biological properties...." (Sternbach, 1978). Sternbach chose the heterocyclic benzoheptoxdiazines (later found actually to be quinazoline 3-oxides) because he had had experience with this ring system in the 1930s. "In place of the rather inert [quinazoline 3-oxide] compounds...which I had formerly studied, I concentrated my efforts on novel derivatives... in which the excocyclic group could be functionalized with a basic side chain" (Sternbach, 1972). Most of the compounds synthesized proved to be inactive. However, by a fortunate set of circum-

Table 1
Profile of Observations and Ideas
Crucial to the Development of Chlordiazepoxide and Diazepam[a]

Sequence: Route to innovative drugs**	Orient- ation	Nature of study	Research institution	National origin	Nature of discovery	Screening involved	Crucial ideas or observations
Chlordiazepoxide**							
Randall et al. (1960)	Pre- clinical	Pharma- cology/ chem- istry	Industry	USA	Orderly	Untargeted	Chlordiazepoxide (methaminodiazep- oxide) is a new psychosedative with unusual properties: a sedative and muscle relaxant with only weak hypnotic effects; qualitatively similar to meproba- mate, but more potent, and exerting marked calming and taming effects on agitated or vicious animals.
Diazepam**							
Sternbach and Reeder (1961b)	Pre- clinical	Chem- istry/ pharma- cology	Industry	USA	Orderly	Targeted	A chemical variation of chlordiazepoxide synthesized; more active as a muscle relaxant, sedative, and anticonvulsant.

[a]Taken from section II. Entries are those contributions without which the discovery of the agent (or additionally, in some cases, a relevant clinical application) would not have taken place or would have been materially delayed.

stances, a crystalline base and its hydrochloride (which had been synthesized several years earlier as part of the program) were test- ed and found to be active. It required several more years to de- termine the correct structure of this active compound, which had undergone an unexpected ring enlargement to become chlordi- azepoxide.

Randall (1983) reminisced,

The BZ molecule [i.e., chlordiazepoxide] had a difficult birth. The chemist made it by accident while preparing an entirely different series of compounds. The discovery of the pharmacological effects resulted from screening for central nervous activity by relatively crude methods which were designed to test hundreds of compounds annually... Initial testing in human subjects failed because of the selection of the wrong type of patient and the wrong doses.

However, the subsequent trials (Symposium, 1960) were rapidly and efficiently carried out. Hines (1960) pointed out, "Clinical appraisal of Librium [chlordiazepoxide] has now been made [over the course of one year] in approximately 16,000 patients seen in private practice, in clinics and hospitals, and in more than half the medical schools of the country."

Regarding the discovery of diazepam, Sternbach (1978) commented that it was surprising to his group that a spontaneously occurring lactam degradation product of chlordiazepoxide, even following removal of its N-oxide oxygen, yielded a compound that was more active than chlordiazepoxide.

Thus, it turned out, that some of the unusual structural features of chlordiazepoxide were not at all needed for its pharmacological activity. The N-oxide function and particularly the basic substituent, which was the cornerstone of our initial working hypothesis, proved to be unnecessary adornments. The only features which were common to these biologically active compounds were the 1,4-benzodiazepine ring system, a chlorine atom in the 7 position and the phenyl group in the 5-position.

As Haefely (1983) pointed out, it would be interesting to know the fate of the work of other chemists who had also been assigned to the project at Hoffman-LaRoche.

IV. Developments Subsequent to Chlordiazepoxide and Diazepam

In addition to chlordiazepoxide and diazepam, there are six benzodiazepines presently used in the USA for the treatment of anxiety: oxazepam, clorazepate, lorazepam, prazepam, alprazolam, and halazepam (Baldessarini, 1985) (Fig. 1). As pointed out by Harvey (1985), all the important benzodiazepines are actually 5-aryl-1,4-benzodiazepines. Many additional benzodiazepines and related agents have been synthesized and studied in humans (Rubinstein and Norman, 1984; Harvey, 1985). Various benzodiazepines are promoted with an emphasis on sedative or hypnotic effects or on muscle relaxant or anticonvulsant effects, but the pharmacological and clinical differences among the entire group seem subtle (Greenblatt and Shader, 1981; Hollister, 1981a, 1984; Rosenbaum, 1982; Greenblatt et al., 1983a; Rubinstein and Norman, 1984; Baldessarini, 1985). According to Rosenbaum (1982), there are only three primary pharmacological criteria that distinguish members of the group from one another: rapidity of absorption, formation of active metabolites, and duration of activity. These differences allow the informed physician some leeway in tailoring his prescription to the specific needs of each patient.

Research continues in the antianxiety area. The ultimate goal is to develop a drug with no propensity at all to produce sedation or tolerance and physical dependence. The availability of many benzodiazepines led to the definition of the benzodiazepine receptor in the brain and to the work regarding its potential physiological and pathological significance (Squires and Braestrup, 1977; Möhler and Okada, 1977).

References

Ayd, F. J., Jr.: Social issues: Misuse and abuse. *Psychosomatics* **21**: 21–25, 1980.

Baldessarini, R. J.: Drugs and the treatment of psychiatric disorders, in *The Pharmacological Basis of Therapeutics*, 7th Ed., A. G. Gilman, L. S. Goodman, T. W. Rall, and F. Murad, eds., pp. 387–445, Macmillan, New York, 1985.

Bowes, H. A.: The role of Librium in an outpatient psychiatric setting. *Dis. Nerv. System* **21** (Suppl.): 20–22, 1960.

Breitner, C.: Drug therapy in obsessional states and other psychiatric problems. *Dis. Nerv. System* **21** (Suppl.): 31–35, 1960.

Burrows, G. D. and Davies, B.: Recognition and management of anxiety, in *Antianxiety Agents*, G. D. Burrows, T. R. Norman, and B. Davies, eds., pp. 1–11, Elsevier, Amsterdam, 1984.

Burrows, G. D., Norman, T. R., and Davies, B., eds.: *Antianxiety Agents*, Elsevier, Amsterdam, 1984.

Cassano, G. B.: What is pathological anxiety and what is not, in *The Benzodiazepines: From Molecular Biology to Clinical Practice*, E. Costa, ed., pp. 287–293, Raven, New York, 1983.

Costa, E., ed.: *The Benzodiazepines: From Molecular Biology to Clinical Practice*, Raven, New York, 1983.

Farb, H. H.: Experience with Librium in clinical psychiatry. *Dis. Nerv. System* **21** (Suppl.): 27–30, 1960.

Greenblatt, D. J. and Shader, R. I.: Clinical use of the benzodiazepines. *Ration. Drug Ther.* **15** (10): 1–6, 1981.

Greenblatt, D. J., Shader, R. I., and Abernethy, D. R.: Current status of benzodiazepines (Part 1). *N. Engl. J. Med.* **309**: 354–358, 1983a.

Greenblatt, D. J., Shader, R. I., and Abernethy, D. R.: Current status of benzodiazepines (Part 2). *N. Engl. J. Med.* **309**: 410–416, 1983b.

Haefely, W.: Alleviation of anxiety—the benzodiazepines saga, in *Discoveries in Pharmacology*, vol. 1, M. J. Parnham and J. Bruinvels, eds., pp. 269–306, Elsevier, Amsterdam, 1983.

Harvey, S. C.: Hypnotics and sedatives, in *The Pharmacological Basis of Therapeutics*, 7th Ed., A. G. Gilman, L. S. Goodman, T. W. Rall, and F. Murad, eds., pp. 339–371, Macmillan, New York, 1985.

Hines, L. R.: Methaminodiazepoxide (Librium): A psychotherapeutic drug. *Curr. Ther. Res.* **2**: 227–236, 1960.

Hollister, L. E.: Benzodiazepines—an overview. *Br. J. Clin. Pharmacol.* **11**: 117S–119S, 1981a.

Hollister, L. E.: Dependence on benzodiazepines, in *Benzodiazepines: A Review of Research Results 1980*, S. I. Szara and J. P. Ludford, eds., pp. 70–82, National Institute on Drug Abuse Res. Monograph Series, US Department of Health and Human Services, Washington, DC, 1981b.

Hollister, L. E.: Clinical aspects of antianxiety agents, in *Antianxiety Agents*, G. D. Burrows, T. R. Norman, and B. Davies, eds., pp. 107–126, Elsevier, Amsterdam, 1984.

Kinross-Wright, J., Cohen, I. M., and Knight, J. A.: The management of neurotic and psychotic states with Ro 5-0690 (Librium). *Dis. Nerv. System* **21**: (Suppl.): 23–26, 1960.

Klein, D. F., Gittelman, R., Quitkin, F., and Rifkin, A.: *Diagnosis and Drug Treatment of Psychiatric Disorders: Adults and Children*, 2nd Ed., Williams & Wilkins, Baltimore, 1980.

Lader, M.: The nature of anxiety. *Br. J. Psychiatry* **121**: 481–491, 1972.

Lewis, A.: Problems presented by the ambiguous word "anxiety" as used in psychopathology, in *Handbook of Studies on Anxiety*, G. D. Burrows and B. Davies, eds., pp. 1–15, Elsevier/North Holland Biomedical, Amsterdam, 1980.

Möhler, H. and Okada, T.: Benzodiazepine receptor: Demonstration in the central nervous system. *Science* **198**: 849–851, 1977.

Randall, L. O.: Pharmacology of Methaminodiazepoxide. *Dis. Nerv. System* **21** (Suppl.): 7–10, 1960.

Randall, L. O.: Discovery of benzodiazepines, in *Pharmacology of Benzodiazepines*, E. Usdin, P. Skolnick, J. F. Tallman, Jr., D. Greenblatt, and S. M. Paul, eds., pp. 15–21, Verlag Chemie, Deerfield Beach, FL, 1983.

Randall, L. O., Schallek, W., Heise, G. A., Keith, E. F., and Bagdon, R. E.: The psychosedative properties of methaminodiazepoxide. *J. Pharmacol. Exp. Ther.* **129:** 163–171, 1960.

Randall, L. O., Heise, G. A., Schalleck, W., Bagdon, R. E., Banziger, R., Boris, A., Moe, R. A., and Abrams, W. B.: Pharmacological and clinical studies on Valium®, a new psychotherapeutic agent of the benzodiazepine class. *Curr. Ther. Res.* **3:** 405–425, 1961.

Rickels, K.: Use of antianxiety agents in anxious outpatients. *Psychopharmacology* **58:** 1–17, 1978.

Rickels, K.: Are benzodiazepines overused and abused? *Br. J. Clin. Pharmacol.* **11:** 17S–83S, 1981a.

Rickels, K.: Benzodiazepines: Clinical use patterns, in *Benzodiazepines: A Review of Research Results 1980,* S. I. Szara and J. P. Ludford, eds., pp. 43–59, National Institute on Drug Abuse Res. Monograph Series, US Department of Health and Human Services, Washington, DC, 1981b.

Rosenbaum, J. F.: The drug treatment of anxiety. *N. Engl. J. Med.* **306:** 401–404, 1982.

Rubinstein, G. and Norman, T. R.: Newer antianxiety agents, in *Antianxiety Agents,* G. D. Burrows, T. R. Norman, and B. Davies, eds., pp. 199–215, Elsevier, Amsterdam, 1984.

Squires, R. F. and Braestrup, C.: Benzodiazepine receptors in rat brain. *Nature* **266:** 732–734, 1977.

Sternbach, L. H.: The discovery of Librium. *Agents Actions* **2:** 193–196, 1972.

Sternbach, L. H.: The benzodiazepines story. *Prog. Drug Res.* **22:** 229–266, 1978.

Sternbach, L. H. and Reeder, E.: Quinazolines and 1,4-benzodiazepines. II. The rearrangement of 6-chloro-2-chloromethyl-4-phenylquinazoline 3-oxide into 2-amino derivatives of 7-chloro-5-phenyl-3H-1,4-benzodiazepine 4-oxide. *J. Org. Chem.* **26:** 1111–1118, 1961a.

Sternbach, L. H. and Reeder, E.: Quinazolines and 1,4-benzodiazepines. IV. Transformations of 7-chloro-2-methylamino-5-phenyl-3H-1,4-benzodiazepine 4-oxide. *J. Org. Chem.* **26:** 4936–4941, 1961b.

Symposium on Chlordiazepoxide. *Dis. Nerv. System* **22** (Suppl.): 1–70, 1961.

Symposium on Newer Antidepressant and Other Psychotherapeutic Drugs. Pt. I. Librium: *Dis. Nerv. System* **21** (Suppl.): 1–60, 1960.

Tobin, J. M., Bird, I. F., and Boyle, D. E.: Preliminary evaluation of Librium (Ro 5-0690) in the treatment of anxiety reactions. *Dis. Nerv. System* **21** (Suppl.): 11–19, 1960.

Trimble, M. R., ed., *Benzodiazepines Divided: A Multidisciplinary Review.* Wiley, Chichester, 1983.

Neurology Group

L-Dopa

Carbamazepine

Diazepam (see Psychiatry Group)

L-Dopa

I. L-Dopa* as an Innovative Therapeutic Agent

Parkinson's disease ("shaking palsy," paralysis agitans) is a disabling disease. Its main clinical features are tremor during rest, rigidity, slowness of movement (bradykinesia, akinesia), and impaired postural and righting reflexes. These abnormalities produce dysarthria, dysphagia, festinant gait, mask-like facies, infrequent blinking, drooling, and seborrhea (Hoehn and Yahr, 1967; Marks, 1974). Parkinson's disease is one of the most common chronic neurologic diseases of late adulthood, striking in the fifth and sixth decade of life (Calne and Sandler, 1970; Perlik et al., 1980). Life expectancy for the untreated patient is only 5–14 yr after diagnosis. Compared to the general population, the untreated Parkinson patient has a shorter life span and a three-times-higher mortality rate. Untreated Parkinsonians are especially susceptible to bronchopneumonia as a consequence of immobilization and debilitation (Hoehn and Yahr, 1967). As the life expectancy of the general population increases, an increase in the number of Parkinson's disease cases is to be expected.

Before L-dopa, belladonna alkaloids and other anticholinergics were the drugs of choice. These drugs controlled tremor, had some effect on rigidity but had no effect on akinesia. Their therapeutic effects were not long-lasting. Amphetamine-like drugs and apomorphine were also used to treat Parkinson's disease. By the oral route, neither apomorphine nor the amphetamine-like drugs were extremely useful. A nonpharmacologic intervention that was exten-

---

*L-Dopa is an acronym for the naturally occurring amino acid levo-dihydroxy-phenylalanine. DL-Dopa is the racemic synthetic form. Endogenous dopa is always the L form.

sively employed was stereotaxic thalamic surgery (Cooper, 1956). This method had some effect against tremor and rigidity, but had no effect on, or aggravated, the akinesia that was responsible for most of the disabling symptoms.

The introduction of L-dopa therapy brought dramatic relief to the Parkinson patient: it improved the quality of life and brought life expectancy in line with the general population. This drug created worldwide enthusiasm not only because it controlled the symptoms of tremor and rigidity, but also because, for the first time, akinesia was improved. L-Dopa is regarded as a milestone in neurological therapeutics because it was the first agent that pharmacologically restored functional loss caused by the destruction of a specific subset of central neurons (Yahr 1975, 1978). However, it is symptomatic therapy and does not cure or stop the progression of Parkinson's disease (Lesser et al., 1979; Shaw et al., 1980). Nonetheless, L-dopa has made self-sufficient existence possible for many Parkinson's patients. Seventy percent of patients respond well to this drug which may provide them with several years of symptomatic relief from their disorder (Bianchine, 1976).

A high-dose regimen of L-dopa is needed to alleviate Parkinson symptoms (as shown by Cotzias; *see* section II). Unfortunately, after several years, such a regimen frequently leads to a range of adverse effects that limit its therapeutic usefulness, including adventitious movements (dyskinesia or chorea), "on–off" phenomena (rapid and seemingly unpredictable fluctuations in motor performance), confusion, hallucinations, and mood disorders (Birkmayer and Riederer, 1983; Hershey, 1985). It is not known whether these problems are the result of long-term L-dopa therapy or of the progression of the disease. Probably both factors play a part (Lesser et al., 1979).

Barbeau (1981) opined that L-dopa, alone or with other compounds, is still the best possible treatment for Parkinson's disease. Some clinicians believe that L-dopa should be withheld until it is absolutely necessary and that patients should be maintained on anticholinergics or dopamine-receptor agonists. Others believe that patients should be treated as soon as possible with the lowest dose of L-dopa that maintains quality of life by permitting reasonable physical activity and psychological well-being. They accept less therapeutic effect in favor of lower side effects.

Many reviews on the role of L-dopa in the management of Parkinson's disease are available; *see,* for example, Cotzias (1971), Calne (1977), Barbeau (1981), and Birkmayer and Riederer (1983).

L-Dopa has also been investigated for the treatment of dementia, manganese intoxication (Bennett, 1983), congestive heart failure (Woodruff, 1986), hepatic encephalopathy, and for diagnosis of pituitary disorders and of presymptomatic Huntington's disease (Yahr, 1975).

Early Clinical Research History

The early clinical research history is intimately involved in the scientific development of L-dopa and will, therefore, be discussed in section II.

II. The Scientific Work Leading to L-Dopa as a Treatment For Parkinsonism

Reserpine was shown to deplete norepinephrine and epinephrine from animal tissues (Bertler et al., 1956; Carlsson and Hillarp, 1956), including brain (Carlsson et al., 1957a). These depletions, especially of norepinephrine from brain, were considered to be responsible for many of the effects of reserpine in animals, e.g., tranquilization, hunched posture, ptosis, lowered body temperature.

Carlsson et al. (1957b) also demonstrated, in animals, that the tranquilization and ptosis induced by reserpine could be antagonized by the administration of the catecholamine precursor, DL-dopa (Fig. 1). Iproniazid, a monoamine oxidase inhibitor, reduced the dose of DL-dopa required, presumably by delaying the catabolism of a catecholamine formed from the DL-dopa.

Using an improved assay technique, Carlsson et al. (1958) went on to demonstrate unequivocally that dopamine (Fig. l) was present in the brain of rabbits. The dopamine concentration was equal to that of norepinephrine. The authors noted that such parity was not to be expected if dopamine were simply a precursor compound. Reserpine treatment depleted these brain dopamine stores, and the administration of L-dopa caused a sharp increase in brain dopamine.

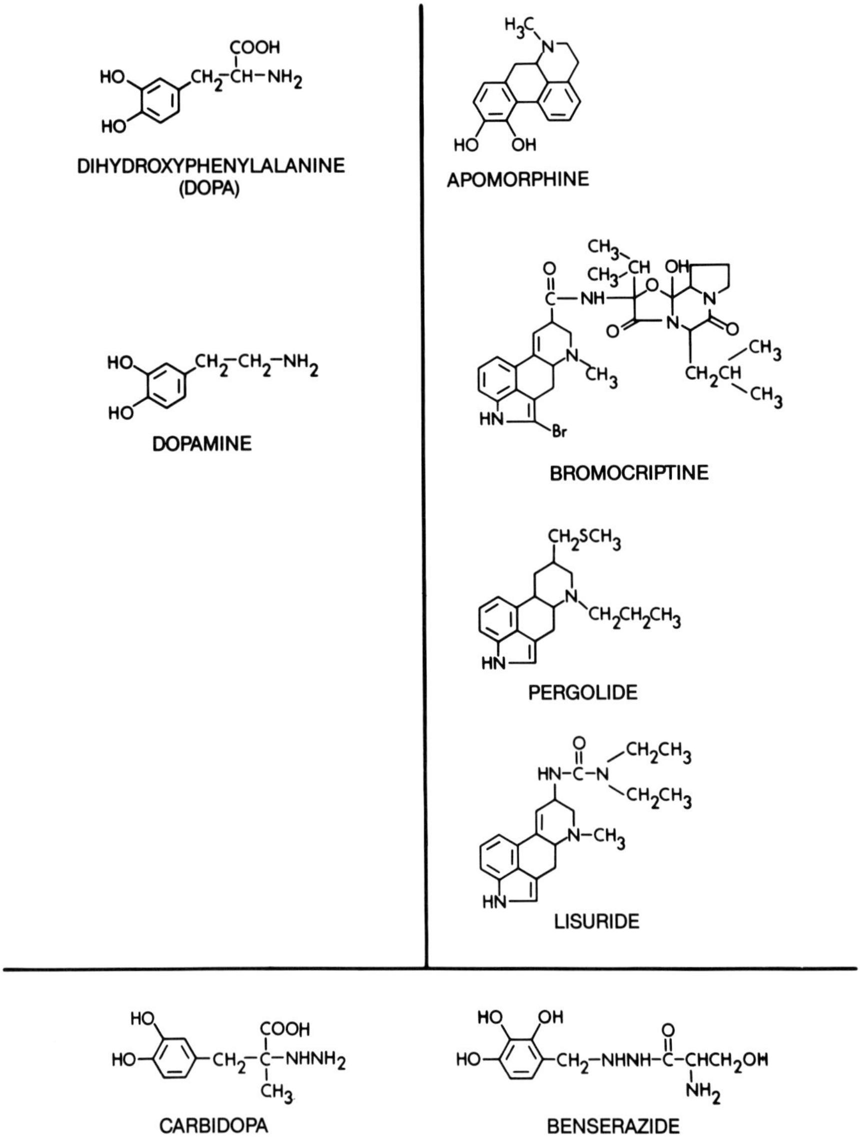

Fig. 1. The structures of dopa and chemically and/or pharmacologically related substances.

Carlsson and his associates concluded that dopamine probably had a function of its own in the brain in addition to acting as a precursor compound.

Bertler and Rosengren (1959) showed in animals, and Sano et al. (1959) in humans, that dopamine and norepinephrine were localized in different parts of the brain, whereas dopa (Sano et al., 1959) had no particular localization. Both groups found dopamine to be mainly in the striatum of the basal ganglia. Both groups of investigators also concluded that the selective presence of dopamine in the extrapyramidal system was evidence for dopamine having functions in the brain separate from its role as a precursor. Finally, both groups commented that the striatum was known to be concerned with central motor function, since it was a part of the extrapyramidal motor system, and that dopamine might be involved in this motor function.

Ehringer and Hornykiewicz (1960) noted that they were stimulated by the results of Carlsson et al. (1958) and Bertler and Rosengren (1959) to examine norepinephrine and dopamine concentrations in the brains of postmortem patients. Patients who had had akinetic syndromes contained low levels of dopamine in their neostriata. Patients who had had hyperkinetic extrapyramidal syndromes, such as Huntington's chorea, contained normal amounts of dopamine in this tissue. These investigators considered it logical to relate the akinetic, hypertonic symptoms seen in Parkinsonism to the deficiency of dopamine in the striatum.

Barbeau (1960, 1961) found that patients with various basal ganglia disorders had a high excretion of a poorly defined catecholamine-like pressor substance in their urine. Barbeau (1960, 1961), who was admittedly influenced by the findings of Carlsson and his associates, suggested that Parkinson's disease and other extrapyramidal diseases might be the result of faulty catecholamine metabolism and, in particular, dopamine catabolism. Subsequently, Barbeau et al. (1961a) demonstrated that 16 Parkinson patients had less dopamine in their urine than did normals.

Birkmayer and Hornykiewicz (1961), and Barbeau et al. (1961b), working independently, used L-dopa to treat Parkinson's disease. Birkmayer and Hornykiewicz (1961) found that intravenous doses of 50–150 mg gave substantial, transient relief from akinesia. Patients walked, ran, and jumped, and their speech became strong and clear. A monoamine oxidase inhibitor prolonged the effect. These authors felt that these findings could be the start of rational therapy for Parkinsonism. Barbeau et al. (1961b) administered 100–200 mg of L-dopa by the oral route. There was a marked effect on rigidity and a lesser effect on tremor. Chronic administration to two Parkinson's disease patients produced "relatively promising" results.

Cotzias et al (1967) treated 16 Parkinson patients with DL-dopa by the oral route for many months. Because several studies using the oral route had led to less-than-convincing results (McGeer et al., 1961; Friedhoff et al., 1963; McGeer and Zeldowicz, 1964; Fehling, 1966), they started with a low dose, and slowly and incrementally increased it to levels that were greatly in excess of those used in earlier studies (i.e., to doses of 3–16 g by mouth, daily). These large, sustained doses of DL-dopa markedly decreased many Parkinson symptoms, including rigidity and tremor. Cotzias et al. (1967) concluded that a long-term investigation with high doses of L-dopa was warranted. Many clinical studies with high doses followed. Marks (1974) noted that since 1967 there had been many studies, involving a total of some 5000 patients. They had received the drug for periods of up to 3–4 yr with good results.

Table 1 defines the critical scientific ideas and experiments leading to L-dopa as an anti-Parkinson agent and categorizes their origin.

Background Contributions
Preceding L-Dopa in Parkinsonism

Work that had been carried out from the 1930s through the 1950s established the biosynthetic pathway—in chromaffin tissue and in adrenergic neurons—that linked dietary amino acids with the catecholamines (Blaschko 1957, 1959). These contributions firmly established a role for dopamine as an immediate precursor to norepinephrine:

	(tyrosine hydroxylase)		(dopa decarboxylase)		(dopamine betahydroxylase)		(N-methyl transferase)	
tyrosine	→	dopa	→	dopamine	→	norepinephine	→	epinephrine

The plant *Rauwolfia serpentina* Benth had been used in folk medicine in India for centuries. Scientific studies by Indian investigators confirmed that extracts of the plant had sedative and hypo-

Table 1
Profile of Observations and Ideas Crucial to the Development of L-Dopa[a]

Sequence: Route to innovative drug**	Orient- ation	Nature of study	Research institution	National origin	Nature of discovery	Screening involved	Crucial ideas or observations
L-Dopa**							
Carlsson et al. (1957a)	Pre- clinical	Pharma- cology	Uni- versity	Sweden	Orderly	No	Reserpine depletes catecholamines from brain.
Carlsson et al. (1957b)	Pre- clinical	Pharma- cology	Uni- versity	Sweden	Orderly	No	CNS effects of reser- pine antagonized by DL-dopa.
Carlsson et al. (1958)	Pre- clinical	Biochem- istry	Uni- versity	Sweden	Orderly	No	Dopamine occurs in brain; dopamine is depleted by reser- pine and replenished by L-dopa.
Bertler and Rosengren (1959)	Pre- clinical	Biochem- istry	Uni- versity	Sweden	Orderly	No	Dopamine localized in striatum in animals; dopamine may act in central motor function; reserpine known to elicit Parkinson-like syndrome in humans.
Ehringer and Horny- kiewicz (1960)	Clinical	Biochem- istry, neur- ology	Uni- versity	Austria	Orderly	No	Striatal dopamine depleted in Parkinsonism.
Birkmayer and Horny- kiewicz (1961)	Clinical	Neur- ology	Hospital, uni- versity	Austria	Orderly	No	Dopa has positive effects in Parkinsonism.

[a]Taken from section II. Entries are those contributions without which the discovery of the agent (or additionally, in some cases, a relevant clinical application) would not have taken place or would have been materially delayed.

tensive properties (summarized by Dikshit, 1980). Reserpine, the active principle of *Rauwolfia*, was isolated by Müller et al. (1952) and later characterized. In the 1950s, reserpine was widely prescribed for the treatment of psychiatric disorders and for hypertension. Reserpine produced Parkinson-like symptoms (Steck, 1954) and de- pression in many of the psychiatric and hypertensive patients that were treated with it. Reserpine was shown to deplete serotonin from the brains of animals (Pletscher et al., 1956).

III. Comments on Events
Leading to L-Dopa

Several investigators point to L-dopa as a clear example of rational drug therapy—a form of replacement therapy—that resulted from the direct application of discoveries in basic research to clinical studies (*see* Hornykiewicz, 1971, 1977; Marks, 1974). Marks (1974) commented, "Although the pathological anatomy [of Parkinsonism] was largely understood by the 1920s,...the next advance...stemmed from...studies in psychopharmacology." Carlsson (1971), looking back, felt that the extrapyramidal side effects of reserpine in humans established a link between higher brain functions and certain biogenic amines. With the benefit of 15 years distance from the events, Carlsson (1972) stated broadly, "Drug-induced Parkinsonism has thus proved to be a useful disease model whereby it has been possible to develop a new pharmacologic principle for treatment of Parkinson's disease."

Hornykiewicz (1977) was of the opinion that the therapeutic efficacy of anticholinergic drugs in improving some symptoms of Parkinson's disease actually "led researchers astray" by making them believe that Parkinson's disease was a disorder of the cholinergic mechanisms of the brain. He credited the Swedish workers (Carlsson and associates) with being responsible for his interest in catecholamines and Parkinsonism. Hornykiewicz (1977) also called attention to the fact that in the 1940s Wilhelm Raab had discovered the pertinent facts about brain dopamine. Raab (1948) and Raab and Gigee (1951) described the occurrence of a new catechol in mammalian brain (including human), located predominantly in the striatal region; Raab called this "encephalin," and he studied the effect of many drugs on this substance. L-Dopa dramatically increased the concentration of encephalin. Hornykiewicz felt that, had Raab studied the brain of Parkinson's disease patients, he would have discovered that they were low in encephalin.

McDowell (1971) remembered that in 1966 clinicians were so disappointed with L-dopa therapy that it seemed to be but another unfounded hope. Symptoms were rarely relieved, and the side effects were pronounced: nausea, vomiting, postural hypotension, infrequent arrhythmias, depression. In like vein, Marks (1974) noted that the results of studies in 1966 were not encouraging. Only a few patients showed a response, and this was usually of a short duration. Barbeau (1981) stated that the many side effects of L-dopa "...almost ruled out further development of the drug," until Cotzias et al. (1967) introduced a stepwise regimen to high doses. Cotzias is widely credited with taking L-dopa out of the theoretical realm and making it a practical treatment. Hornykiewicz (1971) remarked that Cotzias and associates, with their regimen of high oral doses removed the last doubt about the efficacy of L-dopa. Cooper (1971), who had treated tremor and rigidity neurosurgically, after reviewing Cotzias' data agreed that L-dopa was a better choice than surgery for treatment of Parkinson's disease. He had performed 900 operations to alleviate symptoms of Parkinson's disease in 1967. This number was reduced to 50 in 1970.

IV. Developments Subsequent to L-Dopa

A major advance in the therapeutic use of L-dopa was its combination with a dopa-decarboxylase inhibitor. This permitted a substantial reduction in the dose of L-dopa and, as a result, led to a reduction in peripheral side effects, namely, cardiac arrhythmias and nausea. Udenfriend et al. (1966) noticed that a dopa-decarboxylase inhibitor, which would be expected to reduce the production of catecholamines, actually enhanced the dopa-induced increase of brain catecholamines. Likewise, in humans, a decarboxylase inhibitor potentiated and prolonged the ameliorative effect of L-dopa on akinesia (Birkmayer and Mentasti, 1967). Bartholini et al. (1967) showed that a decarboxylase inhibitor, at lower doses, acted as a preferential inhibitor of decarboxylase in the periphery. They demonstrated that, since dopa could not be decarboxylated in peripheral tissue, there was more of it in the peripheral circulation and, therefore, more of it penetrated the brain, where it continued to be decarboxylated. Combining L-dopa with peripherally acting, dopa-decarboxylase inhibitors (carbidopa, benserazide [Fig. 1]) is now routine clinical practice.

The degeneration of dopamine neurons in the substantia nigra of the Parkinson patient leads to progressive loss of the dopa-decarboxylase within the striatum (Lloyd and Hornykiewicz, 1970). Reduction in the rate of conversion of L-dopa to dopamine occurs, as well as reduction in the capacity for storage of dopamine (Hornykiewicz, 1973). However, the receptors for dopamine, which are located postsynaptically, remain sensitive to direct-acting dopamine-like agonists. Two classes of dopamine agonists have been discovered. These are the aporphines (apomorphine) and the ergolines (bromocriptine, lisuride, and pergolide) (Fig. 1). Bromocriptine is the drug most often used in humans as a dopamine-receptor agonist. Unfortunately, it does not stimulate the neostriatum selectively. It can be used alone when patients should no longer receive L-dopa, or before L-dopa therapy is initiated in the early stages of Parkinson's disease. However, this drug is most effective when used as adjuvant therapy with L-dopa (Lieberman et al., 1979). The ideal dopamine agonist would be one that selectively stimulates those dopamine receptors in the neostriatum that restore motor function, but has no effect on those dopamine receptors that mediate unwanted effects, such as dyskinesia, confusion, and nausea. Such an agent is yet to be found.

The development of L-dopa led to the recognition that neurological disorders have biochemical correlates that can be influenced and improved by drugs; this in turn has stimulated research into the biochemical pharmacology of the brain (Birkmayer and Riederer, 1983).

References

Barbeau, A.: Preliminary observations on abnormal catecholamine metabolism in basal ganglia diseases. *Neurology* **10**: 446–451, 1960.

Barbeau, A.: Dopamine and basal ganglia diseases. *Arch. Neurol.* **4**: 109–114, 1961.

Barbeau, A.: The use of L-dopa in Parkinson's disease: A 20 year follow up. *Trends Pharm. Sci.* **2**: 297–299, 1981.

Barbeau, A., Murphy, G. F., and Sourkes, T. L.: Excretion of dopamine in diseases of basal ganglia. *Science* **133**: 1706, 1707, 1961a.

Barbeau, A., Sourkes, T. L., and Murphy, G. F.: Les catecholamines dans la maladie de Parkinson, in *Monoamines et Systemes Nerveaux Central,* pp. 247–262, Symp. de Bel Air, Geneva, Sept., 1961b.

Bartholini, G., Burkard, W. P., and Pletscher, A.: Increase of cerebral catecholamines caused by 3,4-dihydroxyphenylalanine after inhibition of peripheral decarboxylase. *Nature* 215: 852, 853, 1967.

Bennett, D. R., ed.: *AMA Drug Evaluations,* 5th Ed., pp. 284, 1144, American Medical Association, Chicago, 1983.

Bertler, A. and Rosengren, E.: Occurrence and distribution of dopamine in brain and other tissues. *Experientia* 15: 10, 11, 1959.

Bertler, A., Carlsson, A., and Rosengren, E.: Release by reserpine of catecholamines from rabbit hearts. *Naturwissenschaften* 43: 521, 1956.

Bianchine, J. R.: Drug therapy of Parkinsonism. *N. Engl. J. Med.* 295: 814–818, 1976.

Birkmayer, W. and Hornykiewicz, O.: Der L-3,4-Dioxyphenylalanine (=Dopa)-Effekt bei der Parkinson-Akinese. *Wien. Klin. Wochenschr.* 45: 787, 788, 1961.

Birkmayer, W. and Mentasti, M.: Weitere experimentelle untersuchungen über den catecholaminstoffwechsel bei extrapyramidalen erkrankungen (Parkinson- und Chorea Syndrom). *Arch. Psychiatric Nerven Kr.* 210: 29–35, 1967.

Birkmayer, W. and Riederer, P.: *Parkinson's Disease. Biochemistry, Clinical Pathology, and Treatment,* Springer-Verlag, New York, 1983.

Blaschko, H.: Metabolism and storage of biogenic amines. *Experientia* 13: 9–12, 1957.

Blaschko, H.: The development of current concepts of catecholamine formation. *Pharmacol. Rev.* 11: 307–316, 1959.

Calne, D. B.: Developments in the pharmacology and therapeutics of parkinsonism. *Ann. Neurol.* 1: 111–119, 1977.

Calne, D. B. and Sandler, M.: L-dopa and parkinsonism. *Nature* 226: 21–24, 1970.

Carlsson, A.: L-Dopa: The pharmacological rationale, in *Developments in Treatment for Parkinson's Disease.,* G. C. Cotzias and F. H. McDowell, eds., pp. 65–77, Medcom, New York, 1971.

Carlsson, A.: Biochemical and pharmacological aspects of parkinsonism. *Acta Neurol. Scand. (Supp.)* 51: 11–42, 1972.

Carlsson, A. and Hillarp, N. A.: Release of adrenaline from the adrenal medulla of rabbits produced by reserpine. *Kgl. Fysiogr. Sallsk. Lund Forh.* 26: Nr8, 1956.

Carlsson, A., Lindqvist, M., and Magnusson, T.: 3,4-Dihydroxyphenylalanine and 5-hydroxytryptophan as reserpine antagonists. *Nature* 180: 1200, 1957b.

Carlsson, A., Lindqvist, M., Magnusson, T., and Waldeck, B.: On the presence of 3-hydroxytyramine in brain. *Science* **127**: 471, 1958.

Carlsson, A., Rosengren, E., Bertler, A., and Nilsson, J.: Effect of reserpine on the metabolism of catecholamines, in *Psychotropic Drugs*, S. Garattini and V. Ghetti, eds., pp. 363–372, Elsevier, New York, 1957a.

Cooper, I. S.: *The Neurosurgical Alleviation of Parkinsonism*, Charles C. Thomas, Springfield, IL, 1956.

Cooper, I. S.: L-Dopa from a neurosurgeon's point of view, in *Developments in Treatment for Parkinson's Disease*, G. C. Cotzias and F. H. McDowell, eds., p. 56, Medcom, New York, 1971.

Cotzias, G. C.: Levodopa in the treatment of parkinsonism. *JAMA* **218**: 1903–1908, 1971.

Cotzias, G. C., Van Woert, M. H., and Schiffer, L. M.: Aromatic amino acids and modification of parkinsonism. *N. Engl. J. Med.* **276**: 374–379, 1967.

Dikshit, R. K.: The story of rauwolfia. *Trends Pharm.* I(16): viii–x, 1980.

Ehringer, H. and Hornykiewicz, O.: Verteilung von noradrenalin und dopamin (3-hydroxytryramin) im gehirn des menschen und ihr verhalten bei erkrankungen des extrapyramidalen systems. *Wien. Klin. Wochenschr.* **38**: 1236–1239, 1960.

Fehling, C.: Treatment of Parkinson's syndrome with L-dopa. A double blind study. *Acta Neurol. Scand.* **42**: 367–372, 1966.

Friedhoff, A. J., Hekimian, L., Alpert, M., and Tobach, E.: Dihydroxyphenylalanine in extrapyramidal disease. *JAMA* **184**: 285, 286, 1963.

Hershey, L. A.: Controversies in the treatment of Parkinson's disease. *Ration. Drug Ther.* **19**: 1-7, 1985.

Hoehn, M. M. and Yahr, M. D.: Parkinsonism: Onset, progression and mortality. *Neurology* **17**: (5) 427–442, 1967.

Hornykiewicz, O.: Advances in neurochemistry and pharmacology of Parkinson's disease, in *Developments in Treatment for Parkinson's Disease*, G. C. Cotzias and F. H. McDowell, eds., pp. 25–31, Medcom, New York, 1971.

Hornykiewicz, O.: Dopamine in the basal ganglia. *Br. Med. Bull.* **29**: 172–178, 1973.

Hornykiewicz, O.: Historical aspects and frontiers of Parkinson's disease research, in *Parkinson's Disease. Neurological, Clinical and Related Aspects.* F. S. Messiha and A. D. Kenny, eds., pp. 1–8, Plenum, New York, 1977.

Lesser, R. P., Fahn, S., Snider, S. R., Cote, L. J., Isgreen, W. P., and Barrett, R. E.: Analysis of the clinical problems in parkinsonism and the complications of long-term levodopa therapy. *Neurology* **29**: 1253–1260, 1979.

Lieberman, A., Neophytides, A., Kupersmith, M., Casson, I., Durso, R., Hoo Foo, S., Khayali, M., Tartaro, T., and Goldstein, M.: Treatment of Parkinson's disease with dopamine agonists: A review. *Am. J. Med. Sci.* **278**: 65–76, 1979.

Lloyd, K. and Hornykiewicz, O.: Parkinson's Disease: Activity of L-dopa decarboxylase in discrete brain regions. *Science* **170:** 1212, 1213, 1970.
McDowell, F. H.: *Developments in Treatment for Parkinson's Disease,* G. C. Cotzias and F. H. McDowell, eds., p. 9, Medcom, New York, 1971.
McGeer, P. L., Boulding, J. E., Gibson, W. C., and Foulkes, R. G.: Drug-induced extrapyramidal reactions. *JAMA* **177:** 665–670, 1961.
McGeer, P. L. and Zeldowicz, L. R.: Administration of dihydroxyphenylalanine to parkinsonian patients. *J. Can. Med. Assoc.* **90:** 463–466, 1964.
Marks, J.: Trials of oral therapy, in *The Treatment of Parkinsonism with L-Dopa,* pp. 81–83, American Elsevier, New York, 1974.
Müller, J. M., Schlittler, E., and Bein, H. J.: Reserpin, der sedative Wirkstoff aus Rauwolfia serpentina Benth. *Experientia* **8:** 338, 1952.
Perlik, S. J., Koller, W. C., Weiner, W. J., Nausieda, P., and Klawans, H. L.: Parkinsonism: Is your treatment appropriate? *Geriatrics* **35:** (II) 65–74, 1980.
Pletscher, A., Shore, P. A., and Brodie, B. B: Serotonin as a mediator of reserpine action in brain. *J. Pharmacol. Exp. Ther.* **116:** 84–89, 1956.
Raab, W.: Specific sympathomimetic substance in the brain. *Am. J. Physiol.* **152:** 324–339, 1948.
Raab, W. and Gigee, W.: Concentration and distribution of "encephalin" in the brain of humans and animals. *Proc. Soc. Exp. Biol. Med.* **76:** 97–100, 1951.
Sano, I., Gamo, T., Kakimoto, Y., Taniguchi, K., Takesada, M., and Nishinuma, K.: Distribution of catechol compounds in human brain. *Biochim. Biophys. Acta* **32:** 586, 587, 1959.
Shaw, K. M., Lees, A. J., and Stern, G. M.: The impact of treatment with levodopa on Parkinson's disease. *Q. J. Med.* **195:** 283–293, 1980.
Steck, H. Le syndrome extra-pyramidal et diencéphalique au cours des traitements au Largactil et au Serpasil. *Ann. Méd. Psychol. (Paris)* **112**(2): 737–743, 1954.
Udenfriend, S., Zaltzman-Nirenberg, P., Gordon, R., and Spector, S.: Evaluation of the biochemical effects produced *in vivo* by inhibitors of the three enzymes involved in norepinephrine biosynthesis. *Mol. Pharmacol.* **2:** 95–105, 1966.
Woodruff, G. N.: Dwindling dopamine receptors. *Trends Pharm. Sci.* **7:** 252, 253, 1986.
Yahr, M. D.: Levodopa. *Ann. Intern. Med.* **83:** 677–682, 1975.
Yahr, M. D.: Overview of present day treatment of Parkinson's disease. *J. Neural Transm.* **43:** 227–238, 1978.

Carbamazepine

I. Carbamazepine as an Innovative Therapeutic Agent

Epilepsies are a group of diverse chronic disorders of the brain, characterized by frequent recurring seizures (i.e., transient, reversible disturbances of movement, sensation, behavior, perception, and/or consciousness) that are caused by abnormal, excessive discharges of a population of hyperexcitable neurons within the brain (Gastaut and Broughton, 1973; Sutherland et al., 1974; Gallagher, 1977; Penry and Porter, 1979).

There are two major categories of seizures (Dreifuss, 1981; Rall and Schleifer, 1985):

1. Partial seizures (also called focal or local), which originate in a restricted pool of abnormal neurons, limited initially to one hemisphere of the brain. Partial seizures are further categorized as "complex" or "simple" depending on whether consciousness is lost (complex) or is not lost (simple). Complex partial seizures are commonly called "psychomotor epilepsy" or "temporal lobe epilepsy," and frequently involve both cerebral hemispheres. A simple partial seizure may progress to a complex partial seizure. Furthermore, a complex partial seizure may also progress to a generalized motor seizure.
2. Generalized seizures, which reflect widespread neuronal discharge in both cerebral hemispheres. Prominent members of this category are (a) tonic-clonic seizures (grand mal), characterized by tonic-clonic convulsions and by prolonged depression of all central functions, and (b) absence seizures (petit mal), characterized by brief, abrupt losses of consciousness and by some clonic motor activity.

Patients with convulsive seizures of generalized epilepsy or with some forms of partial epilepsies compose 85–90% of all the classifiable instances of epilepsy (Eadie, 1980).

Epilepsy is a serious health problem. According to Hauser (1978) the worldwide prevalence of this disease is about 5/1000 of the population. Porter et al. (1984) commented that 2.5 million (1%) of all Americans have epilepsy and 200,000 have more than one seizure per month. Eadie and Tyrer (1980) pointed out that although epilepsy is not usually a life-threatening disease, it has very detrimental effects on the quality of life. This detriment increases as society becomes more complex and technological (e.g., problems in driving automobiles or operating machinery).

Carbamazepine (Fig. 1) is a major antiepileptic drug with a broad spectrum of activity that benefits all the more common forms of epilepsy. It is most effective in tonic-clonic seizures and partial seizures, whether the seizures become secondarily generalized or not (Alvin and Bush, 1977; Gallagher, 1977; Lander and Eadie, 1987). It should be noted that although the "classic" antiepileptic drugs, phenobarbital and phenytoin (diphenylhydantoin) (Fig. l), are used in complex partial seizures, carbamazepine is considered by many clinicians to be the drug of choice for this condition (Delgado-Escueta, 1983; Lampe, 1986). Like phenobarbital and phenytoin, carbamazepine is not effective in absence seizures.

In addition to being outstandingly effective in partial seizures, carbamazepine ranks as an innovative therapeutic agent because, unlike phenobarbital and phenytoin, it lacks debilitating side effects. Phenobarbital has the disadvantages of producing sedation, lethargy, and mental dullness, and causing hyperactivity and short attention span in children (Gallagher, 1977). In a similar vein, although phenytoin is an effective anticonvulsant and lacks the sedative side effects of phenobarbital, it causes hirsutism and gum hypertrophy, coarsens the face, and affects mental function (Penry and Porter, 1979). Carbamazepine does not interfere with cognitive functions and learning; for this reason, it is especially useful in children. Additionally, it has been found to be particularly useful in females approaching puberty and in women, since it does not cause cosmetic disfigurement (Bladin, 1987; Vajda, 1987).

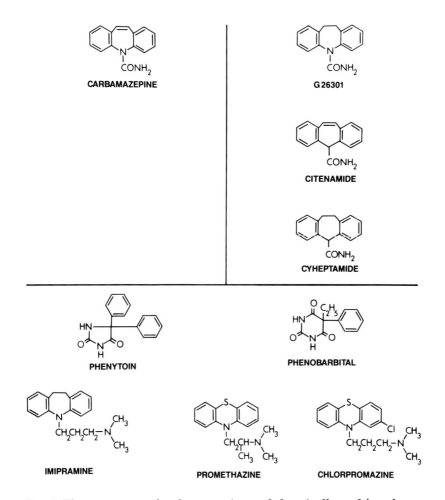

Fig. 1. The structures of carbamazepine and chemically and/or pharmacologically related substances.

According to Reynolds (1981), carbamazepine may be the drug of choice in epileptic patients with psychological disorders. Because it did not interfere with mental functions, as did phenobarbital and phenytoin, replacement of these agents with carbamazepine led to striking improvement in some chronic epileptic patients with intellectual, personality, or psychiatric problems. Post et al. (1983) found carbamazepine to have therapeutic effect in the control of mania, and, by analogy to epileptic seizures, considered that manic-depressive illness might be a "paroxysmal affective disregulation." These investigators suggested using carbamazepine in nonepileptic, manic-depressive patients who did not respond to lithium. Post and Uhde (1987) believed that, in addition to the future role of carbamazepine as an antimanic drug, it would be useful in dissecting the biochemical and pharmacological hypotheses of affective disorders.

Carbamazepine is also used for the treatment of pain from trigeminal neuralgia (Blom, 1962). It is almost universally accepted as the drug of choice for this indication (Taylor et al., 1981) and for glossopharyngeal neuralgia (Rall and Schleifer, 1985).

Early Clinical Research History

Bonduelle et al. (1964a), at an international congress in 1962, reported on the treatment of 89 epileptic patients, 65 adults and 24 children, with carbamazepine. Of 40 patients who had temporal lobe epilepsy (i.e., complex partial seizures), 20 were almost completely relieved of their seizures, 12 others showed different degrees of improvement, and eight responded poorly or got worse. Thirty-eight patients had psychological problems and, interestingly, 32 of these showed remarkable improvement with carbamazepine therapy. Some of this effect was attributed to the reduction in barbiturate dosage and to the elimination of secondary drugs, but an inherent psychotropic action was also suggested. The investigators concluded that, except for petit mal (absence) seizures, carbamazepine controlled various forms of epileptic seizures better than any of the treatments that existed before it. In most cases the patients were also on phenobarbital; however, during treatment with carbamazepine, it was possible to eliminate or reduce other drugs. Carbamazepine was well tolerated and had only minor side effects.

Bonduelle et al. (1964b) updated their report of their experience with carbamazepine (which had grown to 100 patients, many of whom had been observed for over three years). As noted earlier (Bonduelle et al., 1964a), barbiturate treatment was maintained in most cases; however, it was reduced or, sometimes, eliminated as treatment with carbamazepine progressed. Carbamazepine replaced other antiepileptic drugs, such as hydantoins, primidone, and phenylacetylurea. Of the 100 patients with various forms of epilepsy, 69% had good results with carbamazepine; 31% were either complete or partial failures. Carbamazepine was particularly effective in psychomotor epilepsy (i.e., complex partial seizures); 34 out of 48 benefited from this therapy. Moreover, four out of six patients who had not previously been treated with other antiepileptic drugs had their seizures controlled with carbamazepine alone. Seventy-one percent of the patients showed improvement in mental function, anxiety, depression, aggressiveness, and irritability, in part as a result of the removal of previous medications.

Lorge (1964) used carbamazepine in the treatment of 66 inpatients and outpatients for over three years. He reported that it "...seems to act unspecifically on all forms of seizures with approximately the same intensity...." Carbamazepine also had pronounced beneficial psychotropic effects in their epileptic patients.

A flood of clinical trials of carbamazepine followed in Europe, England, and, eventually, in the USA. According to Cereghino et al. (1974) over 250 articles—almost all uncontrolled studies—were published worldwide. This investigator from the National Institute of Neurological Diseases and Stroke (Bethesda) and collaborators evaluated the anticonvulsant efficacy of carbamazepine in a prospective, double-blind study in 45 patients who were not well controlled by other anticonvulsants. Carbamazepine was found to be effective, and the positive findings of the many earlier, uncontrolled clinical reports were scientifically confirmed (Cereghino et al., 1974).

Many original articles, reviews and books discuss the evidence that substantiated these early clinical findings with carbamazepine (*see*, for example, Bird et al., 1966; Livingstone et al., 1967; Mercier, 1973; Penry and Daly, 1975; Vida, 1977; Kosteljanetz et al., 1979; Penry and Newmark, 1979; Glaser et al., 1980; Tyrer, 1980; Mikkelsen et al., 1981; Niedermeyer, 1983; Burrows et al., 1987).

II. The Scientific Work
Leading to Carbamazepine

Schindler (1961) synthesized 5-carbamoyl dibenzazepine (G 32883, later named carbamazepine) (Fig. l) by converting 5H-dibenz [b, f] azepine into the 5-(chlorocarbonyl) derivative and then treating this compound with ammonia. By using various amines in place of ammonia, additional, more elaborately 5-substituted derivatives were made. The author noted in his abstract that these substances had anticonvulsant activity.

Theobald and Kunz (1963), colleagues of Schindler, reported their studies concerning the anticonvulsant effects of carbamazepine in several animal species. Seizures induced by electric shock in rats came under control after oral administration of carbamazepine. In this test carbamazepine was approximately as effective as phenobarbital, and considerably more potent than diphenylhydantoin. Carbamazepine was also effective against strychnine convulsions in mice, but not very effective against pentetrazole or picrotoxin seizures. The compound had low toxicity as well as a slight tranquilizing and sedative effect. It should be noted that, in the brief introduction to their work, these authors commented, without documentation, that N-carbamoyl iminodibenzyl (G 26301) (Fig. 1)—the ring-saturated analog of carbamazepine—had been synthesized by Morel and shown to have anticonvulsant activity by Domenjoz as early as 1953. Theobald and Kunz (1963) also stated that clinical confirmation of the antiepileptic action of G 26301 led to the synthesis of additional carbamoyl compounds, culminating in the synthesis of carbamazepine by Schindler (1961).

Hernandez-Peon (1964), in work originally presented at a conference in 1962, reported implanting multipolar electrodes in the basolateral complex of the amygdala, the dorsal hippocampus, the posteromedial hypothalamus, and the precruciate gyrus (motor cortex) of 18 cats and studying the effects of carbamazepine on seizures evoked by electrical stimulation of the different areas when the animals were awake and unrestrained. He found that carbamazepine "...remarkably depressed or abolished amygdaloid and hippocampal after-discharges as well as their propagated activity to the hypothalamus." He suggested that these regions were probably involved in temporal lobe epilepsy. Carbamazepine was not as effective in bringing under control the seizures induced by the stimulation of the motor cortex. Hernandez-Peon wondered if, clinically, carbamazepine would be more selective for temporal lobe epilepsy (complex partial seizures) than for more generalized cortical seizures.

Table 1 defines the critical scientific ideas and experiments leading to carbamazepine and categorizes their origin.

Background Contributions Preceding Carbamazepine

From the turn of the twentieth century onward, there was a slowly burgeoning collaboration of synthetic organic chemistry and animal and/or clinical testing that led to the development of most modern drugs, including antiepileptic therapies. Von Baeyer had synthesized barbituric acid in 1864, and in 1912 a derivative of this substance, phenobarbital, was found, apparently by accident, to be useful in epilepsy (Hauptmann, 1912). In the 1930s, other structurally related compounds became available, namely, mephobarbital and phenytoin. Phenytoin was discovered through the use of a new experimental procedure for inducing seizures in cats via mouth-occipital electrodes (Putnam and Merritt, 1937; Merritt et al., 1938; Merritt and Putnam, 1938). Sodium phenytoin exhibited excellent anticonvulsant activity and few sedative side effects. Additional methods for producing experimental electroconvulsions were subsequently developed (see Toman and Goodman, 1946; Toman et al., 1947), as were additional methods for eliciting chemical convulsions. During the 1940s, 1950s, and early 1960s, new drugs followed, e.g., the acylureas, oxazolidinediones, succinamides, and benzodiazepines. Carbamazepine arrived on the therapeutic scene in Europe in the early 1960s.

Carbamazepine has a tricyclic ring system (referred to as either dibenzazepine or iminostilbene) that is similar to the tricyclic ring system (referred to as either dihydrodibenzazepine or iminodibenzyl) of the antidepressant drug imipramine (Fig. 1). This similarity of ring systems is a reflection of the fact that many tricyclic compounds, including imipramine, had been synthesized at the Geigy

Table 1
Profile of Observations and Ideas Crucial to the Development of Carbamazepine[a]

Sequence: Route to innovative drug**	Orient-ation	Nature of study	Research institution	National origin	Nature of discovery	Screening involved	Crucial ideas or observations
Carbamazepine**							
Schindler (1961)	Pre-clinical	Chem-istry/ pharma-cology	Industry	Switzer-land	Orderly	Targeted	Carbamazepine synthesized; anti-convulsant proper-ties recognized.

[a]Taken from section II. Entries are those contributions without which the discovery of the agent (or additionally, in some cases, a relevant clinical application) would not have taken place or would have been materially delayed.

Co. from 1948 onward as structural mimics of Rhone Poulenc's clinically successful phenothiazine compounds—the antihistamine, promethazine, and the neuroleptic, chlorpromazine (Fig. 1) (Schindler and Häfliger, 1954) (for details, *see* section II of the chapter on imipramine). The statement of Domenjoz and Theobald (1959) of Geigy Co., "We began a systematic pharmacological work on imi-nodibenzyls already 10 years ago," substantiates Geigy's early inter-est in tricyclic compounds. Carbamazepine had its origins in this general exploration of the iminodibenzyl ring system and its N-substitutions.

III. Comments on Events Leading to Carbamazepine

In 1962 the Kefauver-Harris Drug Amendment was enacted by the United States Congress. It required that, in addition to their safety, the efficacy of all new drugs had to be established. The very high costs of the comprehensive clinical trials that such an efficacy requirement demanded had a serious negative impact on the devel-opment of drugs for diseases that affected a limited population—the market was correspondingly small and the return on corporate investment doubtful (Swinyard, 1980; Porter et al., 1984). Epilepsy fell into this category. Furthermore, according to these authors, there were other problems specific to developing drugs for epilepsy:

1. There was an almost total lack of a patient population whose seizure types and frequencies were well defined.
2. The common use of multiple drugs complicated the design of suitable controlled clinical trials to establish efficacy of a new drug.
3. Many clinicians did not believe that controlled trials were necessary, resulting in a lack of the required scientific data on new antiepileptic drugs.

As Porter et al. (1984) pointed out, "A 1967 survey of pharmaceutical firms revealed that most had no new antiepileptic drugs under development due to prohibitive cost, while several drugs had not gained the approval of the U.S. Food and Drug Administration (FDA) because of inadequate proof of efficacy." These authors felt that, as a consequence, it took from 1960 until 1974 (except for the introduction of diazepam in 1968 as an adjunct agent) for the next agent, carbamazepine, to be introduced as an antiepileptic therapy in the USA.

In 1968 the Epilepsy Branch of the National Institute of Neurological and Communicative Disorders and Stroke (NINCDS) initiated and subsidized controlled clinical trials of seven drugs that required proof of efficacy before they could be used in therapy in the USA. The resulting data, according to Porter et al. (1984), supported the new drug applications (NDAs) for three agents, one of which was carbamazepine (Cereghino et al., 1974).

Carbamazepine, as noted above, has a tricyclic ring structure that closely resembles that of impramine and other tricyclic antidepressants; however, it has no antidepressant activity (Eadie and Tyrer, 1980). Furthermore, as a tricyclic compound, carbamazepine appears structurally unrelated to any other anticonvulsant drug (Livingstone et al., 1967). In this regard, Julien and Hollister (1975) pointed out that, although the formal two-dimensional structure of carbamazepine is very different from that of phenytoin (Fig. 1), a consideration of their three-dimensional structures (i.e., conformational possibilities) allowed for very significant superimposition of key components of the molecules. It seemed to these authors (with all the advantage that hindsight allows in these matters) that it was not surprising that both compounds had similar pharmacologic properties.

IV. Developments
Subsequent to Carbamazepine

Two tricyclic agents related to carbamazepine are mentioned in the literature as anticonvulsants: citenamide (Csáky and Barnes, 1984) (Fig. 1) and cyheptamide, noted by Csáky and Barnes (1984) and in *The Merck Index* (Windholz, 1983) (Fig. 1). However, these agents are not discussed in clinical compendia such as *Drug Evaluations* (Lampe, 1986) or *The Merck Manual* (Berkow, 1982).

Although considerable research has been carried out with antiepileptic drugs, including carbamazepine, it is not really understood how they work (Deupree, 1980). Suria and Killam (1980) discussed possible mechanisms for carbamazepine, but concluded that "...none of these satisfactorily and fully explains the molecular mechanism of action and the observed clinical efficacy of this extremely important and interesting drug."

Swinyard (1980) commented,

Until research workers can identify the underlying biochemical defect(s) in epilepsy and neuroscientists can precisely define the biochemical basis of convulsions, it will be difficult to design more selective laboratory models. Consequently, the discovery of drugs with really novel mechanisms of antiepileptic action will be difficult and perhaps largely a matter of chance.

It seems that, for the present at least, the search for new antiepileptic agents will have to continue to rely on screening a broad sampling of the prolific output of organic chemists in the few available, reliable seizure models. The Epilepsy Branch of the NINCDS continues to carry out an active program of preclinical screening and clinical testing, in collaboration with academia and industry, to encourage the development of new antiepileptic drugs (Porter et al., 1984).

References

Alvin, J. D. and Bush, M. T.: Physiological disposition of anticonvulsants in *Anticonvulsants*, J. A. Vida, ed., pp. 113–150, Academic, New York, 1977.

Berkow, R., ed.: *The Merck Manual,* 14th Ed., Merck Sharp & Dohme Research Laboratories, Rahway, NJ, 1982.

Bird, C. A. K., Griffin, B. P., Miklaszewska, J. M., and Galbraith, A. W.: Tegretol, carbamazepine: A controlled trial of a new anticonvulsant. *Br. J. Psychiatry* **112**: 737–742, 1966.

Bladin, P. F.: Anticonvulsants in children, in *Drugs in Psychiatry,* vol. 4: *Antimanics, Anticonvulsants and Other Drugs in Psychiatry,* G. D. Burrows, T. R. Norman, and B. Davies, eds., pp. 131–159, Elsevier, Amsterdam, 1987.

Blom, S.: Trigeminal neuralgia: Its treatment with a new anticonvulsant drug (G-32883). *Lancet* **1**: 839, 840, 1962.

Bonduelle, M., Bouygues, P., Sallou, C., and Chemaly, R.: Bilan de l' Experimentation Clinique de l' Anti-epileptique G 32883, in *Neuropsychopharmacology,* vol. 3: *Proceedings of the Third Meeting of the Collegium Internationale Neuro-psychopharmacologicum,* P. Bradley, F. Flugel, and P. Hock, eds., pp. 312–316, Elsevier, Amsterdam, 1964a.

Bonduelle, M., Bouygues, Sallou, C., and Grobius, S.: Experimentation clinique de l' anti-epileptique G 32883 (Tegretol): Resultants portant sur 100 cas observes en trois ans. *Rev. Neurol.* **110**: 209–215, 1964b.

Burrows, G. D., Norman, T. R., and Davies, B., eds.: *Drugs in Psychiatry,* vol. 4; *Antimanics, Anticonvulsants and Other Drugs in Psychiatry,* Elsevier, Amsterdam, 1987.

Cereghino, J. J., Brock, J. T., Van Meter, J. C., Penry, J. K., Smith, L. D., and White, B. G.: Carbamazepine for epilepsy. A controlled prospective evaluation. *Neurology* **24**: 401–410, 1974.

Csáky, T. Z. and Barnes, B. A.: *Cutting's Handbook of Pharmacology,* 7th Ed., Appleton-Century-Crofts, Norwalk, CT, 1984.

Delgado-Escueta, A. V.: Epilepsy in adolescents and adults, in *Current Therapy,* H. Conn, ed., pp. 707–717, W. B. Saunders, Philadelphia, 1983.

Deupree, J. D.: Mode of action of anticonvulsant drugs: Membrane effects, in *The Treatment of Epilepsy,* J. H. Tyrer, ed., pp. 1–28, J. B. Lippincott, Philadelphia, 1980.

Domenjoz, R. and Theobald, W.: Zur Pharmakologie des Tofranil. (N-(3-dimethyl-aminopropyl)-iminodibenzyl hydrochloride). *Arch. Int. Pharmacodyn.,* **25**: 450–489, 1959.

Dreifuss, F. E., chmn.: Proposal for revised clinical and electroencephalographic classification of epileptic seizures: From the commission on classification and terminology of the international league against epilepsy. *Epilepsia* **22**: 489–501, 1981.

Eadie, M. J.: Pharmacokinetics of the anticonvulsant drugs, in *The Treatment of Epilepsy,* J. H. Tyrer, ed., pp. 61–93, J. B. Lippincott, Philadelphia, 1980.

Eadie, M. J. and Tyrer, J. H.: *Anticonvulsant Therapy: Pharmacological Basis and Practice,* Churchill Livingstone, Edinburgh, 1980.

Gallagher, B. B.: Neuropharmacology and treatment of epilepsy, in *Anticonvulsants*, J. Vida, ed., pp. 11–55, Academic, New York, 1977.

Gastaut, H. and Broughton, R.: Epileptic seizures: Their clinical nature, pathophysiology and differential diagnosis, in *International Encyclopedia of Pharmacology and Therapeutics*, Section 19: *Anticonvulsant Drugs*, vol. I, J. Mercier, section ed., pp. 3–44, Pergamon, Oxford, 1973.

Glaser, G. H., Penry, J. K., and Woodbury, D. M., eds.: *Antiepileptic Drugs: Mechanism of Action*, Raven, New York, 1980.

Hauptmann, A.: Luminal bei Epilepsie. *Munch. Med. Wochenschr.* **59:** 1907–1909, 1912.

Hauser, W. A.: Epidemiology of epilepsy, in *Advances in Neurology*, vol. 19, Schoenberg, B., ed., pp. 313–339, Raven, New York, 1978.

Hernandez-Peon, R.: Anticonvulsant action of G32883, in *Neuropsychopharmacology*, vol. 3: *Proceedings of the Third Meeting of the Collegium International Neuropsychopharmacologicum*, P. Bradley, F., Flugel, and P., Hoch, eds., pp. 303–311, Elsevier, Amsterdam, 1964.

Julien, R. M. and Hollister, R. P.: Carbamazepine: Mechanism of action. *Adv. Neurol.* **11:** 263–277, 1975.

Kosteljanetz, M., Christiansen, J., Dam, A. M., Hansen, B. S., Lyon, B. B., Pederson, H., and Dam, M.: Carbamazepine vs. phenytoin. A controlled clinical trial in focal motor and generalized epilepsy. *Arch. Neurol.* **36:** 22–24, 1979.

Lampe, K. F., ed.: *Drug Evaluations*, 6th Ed., American Medical Association, Chicago, 1986.

Lander, C. M. and Eadie, M. J.: Plasma levels and pharmacokinetics, in *Drugs in Psychiatry*, vol. 4: *Antimanics, Anticonvulsants and Other Drugs in Psychiatry*, G. Burrows, T. Norman, and B. Davies, eds., pp. 83–112, Elsevier, Amsterdam, 1987.

Livingstone, S., Villamater, C., Sakata, Y., and Pauli, L. L.: Use of carbamazepine in epilepsy. *JAMA* **200:** 204–208, 1967.

Lorge, M.: Uber ein neuartiges Antiepilepticum der Iminostilbenreihe (G 32883), in *Neuropsychopharmacology*, vol. 3: *Proceedings of the Third Meeting of the Collegium Internationale Neuropsychopharmacologicum*, P. Bradley, F. Flugel, and P. Hock, eds., pp. 299–302, Elsevier, Amsterdam, 1964.

Mercier, J., section ed.: *International Encyclopedia of Pharmacology and Therapeutics*, Section 19: *Anticonvulsant Drugs*, vol. I, Pergamon, Oxford, 1973.

Merritt, H. H. and Putnam, T. J.: Sodium diphenyl hydantoinate in the treatment of convulsive disorders. *JAMA* **111:** 1068–1073, 1938.

Merritt, H. H., Putnam, T. J., and Schwab, D. M.: A new series of anticonvulsant drugs tested by experiments on animals. *Arch. Neurol. Psychiatry* **39:** 1003–1015, 1938.

Mikkelsen, B., Berggreen, P., Joensen, P., Kristensen, O., Kohler, O., and Mikkelsen, B. O.: Clonazepam (Rivotril®), and carbamazepine (Tegretol®) in psychomotor epilepsy: A randomized multicenter trial. *Epilepsia* **22:** 415–420, 1981.

Niedermeyer, E.: *Epilepsy Guide: Diagnosis and Treatment of Epileptic Seizure Disorders,* Urban and Schwarzenberg, Baltimore, 1983.

Penry, J. K. and Daly, D. D., eds.: *Advances in Neurology,* vol. 11: *Complex Partial Seizures and Their Treatment,* Raven, New York, 1975.

Penry, J. K. and Newmark, M. E.: The use of antiepileptic drugs. *Ann. Intern. Med.* **90:** 207–218, 1979.

Penry, J. K. and Porter, R. J.: Epilepsy: Mechanisms and therapy. *Med. Clin. North Am.* **63:** 801–812, 1979.

Porter, R. J., Cereghino, J. J., Gladding, G. D., Hesse, B. J., Kupferberg, H. J., Scoville, B., and White, B. G.: Antiepileptic drug development program. *Cleveland Clin. Q.* **51:** 293–305, 1984.

Post, R. M., and Uhde, T. W.: The use of carbamazepine in mania, in *Antimanics, Anticonvulsants and Other Drugs in Psychiatry,* G. Burrows, T. Norman, and B. Davies, eds., pp. 49–79, Elsevier, Amsterdam, 1987.

Post, R. M., Uhde, T. W., Rubinow, D. R., Ballenger, J. C., and Gold, P. W.: Biochemical effects of carbamazepine: Relationship to its mechanisms of action in affective illness. *Prog. Neuropsychopharmacol. Biol. Psychiatry* **7:** 263–271, 1983.

Putnam, T. J. and Merritt, H. H.: Experimental determination of the anticonvulsant properties of some phenyl derivatives. *Science* **85:** 525, 526, 1937.

Rall, T. W. and Schleifer, L. S.: Drugs effective in the therapy of the epilepsies, in *The Pharmacological Basis of Therapeutics,* 7th Ed., A. G. Gilman, L. S. Goodman, T. W. Rall, and F. Murad, eds., pp. 446–472, Macmillan, New York, 1985.

Reynolds, E. H.: The management of seizures associated with psychological disorders, in *Epilepsy and Psychiatry,* E. H. Reynolds and M. R. Trimble, eds., pp. 322–336, Churchill Livingstone, Edinburgh, 1981.

Schindler, W.: 5-H-dibenz (b, f) azepines. US patent 2,948,718. *Chem. Abstr.* **55:** 1671, 1961.

Schindler, W., and Häfliger, F.: Über derivate des iminodibenzyls. *Helv. Chim. Acta* **37:** 472–483, 1954.

Suria, A. and Killam, E. K.: Antiepileptic drugs, in *Antiepileptic Drugs: Mechanism of Action,* G. Glaser, J. Penry, and D. Woodbury, eds., pp. 563–575, Raven, New York, 1980.

Sutherland, J. M., Tait, H., and Eadie, M. J.: *The Epilepsies: Modern Diagnosis and Treatment,* 2nd Ed., Churchill Livingstone, Edinburgh, 1974.

Swinyard, E. A.: History of antiepileptic drugs, in *Antiepileptic Drugs:*

Mechanism of Action, G. Glaser, J. Penry, and D. Woodbury, eds., pp. 1–9, Raven, New York, 1980.

Taylor, J. C. Brauer, S., and Espir, M. L. E.: Long-term treatment of trigeminal neuralgia with carbamazepine. *Postgrad. Med. J.* **57:** 16–18, 1981.

Theobald, W. and Kunz, H. A.: Zur pharmacologie des antiepilepticums 5-carbamyl-5H-dibenz(b, f)azepin. *Arzneimittelforsch.* **13:** 122–125, 1963.

Toman, J. E. P. and Goodman, L. S.: Conditions modifying convulsions in animals. *Proc. Assoc. Res. Nerv. Ment. Dis.* **26:** 141–163, 1946.

Toman, J. E. P., Loewe, S., and Goodman, L. S.: Studies on the physiology and therapy of convulsive disorders. I. The effect of anticonvulsant drugs on electroshock seizures in man. *Arch. Neurol. Psychiat.* **58:** 312–324, 1947.

Tyrer, J. D., ed.: *The Treatment of Epilepsy,* J. B. Lippincott, Philadelphia, 1980.

Vajda, F. J. E.: Anticonvulsant drugs: An overview, in *Drugs in Psychiatry,* vol. 4: *Antimanics, Anticonvulsants and Other Drugs in Psychiatry,* G. Burrows, T. Norman, and B. Davies, eds., pp. 161–188, Elsevier, Amsterdam, 1987.

Vida, J. A., ed.: *Anticonvulsants,* Academic, New York, 1977.

Windholz, M., ed.: *The Merck Index,* 10th Ed., Merck & Co., Rahway, NJ, 1983.

Rheumatology Group

Indomethacin

D-Penicillamine

Hydroxychloroquine

Methotrexate

Cyclophosphamide

Azathioprine (see Cardiovascular
and Renal Group)

Indomethacin

I. Indomethacin as an Innovative Therapeutic Agent

Nonsteroidal antiinflammatory drugs (NSAIDs) are used for the treatment of inflammation—a response to tissue injury already characterized in ancient times as consisting of redness, heat, swelling, and pain (Brune, 1984). This group of agents, which has aspirin as its prototype, shares several pharmacological properties, namely, antiinflammatory, antipyretic, and peripheral analgesic actions, all of which are useful for the relief of inflammation and pain (Shen, 1984).

NSAIDs find their heaviest use in the acute and chronic symptomatic treatment of arthritic (rheumatic) diseases, namely, rheumatoid arthritis, ankylosing spondylitis, psoriatic arthritis, and Reiter's syndrome, as well as osteoarthritis. The pathogenesis of most of these degenerative diseases is unknown (Bennett, 1983), but they are associated with a high level of inflammation of the joints. Rheumatoid arthritis is the most crippling of the rheumatic diseases. It is a generalized disease that may go beyond the joints and damage all connective tissue structures, including vital organs (Calabro, 1975). It has been estimated that 7% of the population of the world suffers with various forms of arthritis (Shen, 1984) and that as many as 20 million Americans are afflicted, with 5 million of these suffering from rheumatoid arthritis (Calabro, 1975). The primary use for NSAIDs "...is to ease joint pain and stiffness so that the patient can comfortably begin an individually prescribed program of exercises or other long-term measures" (Calabro, 1975). NSAIDs are the mainstay of therapy in rheumatoid arthritis (Katz, 1985).

Most NSAIDs act by blocking the production, or action, of local mediators of the inflammatory response, e.g., prostaglandins, polypeptides of the kinin system, lysosomal enzymes, and mediators of cellular activity, such as lympkokines (Mills, 1974). Other actions may also be involved, such as interference with migration of leukocytes and inhibition of phosphodiesterase (Bennett, 1983). Some investigators have stressed the complex interrelationship of prostaglandins, the immune response and NSAIDs and suggest that the action of these drugs could be related to increased T-suppressor cell function, inhibition of the release of monocyte collagenase, and inhibition of neutrophil migration and activation (Goodwin, 1984; Hess and Tangnijkul, 1986).

The term "NSAIDs" distinguishes this group of agents from the adrenal corticosteroids (that is, the endogenous glucocorticoids, e.g., cortisone, hydrocortisone, and their semisynthetic congeners, such as prednisolone and dexamethasone) (Fig. 1), which are highly effective antiinflammatory agents. Unfortunately, long-term administration of glucocorticoids leads to serious toxicities (Cochrane, 1983; Haynes and Murad, 1985): (1) osteoporosis and vertebral compression fractures; fluid and electrolyte disturbances; hyperglycemia and glycosuria; increased susceptibility to infections; hemorrhagic and perforating peptic ulcers; myopathy; behavioral disturbances; cataracts; other problems and (2) a suppression of the pituitary–adrenal system that is slow to recover: this suppression may result in adrenal insufficiency on rapid withdrawal of the corticosteroids or may leave patients quite vulnerable to stress and infection for many months following a more measured withdrawal.

The introductions of aspirin and phenylbutazone (Fig. 1) as therapeutic agents preceded that of indomethacin (Fig. 1). Aspirin, the oldest and most established NSAID, is still considered by many investigators to be one of the most effective (Mills, 1974; Hadler, 1984; Katz, 1985). Phenylbutazone, although undoubtedly an effective drug, is less safe than most other NSAIDs. Long-term use is accompanied by the relatively high risk of serious side effects, i.e., bone marrow depression (leukopenia, pancytopenia, agranulocytosis, aplastic anemia). Some deaths have been related to its use. It is not widely considered as a first-line agent in therapy (Katz, 1985; Flower et al., 1985; Hess and Tangnijkul, 1986).

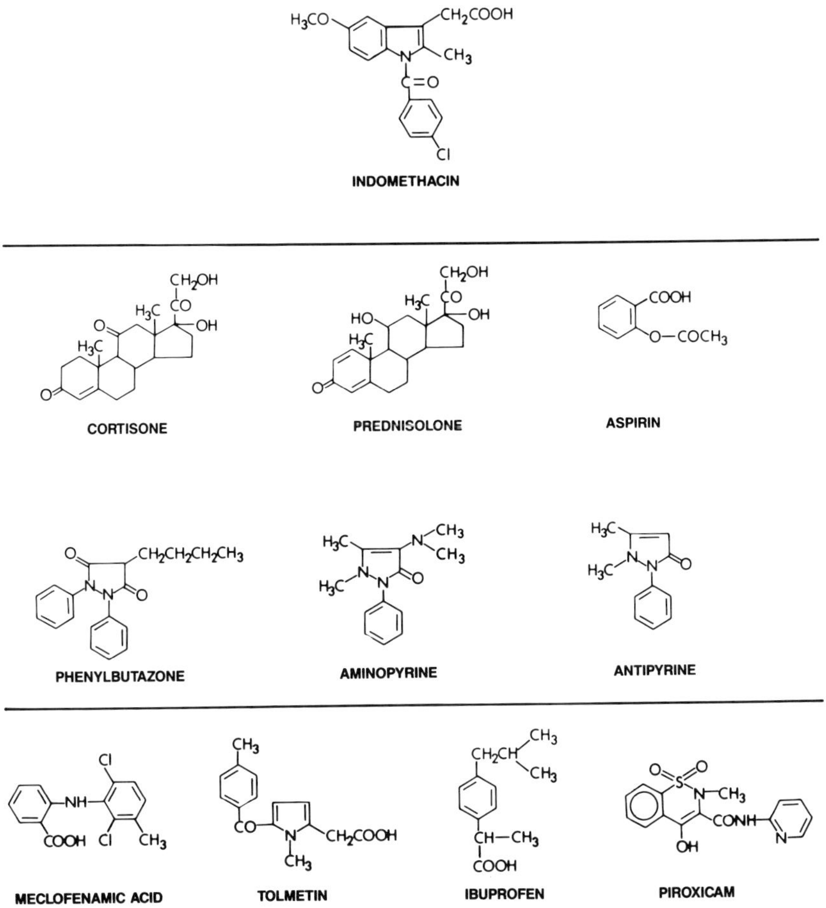

INDOMETHACIN

CORTISONE   PREDNISOLONE   ASPIRIN

PHENYLBUTAZONE   AMINOPYRINE   ANTIPYRINE

MECLOFENAMIC ACID   TOLMETIN   IBUPROFEN   PIROXICAM

Fig. 1. The structures of indomethacin and chemically and/or pharma-cologically related substances.

Indomethacin was the first of the very potent, newer NSAIDs to be introduced into therapy. It was an innovation because it was so much more potent than aspirin or phenylbutazone (Winter et al., 1963) and because it had a unique chemical structure (Shen et al., 1963). Indomethacin is considered to be the drug of choice in acute crystal-induced arthritis and in seronegative spondyloarthropa-thies, such as ankylosing spondylitis (Bennett, 1983), Reiter's syndrome, and psoriatic arthritis (Hess and Tangnijkul, 1986). Indomethacin is also extremely useful in acute attacks of gouty arthritis and in osteoarthritis of the hip joint, where it rapidly and dramatically reduces pain (Calabro, 1975). According to Katz (1985), "...indomethacin remains one of the most established agents for the treatment of rheumatoid arthritis." This is particularly so for acute flares in moderate to severe forms of the disease. Fifty to sixty percent of patients with rheumatoid arthritis experience striking or worthwhile relief of pain and stiffness and a decrease in joint swelling when treated with indomethacin (Calabro, 1975; Katz, 1985). Unfortunately, indomethacin is burdened with a large number of side effects. Most serious are gastrointestinal bleeding, ulceration, and perforation and, less ominously, diarrhea. Much less serious, but fairly frequent in incidence, are headache and gastric upset (Calabro, 1975).

Some controversy still remains over the therapeutic status of indomethacin (and the newer NSAIDs) vis-á-vis aspirin in rheumatoid arthritis. According to Hadler (1984), "In terms of cost and the convenience of consumer autonomy, ASA [aspirin] has no peer among NSAIDs. There are no data to support that any NSAID is more effective than ASA." However, noting that the effectiveness of high-dose, short-term aspirin treatment in rheumatoid arthritis was unimpeachable, Katz (1985) also pointed out that long-term therapy presented a problem of poor compliance, with few patients willing to take the 10–14 tablets required daily. In addition, Hess and Tangnijkul (1986) maintained that distinctive differences in anti-inflammatory mechanisms, in alterations in cartilage metabolism, and in modulation of the immune system "...remind us that these agents [NSAIDs] are not 'the same' drug that can be used randomly or interchangeably." Flower et al. (1985) noted, "Indomethacin has become an accepted part of the rheumatologist's armamentarium and a standard (together with aspirin) against which to measure the activity of other, newer drugs."

Early Clinical Research History

Norcross (1963) presented the first preliminary report on the efficacy of indomethacin in rheumatic disorders. More than 200 patients were treated for 4–12 mo in an open study. Improvement was reported in 66% of rheumatoid patients, in 75% of osteoarthritic patients, and in over 80% of acute disorders (i.e., gout and tendonitis) and rheumatoid spondylitic patients. The author concluded that "...indomethacin was more effective and associated with less toxicity than phenylbutazone or adrenal steroids in the long-term management of rheumatoid or osteoarthritic patients." Headache, nausea, and vomiting were noted as principal side effects.

Rothermich (1963), in a preliminary report of an 18–mo open study, found that "...a high rate of significant improvement has been achieved with its [indomethacin's] use" in peripheral and spinal rheumatoid arthritis. Indomethacin could be readily substituted for phenylbutazone and was less toxic.

Indomethacin was administered to 99 patients with various arthritic disorders for periods of 14 d–1 yr (Hart and Boardman, 1963). Thirteen of 15 acute gout patients, 11 of 14 ankylosing spondylitis patients, 22 of 52 rheumatoid arthritis patients, and six of seven osteoarthritis patients showed dramatic to good clinical improvement. At least two of the following side effects were seen in 45% of the patients: headache, giddiness, muzziness, mental change, anorexia, nausea and vomiting, dyspepsia, diarrhea, drowsiness and blurred vision. The authors considered indomethacin to be an effective antiinflammatory agent, but less effective than corticosteroids and corticotrophin. It was superior to phenylbutazone in acute gout attacks because of its rapid onset.

In a preliminary study of 10 patients with acute gouty arthritis who were treated for up to 5 d, indomethacin was found to be "...a quick acting and strikingly effective anti-inflammatory agent" (Smyth et al., 1963).

Many studies, reviews, and books are available that generally confirm the usefulness of indomethacin in ankylosing spondylitis, acute gouty arthritis, and osteoarthritis of the hip (e.g., *see* Bird and Wright, 1982; Huskisson, 1983; Bennett, 1983; Haynes and Murad, 1985). However, as already noted, there has been, and remains, some controversy as to whether indomethacin (and the other NSAIDs as well) is in any way superior to aspirin in the management of rheumatoid arthritis (*see*, for example, Cooperating Clinics Report, 1967; Healey, 1967; Boardman and Hart, 1967; O'Brien, 1968; Smyth, 1970; Calabro, 1975; Hadler, 1984; Katz, 1985).

II. The Scientific Work
Leading to Indomethacin

Shen et al. (1963) described the synthesis of indomethacin and gave a preliminary statement of its antiinflammatory activity; Winter et al. (1963) presented the pharmacology in some detail.

By the oral route, indomethacin was a very potent inhibitor of the granuloma induced in rats by the subcutaneous implant of a cotton pellet: it had a potency approximately 85 times greater than phenylbutazone and four times greater than hydrocortisone. It was also active in the granuloma test in the absence of the adrenal glands, and when applied locally in the pellet. In addition, indomethacin proved to be 2, 20, and 30 times more potent than hydrocortisone, phenylbutazone and aspirin, respectively, by the oral route, in inhibiting the edema of the hind paw of the rat induced by the subplantar injection of carageenin. Indomethacin was also a very potent antipyretic agent in rats and rabbits (Winter et al., 1963).

Table 1 defines the critical scientific ideas and experiments leading to indomethacin and categorizes their origin.

Background Contributions
Preceding Indomethacin

Aspirin was synthesized as an improved form of sodium salicylate, studied pharmacologically, and introduced into therapy in the last decade of the 19th century (Dreser, 1899; *see* Collier, 1984).

The antiinflammatory pyrazalone derivatives, antipyrine (Knorr, 1884) and aminopyrine (Fig. 1), were also synthesized in the late 19th century and used as antipyretics. More recently, after decades of clinical use as an analgesic and antiinflammatory agent, aminopyrine fell into disfavor when it was shown to produce agranulocytosis. Neither drug is now used therapeutically in the USA. Phenylbutazone was developed as an acidic solubilizing agent for the poorly soluble aminopyrine, and the mixture was introduced in 1948 (Wilhelmi, 1949). It is structurally related to aminopyrine (Fig. 1) and was found to have potent antiinflammatory properties of its own (Wilhelmi, 1950). Aspirin and phenylbutazone were the mainstay NSAIDs of the 1950s.

Table 1
Profile of Observations and Ideas Crucial to the Development of Indomethacin[a]

Sequence: Route to innovative drug**	Orient- ation	Nature of study	Research institution	National origin	Nature of discovery	Screening involved	Crucial ideas or observations
Indomethacin**							
Winter et al. (1963)	Pre- clinical	Pharma- cology/ chemistry	Indus- try	USA	Orderly	Untargeted	Indomethacin discovered: anti- inflammatory and antipyretic actions; much greater potency than aspirin and phenylbutazone; novel structure.

[a]Taken from section II. Entries are those contributions without which the discovery of the agent (or additionally, in some cases, a relevant clinical application) would not have taken place or would have been materially delayed.

Hench et al. (1949) had observed, in a series of studies over many years, that remissions of active rheumatic arthritis occurred during pregnancy and during jaundice. They reasoned that this was possibly attributable to increased secretion of the adrenal steroid, Compound E (cortisone), since stressful procedures were known to stimulate the adrenal cortices. These ideas led Hench and coworkers to the successful treatment of rheumatoid arthritis with cortisone.

The dramatic positive effects of phenylbutazone and the steroids in treating rheumatic conditions, coupled with their equally dramatic shortcomings, prompted further discovery efforts in the area of NSAIDs (Shen, 1984). Unlike aspirin, the more potent agents—phenylbutazone and the steroids—could be demonstrated to have some specific antiinflammatory activity in animal models (Meier et al., 1950) and, thereby, encouraged the development of more sensitive assay procedures (Winter and Porter, 1957; Winter et al., 1962).

III. Comments on Events Leading to Indomethacin

According to Shen and Winter (1977), a group of indole deriva-tives, synthesized earlier as part of a serotonin antagonist program at the Merck Sharp and Dohme laboratories, were available for a limited random screening. Positive results with one of these compounds in a granuloma test known to be responsive to cortisone led to a program of synthesis and testing of more than 2000 compounds, including over 350 indoles, before significant activity was found. Of the three compounds that were eventually tested in humans, MK615 (indomethacin) was the best. Shen and Winter (1977) and Shen (1984) maintained that they had a rationale in testing indoles because, at the time, there was much discussion of the role of serotonin, an indole, as a mediator of inflammation. Moreover, evidence existed that abnormalities in the metabolism of the serotonin precursor substance, tryptophan, occurred in some rheumatic patients. Although these notions concerning a causative role of serotonin in inflammation were later found to be untenable, they served a useful purpose (Shen and Winter, 1977).

Shen (1984) states that in the mid-1950s

> ...the experimental approach to find non-steroidal agents, hopefully with steroid-like anti-inflammatory actions but without hormonal side effects, had to rely much on serendipitous clinical observations or direct *in vivo* screening....The perseverance of the research and medical management [of the pharmaceutical companies involved], especially in the face of some early discouraging side effects, clearly played an important role in the successful development of this class [i.e., NSAIDs] of therapeutic agents...

IV. Developments
Subsequent to Indomethacin

Following the introduction and clinical success of indomethacin in 1965, a plethora of NSAIDs has been introduced into medicine throughout the world. Shen (1984) classified the NSAIDs into six categories, as follows (with a few examples for each class):

1. *Carboxylic acids*—aspirin, mefenamic acid, meclofenamic acid (Fig. 1), diflunisal;
2. *Acetic acids*—indomethacin, sulindac, tolmetin (Fig. 1);
3. *Propionic acids*—ibuprofen (Fig. 1), naproxen, fenoprofen;
4. *Acidic enols*—phenylbutazone, oxyphenbutazone, piroxicam (Fig. 1);
5. *Butryric acids*—fenbufen;
6. *Nonacidic agents*—ditazole.

According to Mills (1974), none of the large number of NSAIDs introduced up to 1974 had any great advantage over salicylate except that they were claimed to produce less gastric problems; they did not compare with phenylbutazone or indomethacin in potency. Bird and Wright (1982) felt that the propionic acid derivatives had bypassed the gastric side effects of the earlier families of drugs, but possibly at the cost of decreased potency.

Hess and Tangnijkul (1986) made the judgment,

Although the overall profile of the newer NSAIDs may not be superior to those already available, the fact that there are differences in patient response and mechanisms of action would favor introduction of these newer agents. Some of their selected beneficial features may help in improving the treatment outcome of different rheumatic conditions. At the current rate of research in cell biology, immunology and biochemistry, there will be better understanding of the pathogenesis and pathophysiology of different rheumatic pathways. This will hopefully result in the production of more disease-specific or even disease-modifying NSAIDs.

References

Bennett, D. R., ed.: *AMA Drug Evaluations,* 5th Ed., pp. 107–138, W. B. Saunders, Philadelphia, 1983.

Bird, H. A. and Wright, V.: *Applied Drug Therapy of the Rheumatic Diseases,* Wright PSG, Bristol, 1982.

Boardman, P. L., and Hart, F. D.: Side-effects of indomethacin. *Ann. Rheum. Dis.* 26: 127–132, 1967.

Brune, K.: The concept of inflammatory mediators, in *Discoveries in Pharmacology,* vol. 2, *Haemodynamics, Hormones and Inflammation,* M. J. Parnham and J. Bruinvels, eds., pp. 487–521, Elsevier, Amsterdam, 1984.

Calabro, J. J.: Long-term reappraisal of indomethacin. *Drug Ther.* 5: 46–60, 1975.

Cochrane, G. M.: Systemic steroids in asthma, in *Steroids in Asthma,* T. Clark, ed., pp. 103–120, Adis, Auckland, 1983.

Collier, H. O. J.: The story of aspirin, in *Discoveries in Pharmacology,* vol. 2, *Haemodynamics, Hormones and Inflammation,* M. J. Parnham and J. Bruinvels, eds., pp. 555–593, Elsevier, Amsterdam, 1984.

Cooperating Clinics Committee of the American Rheumatism Association: A three month trial of indomethacin in rheumatoid arthritis, with special reference to analysis and inference. *Clin. Pharmacol. Ther.* 8: 11–37, 1967.

Dreser, H.: Pharmakologisches über Aspirin (Acetylsalicylsäure). *Pflügers Arch. Ges. Physiol.* **76:** 306–318, 1899.

Flower, R. J., Moncada, S., and Vane, J. R.: Analgesic-antipyretics and antiinflammatory agents; drugs employed in the treatment of gout, in *The Pharmacological Basis of Therapeutics,* 7th Ed., A. G. Gilman, L. S. Goodman, T. W. Rall, and F. Murad, eds., pp. 674–715, Macmillan, New York, 1985.

Goodwin, J. S.: Immunologic effects of nonsteroidal antiinflammatory drugs. *Am. J. Med.* 77(4B), 7–15, 1984.

Hadler, N. M.: The argument for aspirin as the NSAID of choice in the management of rheumatoid arthritis. *Drug Intell. and Clin. Pharm.* **18:** 34–38, 1984.

Hart, F. D. and Boardman, P. L.: Indomethacin: A new non-steroid anti-inflammatory agent. *Br. Med. J.* **2:** 965–970, 1963.

Haynes, R. C. Jr. and Murad, F.: Adrenocorticotrophic hormone; adreno-cortical steroids and their synthetic analogs; inhibitors of adrenocortical steroid biosynthesis, in *The Pharmacological Basis of Therapeutics,* 7th Ed., A. G. Gilman, L. S. Goodman, T. W. Rall, and F. Murad, eds., pp. 1459–1489, Macmillan, New York, 1985.

Healey, L. A.: An appraisal of indomethacin. *Bull. Rheum. Dis.* **18:** 483–486, 1967.

Hench, P. S., Kendall, E. C., Slocumb, C. H., and Polley, H. F.: The effect of a hormone of the adrenal cortex (17-hydroxy-11-dehydrocorticosterone: Compound E) and of pituitary adrenocorticotropic hormone on rheuma-toid arthritis; preliminary report. *Proc. Staff Mtg. Mayo Clinic* **24:** 181–197, 1949.

Hess, E. V., and Tangnijkul, Y.: A rational approach to NSAID therapy. *Ration. Drug Ther.* **20:** 1–6, 1986.

Huskisson, E. C., ed.: *Anti-Rheumatic Drugs,* Praeger, Westport, CT, 1983.

Katz, W. A.: Modern management of rheumatoid arthritis. *Am. J. Med.* **79** (Suppl. 4C): 24–31, 1985.

Knorr, L.: Einwirkung von Acetessigester auf Hydrazinchinizinderivate. *Chemische Berichte* **17:** 546–552, 1884.

Meier, R., Schuler, W., and Desaulles, P.: Zur Frage des Mechanismus der Hemmung des Bindegewebswachstums durch Cortisone. *Experientia* **6:** 469–471, 1950.

Mills, J. A.: Nonsteroidal anti-inflammatory drugs (in two parts). *N. Engl. J. Med.* **290:** 781–784; 1002–1005, 1974.

Norcross, B. M.: Treatment of connective tissue diseases with a new non-steroidal compound (indomethacin). *Arthritis Rheum.* **6:** 290 (abs.), 1963.

O'Brien, W. M.: Indomethacin: a survey of clinical trials. *Clin. Pharmacol. Ther.* **9:** 94–107, 1968.

Rothermich, N. O.: Indomethacin: a new pharmacologic approach to the management of rheumatoid disease. *Arthritis Rheum.* **6:** 295 (abs.), 1963.

Shen, T. Y.: The proliferation of non-steroidal anti-inflammatory drugs (NSAIDs), in *Discoveries in Pharmacology*, vol. 2, *Haemodynamics, Hormones and Inflammation.* M. J. Parnham and J. Bruinvels, eds., pp. 523–553, Elsevier, Amsterdam, 1984.

Shen, T. Y. and Winter, C. A.: Chemical and biological studies on indomethacin, sulindac and their analogs. *Adv. Drug Res.* **12:** 90–245, 1977.

Shen, T. Y., Windholz, T. B., Rosegay, A., Witzel, B. E., Wilson, A. N., Willet, J. D., Holtz, W. J., Ellis, R. L., Matzuk, A. R., Lucas, S., Stammer, C. H., Holly, F. W., Sarrett, L. H., Risley, E. A., Nuss, G. W., and Winter, C. A.: Nonsteroid anti-inflammatory agents. *J. Am. Chem. Soc.* **85:** 488, 489, 1963.

Smyth, C. J.: Indomethacin—its rightful place in treatment (editorial). *Ann. Intern. Med.* **72:** 430–432, 1970.

Smyth, C. J., Velayos, E. E., and Amoroso, C.: A method for measuring swelling of hands and feet. Part II. Influence of new anti-inflammatory drug, indomethacin, in acute gout. *Acta Rheum. Scand.* **9:** 306–322, 1963.

Wilhelmi, G.: Ueber die pharmakologischen Eigenschaften von Irgapyrin, einem neuen Präparat aus der Pyrazolreihe. *Schweiz. Med. Wochenschr.* **79:** 577–582, 1949.

Wilhelmi, G.: Ueber die antiphlogistische Wirkung von Pyrazolen, speziell von Irgapyrin, bei peroraler und parenteraler Verabreichung. *Schweiz. Med. Wochenschr.* **80:** 936–942, 1950.

Winter, C. A. and Porter, C. C.: Effect of alterations in side chain upon anti-inflammatory and liver glycogen activities of hydrocortisone esters. *J. Am. Pharmaceut. Assoc.* **46:** 515–519, 1957.

Winter, C. A., Risley, E. A., and Nuss, G. W.: Carrageenin-induced edema in hindpaw of the rat as an assay for antiinflammatory drugs. *Proc. Soc. Exp. Biol. Med.* **111:** 544–547, 1962.

Winter, C. A., Risley, E. A., and Nuss, G. W.: Anti-inflammatory and antipyretic activities of indomethacin, 1-(p-chlorobenzoyl)-5-methoxy-2-methylindole-3-acetic acid. *J. Pharmacol. Exp. Ther.* **141:** 369–376, 1963.

D-Penicillamine

I. D-Penicillamine as an Innovative Therapeutic Agent

According to Lipsky (1985), rheumatoid arthritis in most patients is a mild to moderate and intermittent affliction with little permanent destruction of articular structures. However, in a small percentage of sufferers, the course of the disease can be "aggressively destructive" with severe damage to articular structures and consequent deformation and reduced function. The first-line agents for most cases of rheumatoid arthritis, the nonsteroidal antiinflammatory drugs (NSAIDs), are not adequate for sustaining this small group of severely-afflicted patients, since their main role is only to ease joint pain and stiffness, thus enabling patients to begin exercise programs or other long-term measures (Calabro, 1975). D-Penicillamine, along with gold compounds and antimalarials (and possibly the antiproliferative agents, azathioprine, methotrexate, and cyclophosphamide), compose a group of agents that have become known as disease-modifying antirheumatic drugs (DMARDs). Unlike NSAIDs (which are demonstrably potent, specific, acutely acting antiinflammatory and analgesic agents), DMARDs elicit, at most, only minimal, nonspecific, acute antiinflammatory or analgesic effects. Instead, with slow onset, they exert clinical benefit that is often associated with improvement of serologic abnormalities and, on occasion, even with improvement of joints. The mechanisms of action of DMARDs are unknown, although considerable evidence suggests that they all interfere in some way with the immunological aspects of the disease (Lipsky and Ziff, 1982; Jaffe, 1983; Lipsky, 1985; Muirden, 1986).

221

Thus, D-penicillamine is a slow-acting drug in rheumatoid arthritis, with the first clinical signs of improvement being seen only after 8–12 wk of therapy. These signs include reduction in the degree of inflammation of synovia and an associated reduction in the level of rheumatoid factor and immune complexes in the synovial fluid and in the serum. Vasculitis may also be attenuated, and after 2–3 yr of treatment there may be radiographic evidence for modest healing of erosive lesions (Jaffe, 1983). Although many physicians prefer to turn to gold compounds as the first choice among the second-line agents because of a longer experience with them, D-penicillamine, which is as effective as gold compounds, is used very commonly, with some physicians preferring to give it before gold compounds (Lampe, 1986).

D-Penicillamine is widely accepted as an effective agent, but, unfortunately, as is the case with other DMARDs, a long list of side effects has prevented unqualified recommendations for its use, and has relegated it (and all DMARDs) to second-line therapeutic status behind NSAIDs, despite its higher "remitting" potential. According to Muirden (1986), side effects occur in 50–75% of patients receiving the drug, and in approximately 25–40% of cases the drug has to be discontinued because of the severity of the adverse reactions. Similar figures are quoted by Lipsky (1985). The side effects include rashes, fever, pruritus, anorexia, epigastric pain, nausea, vomiting, occasional diarrhea, oral ulcers, and loss of taste. More serious are lymphadenopathy, leukopenia, thrombocytopenia, agranulocytosis and aplastic anemia, and renal problems such as hypoalbuminemia, as well as proteinuria and hematuria, which may progress to nephrotic syndrome. The majority of side effects appear in the first 6 mo; thrombocytopenia and proteinuria appear later (Lipsky, 1985; Lampe, 1986; Muirden, 1986).

Several autoimmune syndromes, such as lupus-like diseases, Goodpasture's syndrome, polymyositis, and myasthenia gravis have been observed as rare side effects of D-penicillamine (St. Clair and Polisson, 1986). Jaffe (1983) was of the opinion that the induction of all these autoimmune syndromes by D-penicillamine is unique in clinical medicine and that understanding of the mechanisms responsible for the induction of these syndromes could provide insight into the mode of action of D-penicillamine in rheumatoid arthritis.

It is considered that much of the toxicity of D-penicillamine is caused by the use of high doses of the drug and/or by too rapid escalation of doses. Jaffe (1975) suggested a "go slow—go low" policy that is now widely accepted. Most investigators agree that at lower doses and slower increments, with careful monitoring of the patient, severe complications can be reduced.

D-Penicillamine, aside from its use in rheumatoid arthritis, is the drug of choice for the treatment of symptomatic and asymptomatic individuals with Wilson's disease, a rare genetic disorder of chronic copper toxicosis caused by faulty metabolism of dietary copper. D-Penicillamine, since it is a sulfhydryl compound (Fig. 1), acts as a metal-chelating agent and, by binding to the excess copper in the body, facilitates its excretion by the kidney (Scheinberg and Sternlieb, 1960,1984; Scheinberg et al., 1987).

D-Penicillamine also combines with iron, mercury, lead, gold, and arsenic to form soluble complexes that are readily excreted by the kidneys. It is as effective as dimercaprol (BAL) (Fig. 1) for arsenic poisoning. Although not as effective as edetate calcium disodium or dimercaprol for lead poisoning, it has the advantage of being effective by the oral route (Lampe, 1986).

In addition, because of its sulfhydryl nature, D-penicillamine is used for the treatment of cystinuria. Cystinuria results from an inherited defect in the renal tubular reabsorption of the amino acid cystine (the disulfide combination of two cysteine molecules) (Fig. 1). D-Penicillamine combines with cysteine to form the disulfide penicillamine-cysteine (Fig. 1), which is more water-soluble than cystine. Therefore, it can prevent the formation of new cystine stones in the urinary tract and permit gradual dissolution of existing stones that are secondary to the occurrence of large quantities of cystine in an acid urine (Walshe, 1963; Berkow, 1982). Although it is a degradation product of penicillin, D-penicillamine has no antibacterial activity.

The efficacy of D-penicillamine as a DMARD in the treatment of rheumatoid arthritis has been chronicled in many reviews and chapters (e.g., Milne, 1968; Multicentre Trial Group, 1973; Jaffe, 1977,1981; Markenson, 1981; Lipsky and Ziff, 1982; Jaffe, 1983; Brooks et al., 1984; Parnham, 1984; Lipsky, 1985; Rothermich et al., 1985).

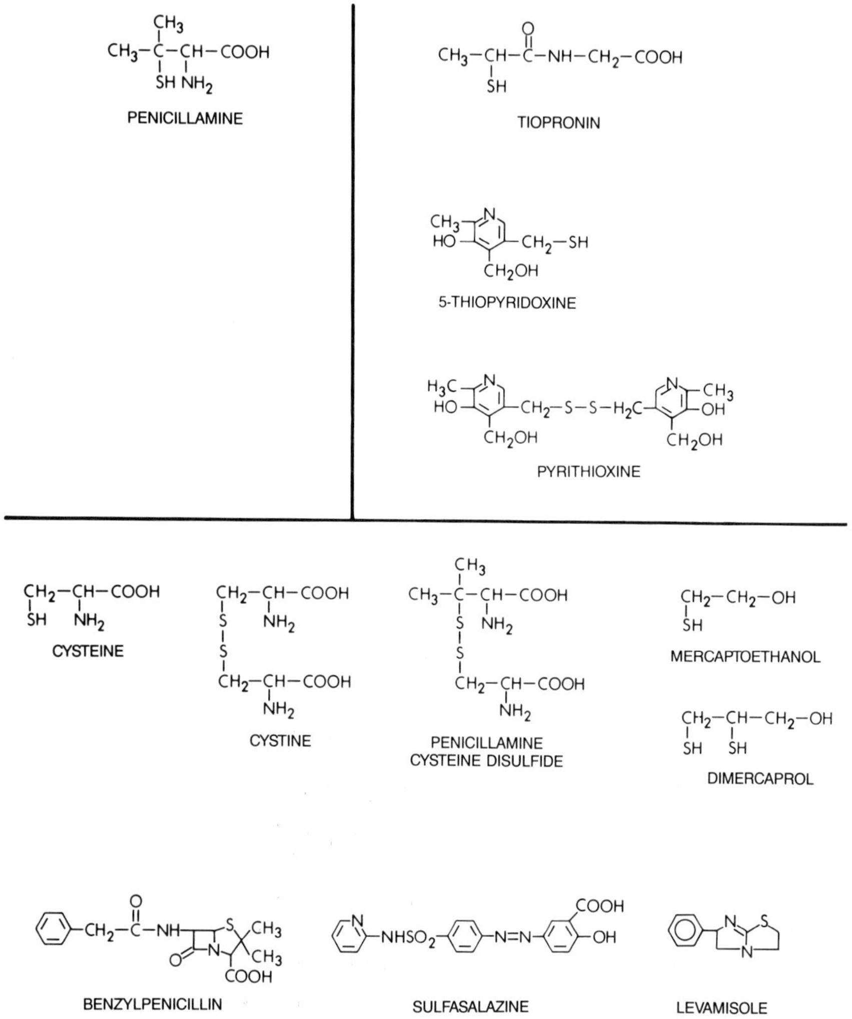

Fig. 1. The structures of penicillamine and chemically and/or pharmacologically related substances.

Early Clinical Research History

In the case of penicillamine, the early clinical research is intimately involved with the discovery of its usefulness in rheumatoid arthritis, and is discussed in section II.

II. The Scientific Work
Leading to D-Penicillamine
as an Antirheumatic Agent

Franklin et al. (1957) demonstrated that, in contrast to the globulin preparations of normal sera (and of joint fluid), which contained two ultracentrifugal fractions—one having a sedimentation constant of seven Svedberg units (S) and the other of 19S—similar preparations from some rheumatoid arthritis patients contained, in addition, a fraction with a constant of 22S. Urea dissociated this high-molecular-weight material into two components with sedimentation rates of 19S and 7S, clearly suggesting a group of proteins or protein aggregates. The authors felt that their observations favored the possibility that the 22S component was a complex of 19S material and some lower-molecular-weight protein, and that the complex existed in a soluble state in the sera of some rheumatoid arthritis patients. This complex precipitated readily under various conditions, especially upon the addition of small amounts of slightly altered γ-globulin.

Deutsch and Morton (1957) demonstrated that adding sulfhydryl compounds, such as mercaptoethanol and cysteine (Fig. 1), led to the conversion of macroglobulin fractions from macroglobulinemic sera (a mixture of molecules with ultracentrifuge sedimentation constants of 18, 25, and 32S units) into a single molecular entity with an S value the same as that of γ-globulin, 6.5. These authors suggested, therefore, that macroglobulins might actually be aggregates of normal serum globulins and that they were depolymerized as a result of the breaking of disulfide bonds via reduction by the sulfhydryl agents.

Noting the work of Franklin et al. (1957) and Deutsch and Morton (1957), Heimer and Federico (1958) treated serum preparations from patients with rheumatoid arthritis with cysteine, and compared these with untreated preparations. Cysteine treatment depolymerized the 19S and 22S components and increased the amount of the 7S component.

Ritzmann et al. (1960) administered (*inter alia*) the sulfhydryl compound DL-penicillamine to a patient with Waldenström's macroglobulinemia, and observed a marked sustained decrease of relative serum viscosity and an increase of sedimentation rate. They suggested that DL-penicillamine dissociated the macroglobulin that was responsible for the increased serum viscosity (and the consequent poor circulation and abnormal clotting) seen in this macroglobulinemia. Clinical improvement of the patient was reported. Bloch et al. (1960) also showed that DL-penicillamine depolymerized the macroglobulin of two patients with Waldenström's macroglobulinemia in vitro, and that its oral administration decreased total protein and γ-globulin concentrations in their sera. Griffin et al. (1960) and Dresner and Trombly (1960) (in abstracts) reported treating seven rheumatoid arthritis patients, each, with D-penicillamine by mouth. They stated that there was evidence of a decrease in the serum rheumatoid factor in these short-term studies (1–10 d). Clinical improvement was reported by Griffin et al. (1960).

Jaffe (1962) cited all of the above work and went on to confirm that D-penicillamine was capable of dissociating the rheumatoid factor in vitro, but found that oral administration of the compound for 14 d to four patients with advanced rheumatoid arthritis did not result in dissociation. On the other hand, when D-penicillamine was injected directly into the joint space, depolymerization of the macroglobulin in synovial fluid was achieved. Jaffe (1962) suggested that perhaps a systemic effect could be realized if more potent sulfhydryl compounds were available. Following up on this work, Jaffe (1963) compared the effects of plasmapheresis (physical removal of plasma protein) with those of protracted DL-penicillamine therapy in two rheumatoid patients. Plasmapheresis elicited prompt and transient reduction in rheumatoid factor, but was clinically ineffective. In contrast, the decline in rheumatoid factor caused by penicillamine was slow in onset and more lasting in duration. Furthermore, following 3–6 wk of DL-penicillamine therapy, there appeared to be subjective and objective signs of gradual clinical improvement. Jaffe (1963) noted that, "There appeared to be a favorable clinical change associated with prolonged drug administration which merits a larger clinical trial." Because of the differences between plasmapheresis and penicillamine therapy, the author concluded that penicillamine was "...not exerting its effect on RF [rheumatoid factor] by sulfhydryl dissociation of the macroglobulin within the vascular compartment." He suggested, among other ideas, that penicillamine might act by "...a more basic effect on the underlying disease process which was then reflected by a secondary decrease in the titre [of rheumatoid factor]."

Jaffe (1965) went on to study the effect of 4–6 mo of treatment with D-penicillamine on rheumatoid factor, erythocyte sedimentation rate, and C-reactive protein in 21 patients. An improvement in one or more of these parameters occurred in most patients by the end of the drug administration period. Although the study was not designed to test the therapeutic efficacy of D-penicillamine, a decrease in disease activity occurred and correlated well with a significant fall in erythrocyte sedimentation rate. Subcutaneous nodules, especially new ones, decreased in size, and some had disappeared by end of the drug-testing period. The author considered that the mechanism by which penicillamine influenced rheumatoid factor and the other variables remained in doubt.

Table 1 defines the critical scientific ideas and experiments leading to the use of penicillamine in rheumatoid arthritis and categorizes their origin.

Background Contributions Preceding the Use of Penicillamine in Rheumatoid Arthritis

Penicillamine was discovered as a part of the intensive research on the chemistry of penicillin (Fig. 1) that was carried out during World War II—it was found in acid hydrolysates of this antibiotic by Abraham et al. (1943). These workers described it as an unusual amine base with two acidic centers. Because of its clearly amine nature, it was dubbed penicillamine. Its structure was reported by Chain (1949), who noted that penicillamine was similar to cysteine in many respects, but was much more soluble in water and was not oxidized by enzymes occurring in animal tissues. At approximately the same time, Wilson and duVigneaud (1950) demonstrated that penicillamine had biological activity. The L-isomer inhibited the growth of young rats and eventually led to their deaths, whereas the D-isomer, the naturally occurring form, was apparently not toxic.

Walshe (1956a,b) recognized that there was a need for an orally administered drug that would promote the excretion of excess copper in patients with Wilson's disease. Although parenteral admin-

Table 1
Profile of Observations and Ideas Crucial to the Development of D-Penicillamine[a]

Sequence: Route to innovative drug[**]	Orient- ation	Nature of study	Research institution	National origin	Nature of discovery	Screening involved	Crucial ideas or observations
D-Penicillamine[**]							
Franklin et al. (1957)	Clinical	Bio- chem- istry	Univer- sity	USA	Orderly	No	Rheumatoid factor discovered in serum and joint fluid of rheumatoid arthritic patients.
Heimer and Fed- erico (1958)	Clinical	Bio- chem- istry	Hospi- tal	USA	Orderly	No	The sulfhydryl amino acid cysteine depolymerizes rheumatoid factor in vitro.
Jaffe (1963)	Clinical	Pharma- cology, rheuma- tology	Univer- sity	USA	Orderly	No	Penicillamine, in vivo, lowers serum rheumatoid factor and produces clin- ical improvement; both events very slow in onset and prolonged in dura- tion; effect may not be from direct depolymerization of rheumatoid factor.

[a]Taken from section II. Entries are those contributions without which the discovery of the agen (or additionally, in some cases, a relevant clinical application) would not have taken place or woulc have been materially delayed.

istration of the sulfhydryl compound dimercaprol had proved the most effective form of treatment, causing mobilization of excess copper by chelation and distinct clinical improvement, repeated in- jections of dimercaprol were extremely painful. Penicillamine, also a sulfhydryl compound, which was by then detectable as a metabo- lite of penicillin (and, therefore, presumably safe) was known to be excreted in the reduced sulfhydryl form (Walshe, 1956a). He con- sidered it likely that penicillamine would remain reduced when given by mouth and, thereby, like dimercaprol, be active in chelating and removing excess copper. Upon testing this hypothesis, peni- cillamine was found to be as effective as dimercaprol in promoting copper excretion in two normal patients and six with Wilson's dis- ease (Walshe, 1956a,b).

III. Comments on Events Leading to D-Penicillamine

Lipsky and Ziff (1982) commented that, "Although treatment with D-penicillamine often decreases circulating rheumatoid factor titers, it is unlikely that this effect results directly from D-penicillamine-induced dissociation of serum or synovial fluid IgM rheumatoid factor, since the concentration of D-penicillamine attained in vivo is hundreds-of-folds less than that needed to dissociate macroglobulins." Thus, although the rationale that led to the testing of D-penicillamine in rheumatoid arthritis—the sulfhydryl-induced depolymerization of rheumatoid factor—was erroneous, it none the less led to useful consequences.

Rothermich et al. (1985) pointed out that it took 15 years from the early reports of the efficacy of penicillamine in rheumatoid arthritis till it was approved for this indication in the USA. They expressed the view,

A major [but not the only] impediment from the onset was that penicillamine was manufactured by several pharmaceutical companies and not covered by a patent. This naturally resulted in a reluctance for the pharmaceuticals [pharmaceutical companies] to commit the considerable resources necessary for clinical trials and approval for use in rheumatoid arthritis.

IV. Developments Subsequent to D-Penicillamine

Jaffe (1983) held the opinion,

Despite the lack of a clear understanding of its action, as well as the high incidence of adverse reactions that may attend its use, penicillamine is increasingly accepted as a highly effective remittive agent for this disease [rheumatoid arthritis]. It is anticipated that it will serve as a prototype for disease-modifying drugs of this chemical class, which will afford comparable or even greater efficacy, with a more favorable benefit-to-risk ratio.

Attempts have been made to produce new sulfhydryl compounds that would be as active as penicillamine but less toxic. Three compounds (Fig. 1) have been considered to be active: tiopronin (Camus et al., 1981; Amor et al., 1982; Pasero et al., 1982); 5-thiopyridoxine (Huskisson et al., 1980; Huskisson, 1981); and pyrithioxine, which is the dimer of 5-thiopyridoxine (Camus et al., 1981). Unfortunately, these compounds also displayed toxicities similar to those of penicillamine, with pyrithioxine appearing to be the best tolerated of the three (Huskisson, 1981).

Several nonsulfhydryl agents have DMARD activity. These include sulfasalazine and levamisole (Fig. 1) (and also hydroxychloroquine, which is discussed in a separate chapter). Both of these agents, however, like other DMARDs, produce an array of minor to serious adverse reactions. These range from nausea and vomiting to megaloblastic anemia and leukopenia with the former compound (McConkey et al., 1980; Capell et al., 1988), and from rashes to neutropenia and agranulocytosis with the latter (Multicentre Study Group, 1978; Huskisson and Adams, 1980). Huskisson (1981) concluded,

> The ideal compound of this type [DMARD] has not yet been found. The search continues; meantime, penicillamine offers the possibility of controlling a substantial proportion of patients with persistent or progressive RA [rheumatoid arthritis] and there are a number of alternatives for the intolerant or unresponsive patient.

Lipsky (1985) pointed out,

> The awareness that certain agents have the potential, although only partially realized in most patients, to modify the disease process has begun to change the way physicians approach patients with rheumatoid arthritis. The notion that early treatment with these agents may prevent deformities has begun to supersede the therapeutic nihilism of the past.

This author also felt that these drugs might lead to a better understanding of the pathogenesis of rheumatoid arthritis.

References

Abraham, E. P., Chain, E., Baker, W., and Robinson, R.: Penicillamine, a characteristic degradation product of penicillin. *Nature* **151**: 107, 1943.

Amor, B., Mery, C., and deGery, A.: Tiopronin (N-[2-mercaptopropionyl]-glycin) in rheumatoid arthritis. *Arthritis Rheum.* 25: 698–703, 1982.

Berkow, R., ed.: *The Merck Manual*, 14th Ed., Merck Sharp & Dohme Research Laboratories, Rahway, NJ, 1982.

Bloch, H. S., Prasad, A., Anastasi, A., and Briggs, D. R.: Serum protein changes in Waldenström's macroglobulinemia during administration of a low molecular weight thiol (penicillamine). *J. Lab. Clin. Med.* 56: 212–217, 1960.

Brooks, P. M., Kean, W. F., Kassam, Y., and Buchanan, W. W.: Problems of antiarthritic therapy in the elderly. *J. Am. Geriatr. Soc.* 32: 229–234, 1984.

Calabro, J. J.: Long-term reappraisal of indomethacin. *Drug Ther.* 5: 46–60, 1975.

Camus, J-P., Crouzet, J., Prier, A., and Bergevin, H.: Pyrithioxine and thiopronine: New penicillamine-like drugs in rheumatoid arthritis. *J. Rheum.* 8 (Suppl. 7): 175–177, 1981.

Capell, H. A., Hunter, J. A., and Pullar, T.: Sulphasalazine in the management of rheumatoid arthritis, in *New Perspectives in Antiinflammatory Therapies*, A. Lewis, N. Ackerman, and I. Otterness, eds., pp. 247–255, Raven, New York, 1988.

Chain, E.: Components of the penicillin molecule, in *Antibiotics*, vol. 2, H. W. Florey, E. Chain, N. G. Heatley, M. A. Jennings, A. G. Sanders, E. P. Abraham, and M. E. Florey, eds., pp. 819–870, Oxford University Press, London, 1949.

Deutsch, H. F. and Morton, J. I.: Dissociation of human serum macroglobulins, *Science* 125: 600, 601, 1957.

Dresner, E. and Trombly, P.: Chemical dissociation of the rheumatoid factor *in vitro* and *in vivo*. *Clin. Res.* 8: 16, 1960.

Franklin, E. C., Holman, H. R., Müller-Eberhard, H. J., and Kunkel, H. G.: An unusual protein component of high molecular weight in the serum of certain patients with rheumatoid arthritis. *J. Exp. Med.* 105: 425–438, 1957.

Griffin, S. W., Ulloa, A., Henry, M., Johnston, M. L., and Holley, H. L.: *In vivo* effect of penicillamine on circulating rheumatoid factor. *Clin. Res.* 8: 87, 1960.

Heimer, R. and Federico, O. M.: Depolymerization of the 19S antibodies and the 22S rheumatoid factor. *Clin. Chim. Acta* 3: 496–498, 1958.

Huskisson, E. C.: Other penicillamine-like drugs. *J. Rheumatol.* 8 (Suppl. 7): 180, 181, 1981.

Huskisson, E. C. and Adams, J. G.: An overview of the current status of levamisole in the treatment of rheumatic diseases. *Drugs* 20: 100–104, 1980.

Huskisson, E. C., Jaffe, I. A., Scott, J., and Dieppe, P. A.: 5-Thiopyridoxine in rheumatoid arthritis: Clinical and experimental studies. *Arthritis Rheum.* **23:** 106–110, 1980.

Jaffe, I. A.: Intra-articular dissociation of the rheumatoid factor. *J. Lab. Clin. Med.* **60:** 409–421, 1962.

Jaffe, I. A.: Comparison of the effects of plasmapheresis and penicillamine on the level of circulating rheumatoid factor. *Ann. Rheum. Dis.* **22:** 71–76, 1963.

Jaffe, I. A.: The effect of penicillamine on the laboratory parameters in rheumatoid arthritis. *Arthritis Rheum.* **8:** 1064–1079, 1965.

Jaffe, I. A.: The technique of penicillamine administration in rheumatoid arthritis. *Arthritis Rheum.* **18:** 513, 514, 1975.

Jaffe, I. A.: Actions of gold and penicillamine, in *Rheumatoid Arthritis,* J. L. Gordon and B. L. Hazleman, eds., pp. 131–140, Elsevier/North Holland Biomedical, Amsterdam, 1977.

Jaffe, I. A.: Penicillamine: An antirheumatoid drug. *Am. J. Med.* **75** (6A): 63–68, 1983.

Jaffe, I. A., chmn.: Proceedings of the international symposium on penicillamine. *J. Rheumatol.* **8** (Suppl. 7): 1–181, 1981.

Lampe, K. F., ed.: *Drug Evaluations,* 6th Ed., American Medical Association, Chicago, 1986.

Lipsky, P. E.: Disease-modifying drugs, in *Rheumatoid Arthritis: Etiology, Diagnosis, Management,* P. D. Utsinger, N. J. Zvaifler, and G. E. Ehrlich, eds., pp. 601–634, Lippincott, Philadelphia, 1985.

Lipsky, P. E. and Ziff, M.: The mechanisms of action of gold and D-penicillamine in rheumatoid arthritis, in *Rheumatoid Arthritis,* M. Ziff, G. P. Velo, and S. Gorini, eds., pp. 219–235, Raven, New York, 1982.

McConkey, B., Amos, R. S., Durham, S., Forster, P. J. G., Hubball, S., and Walsh, L.: Sulphasalazine in rheumatoid arthritis. *Br. Med. J.* **280:** 442–444, 1980.

Markenson, J. A.: Antiarthritic drugs: A comparative overview. *Drug Ther.* **11:** 45–57, 1981.

Milne, M. D., chmn.: Proceedings of conference on penicillamine. *Postgrad. Med. J.* **44:** (Suppl.): 1–56, 1968.

Muirden, K. D.: The use of chloroquine and D-penicillamine in the treatment of rheumatoid arthritis. *Med. J. Aust.* **144:** 32–37, 1986.

Multicentre Study Group: Levamisole in rheumatoid arthritis. *Lancet* **2:** 1007–1012, 1978.

Multicentre Trial Group: Controlled trial of D(-)penicillamine in severe rheumatoid arthritis. *Lancet* **1:** 275–280, 1973.

Parnham, M. J.: The pharmacology of antirheumatic drugs. *Agents Actions Suppl.* **14:** 153–169, 1984.

Pasero, G., Pellegrini, P., Ambanelli, U., Ciompi, M. L., Colamussi, V., Ferraccioli, G., Barbieri, P., Mazzoni, M. R., Menegale, G., and Trippi, D.: Controlled multicenter trial of tiopronin and D-penicillamine for rheumatoid arthritis. *Arthritis Rheum.* **25:** 923–929, 1982.

Ritzmann, S. E., Coleman, S. L., and Levin, W. C.: The effect of some mercaptans upon a macrocryogelglobulin; modifications induced by cysteamine, penicillamine, and penicillin. *J. Clin. Invest.* **39:** 1320–1329, 1960.

Rothermich, N. O., Whisler, R. L., Brower, A. C., and Kantor, S. M.: Penicillamine, in *Rheumatoid Arthritis,* pp. 209–216, Grune and Stratton, Orlando, FL, 1985.

St. Clair, E. W. and Polisson, R. P.: Therapeutic approaches to the treatment of rheumatoid disease. *Med. Clin. North Am.* **70:** 285–304, 1986.

Scheinberg, I. H. and Sternlieb, I.: Long term management of hepatolenticular degeneration (Wilson's disease). *Am. J. Med.* **29:** 316–333, 1960.

Scheinberg, I. H. and Sternlieb, I.: *Wilson's Disease.* W. B. Saunders, Philadelphia, 1984.

Scheinberg, I. H., Jaffe, M. E., and Sternlieb, I.: The use of trientine in preventing the effects of interrupting penicillamine therapy in Wilson's disease. *N. Engl. J. Med.* **317:** 209–213, 1987.

Walshe, J. M.: Wilson's disease. New oral therapy. *Lancet* **1:** 25, 26, 1956a.

Walshe, J. M.: Penicillamine. A new oral therapy for Wilson's disease. *Am. J. Med.* **21:** 487–495, 1956b.

Walshe, J. M.: Current therapeutics CXCII—Penicillamine. *Practitioner* **191:** 789–795, 1963.

Wilson, J. E. and duVigneaud, V.: Inhibition of the growth of the rat by L-penicillamine and its prevention by aminoethanol and related compounds. *J. Biol. Chem.* **184:** 63–70, 1950.

Hydroxychloroquine

I. Hydroxychloroquine as an Innovative Therapeutic Agent

The cause of rheumatoid arthritis is unknown and, therefore, therapy remains empirical. Nevertheless, therapeutic advances have taken place in this field, as exemplified by antirheumatic drugs such as gold salts, hydroxychloroquine, and D-penicillamine (Dugowson and Gilliland, 1986). These agents are variously referred to as "slow-acting antiinflammatory drugs," "disease-modifying drugs," "remission-inducing drugs," and "second-line drugs." Lipsky (1985) considered none of these terms to be entirely accurate. However, since all members of this group elicited some clinical, serologic, and, occasionally, radiographic signs of improvement in rheumatoid arthritis, and induction of true remission was very rare, the term "disease-modifying drugs" (DMARDs) seemed the most accurate label. The capacity of DMARDs to act slowly to modify the rate of progression of rheumatoid arthritis sets them apart from non-steroidal antiinflammatory drugs (NSAIDs), which produce prompt clinical alleviation of pain and inflammation, but do not modify the course of the disease.

The mechanism of action of the 4-aminoquinoline antimalarials (chloroquine as well as hydroxychloroquine) in rheumatoid arthritis is not known with certainty, but they have two interactions with cells that could diminish inflammation and autoimmune reactions (Rothermich et al., 1985): (1) they bind to DNA and RNA and presumably intercalate between base pairs, thereby stabilizing nucleotides and inhibiting the prepolymerization and transcription necessary for cellular replication and normal protein synthesis (Allison et al., 1965; Rothermich et al., 1985); (2) in addition, they also accumulate in lysosomes, stabilizing them, and thereby interfering with chemotaxis, phagocytosis, autophagy, and digestion. Mackenzie (1983) and Dugowson and Gilliland (1986) suggested that the action of the 4-aminoquinolines on lysosomes is probably the basis for most of their actions in autoimmune diseases.

The 4-aminoquinolines are less widely used in treating rheumatoid arthritis than they might be, because of deep-rooted concern about ocular toxicity. Although these drugs can be sufficiently concentrated in the cornea to cause punctate or larger opacities, such effects are usually subclinical and reversible, and only rarely interfere with vision. Of greater significance, the potential for inducing a more serious toxicity, retinopathy, has come to stigmatize these agents, since the retinopathy may lead to irreversible loss of vision. Fortunately, in recent years it has become clear that by rigidly restricting the *per diem* dose—in the case of hydroxychloroquine to no greater than 400 mg (6 mg/kg lean body weight)—and by requiring frequent ocular examinations, the occurrence of retinopathy is reduced to an essentially negligible level (Mackenzie and Scherbel, 1980; Scherbel, 1983; Rynes, 1985). Scherbel (1983) noted that "...during the past decade hydroxychloroquine has again gained popularity after it has been demonstrated that ocular toxicity is a dose-related problem that usually can be avoided."

Other side effects of the 4-aminoquinoline agents include frequent but tolerable nausea and dyspepsia, as well as infrequent and reversible skin rashes. At high or excessive doses, bleaching of hair and vitiligo may occur, and, rarely, reversible agranulocytosis or aplastic anemia, and a reversible myopathy may also be seen (Capell et al., 1983; Rothermich et al., 1985).

The 4-aminoquinoline antimalarial drugs are quite widely used as DMARDs. In the USA, hydroxychloroquine is used almost exclusively, being considered to have less potential for eye toxicity than chloroquine (Dugowson and Gilliland, 1986; Rynes, 1985; Rothermich et al., 1985), whereas in England, chloroquine is more widely used. Hydroxychloroquine, today, is considered to be a relatively safe, moderately active DMARD and is frequently administered with an NSAID. It is the only DMARD that is occasionally given in combination with other DMARDs (Katz, 1987), and Scherbel (1983) believed that hydroxychloroquine was unique in this regard, because, when used in combination with other DMARDs or antiproliferative drugs, it rarely caused adverse reactions.

Runge (1983) indicated that hydroxychloroquine was better tolerated than gold, D-penicillamine, or levamisole and was easier to use. Long periods of treatment did not result in the development of retinal toxicity, autoimmune effects, or proteinuria. Consequently, it was considered to be a reasonable first choice among slow acting antirheumatic remittive drugs. Mackenzie and Scherbel (1980) were also of the opinion that "[s]ince comparable efficacy is obtainable with less risk, it is reasonable to administer 4-aminoquinolines [hydroxychloroquine] before the other more hazardous remission-inducing agents."

Rynes (1985) summed up the status of hydroxychloroquine at present: "The effectiveness of antimalarials has withstood the test of time." He felt that a balance had been reached between the initial enthusiasm for chloroquine and hydroxychloroquine and the disappointment over their lower-than-expected effectiveness and potential serious side effects. Rynes (1985) concluded, "Based on effectiveness, toxicity and cost, hydroxychloroquine is the slow acting antirheumatic drug of choice for many patients with RA [rheumatoid arthritis] in 1985."

Hydroxychloroquine, as well as chloroquine, is also used for the treatment of discoid and systemic lupus erythematosus. Both drugs are particularly effective in patients with skin and joint manifestations, (Dubois, 1978, Isaacson et al., 1982). The mechanism of action in discoid and systemic lupus erythematosus remains unknown.

Isaacson et al. (1982) indicated that chloroquine and hydroxychloroquine are powerful weapons in the dermatologist's armamentarium and should not be ignored. They have proved useful in management of porphyria cutanea tarda, polymorphous light eruption, and solar urticaria.

Early Clinical Research History

In the case of hydroxychloroquine, the early clinical research is the scientific work leading to its use in rheumatoid arthritis, and it is, therefore, reported in section II.

II. The Scientific Departure
Leading to the Use of Hydroxychloroquine
in Rheumatoid Arthritis: Quinacrine

Page (1951) noted that there were many remedies recommended for the treatment of lupus erythematosus—a chronic relapsing disorder characterized by face lesions consisting of plaques with erythema, hyperkeratosis, follicular plugging, and dilation of small terminal blood vessels (discoid lupus), which can also exist as a more disseminated, inflammatory, connective tissue disease (systemic lupus). He hesitated to describe yet another treatment, but went on to state, "A chance observation led to the use of mepacrine [the antimalarial quinacrine, also widely known as Atabrine (Fig. 1)] in a case of lupus erythematosus....The result was so dramatic that all cases of lupus erythematosus seen since in the dermatological department of this hospital...have been treated with this drug." Of the 18 cases reported, only one failed to improve. Significantly, Page (1951) went on to note, "In two patients associated changes of rheumatoid arthritis have disappeared as the skin condition has improved."

Freedman and Bach (1952) used the positive findings of Page (1951) in the two lupus patients with rheumatoid symptoms as a rationale for trying quinacrine in rheumatoid arthritis. The 23 patients in their study had active joint inflammation and had had the disease for more than 2 yr. During 6 wk to 8 mo of treatment, soft tissue swellings subsided, movement became free and more vigorous, the need for analgesics was reduced, and all signs of joint inflammation were lost in 22 of the 23 patients. The positive effects were not seen for at least 4 wk. Large doses of the drug caused toxicity. These investigators recognized that their study was uncontrolled and that the course of the disease was remarkably variable, but they concluded that the improvements in the patients may have been caused by quinacrine.

Brennecke et al. (1951), without stating a rationale for their study, reported (in abstract) on the short-term treatment of 38 rheumatoid arthritics with primaquine (Fig. 1) and three other related 8-aminoquinoline antimalarial agents. With only 2 wk of oral administration, 20 patients in this open study were considered to have

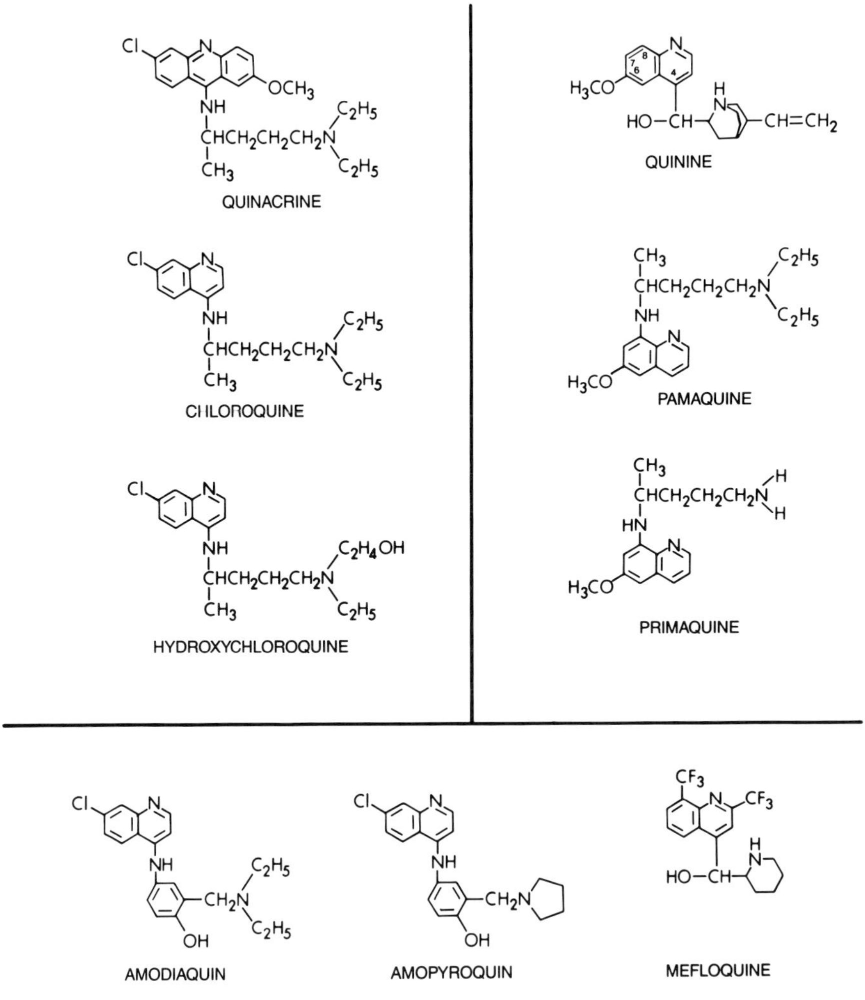

Fig. 1. The structures of hydroxychloroquine and chemically and/or pharmacologically related substances.

shown improvement, whereas 15 were not; three patients with rheumatoid spondylitis appeared to respond well. After the drugs were stopped, some patients continued in remission, but most relapsed. Many patients were continued on small doses of the drug. Brennecke et al. (1951) suggested that 8-aminoquinolines possessed some degree of antirheumatic activity, but because of toxic manifes-

tations (methemoglobinemia, anorexia, abdominal distress, neutropenia) a search should be continued for 8-aminoquinolines with
greater therapeutic potency and less toxicity.

Background Contributions Preceding
the Use of Quinacrine and 4-Aminoquinolines
in Rheumatoid Arthritis

Synthetic antimalarials owe their existence to both real and
potential shortages of the natural product, quinine, during World
War I and World War II. The military operations of both Germany
and the Allies in the malaria-infested parts of the world depended
on adequate supplies of the bark of the cinchona tree (native to South
America but heavily cultivated in southeast Asia), from which quinine was extracted. Since these supplies could be, or were, suddenly
cut off by enemy action, the desirability of having synthetic antimalarials was obvious. The molecular configuration of quinine (Fig. 1),
one part of which is the quinoline nucleus, provided the point of
departure for the synthesis of the quinoline, acridine, and other
chemical series of antimalarials during the 1920s and later (Rollo,
1970). Pamaquine (Fig. 1), the first of the 8-aminoquinoline antimalarials, was prepared in Germany in 1924 (Schulemann, 1932;
Schulemann et al., 1932), and quinacrine, an acridine, was likewise
introduced in Germany in 1930 as an antimalarial (Mauss and
Mietzsch, 1933).

According to Coatney (1963), chloroquine (Fig. 1), a 4-amino-
quinoline, was first synthesized in Germany in 1934 by Andersag of
Bayer, I. G. Farbenindustrie AG. The subsequent confusing and
complex story of the development of this compound as an antimalarial drug, from 1934 through the World War II years to 1946, has
been recounted by Coatney (1963). It involved investigators in six
countries on five continents and embraced chloroquine's initial
discovery, rejection, rediscovery, evaluation, and acceptance. Coatney (1963) remarked that since 1946 chloroquine was the drug of
choice for malaria the world over.

In a continuing chemical exploration of the 4-aminoquinoline
series for better antimalarial compounds, Surrey and Hammer

(1950) synthesized hydroxychloroquine by replacing one of the *N*-ethyl groups of the side chain of chloroquine with an *N*-hydroxyethyl group (Fig. 1).

Significant Events Following the Use of Quinacrine in Rheumatoid Arthritis

Haydu (1953) administered chloroquine three times a week for a period of six months to 28 patients with rheumatoid arthritis. He provided a lengthy, vague rationale based on the concept that the tissues of rheumatoid arthritic patients had an increased requirement for ATP. He noted that compounds related to quinine had ATPase-inhibiting activity and ATP-sparing qualities. He further felt that "...the molecular configuration of antimalarial drugs might be utilized in treatment of rheumatoid arthritis...with the view of inhibiting the tissues' requirement for ATP." Twenty-one of the 28 rheumatoid arthritis patients were reported to have improved considerably. Haydu (1953) noted the work of Page (1951) with quinacrine and that of Brennecke et al. (1951) with primaquine and stated that in a preliminary study he had found primaquine to be inferior to chloroquine in antirheumatic activity.

Forestier and Certonciny (1954), in an open study with quinacrine and chloroquine in 24 cases of rheumatoid arthritis, found that 50% of the patients benefited from the antimalarials. Chloroquine was much better tolerated than quinacrine.

Freedman (1956) carried out the first short-term, double-blind, placebo-controlled study with chloroquine, which he indicated that he had begun in 1953. Thirty-four patients received chloroquine and 32 received placebo for 16 wk. Moderate, gradual improvement was seen only in the chloroquine-treated patients. A total of 50 patients were treated with chloroquine on a long-term basis after the trial ended; 43 of these eventually had no stiffness or joint inflammation and had little or no need for analgesics. Furthermore, no significant toxicity was observed in patients who had been treated for as long as 2 yr. The author suggested that a larger investigation was warranted. Other clinical studies followed in rapid succession. Bagnall (1957) reported on a long-term study of chloroquine and stressed that there was no early response to this agent, but that it was eventually so effective that he could not "...ethically substantiate administration of placebo to seriously affected patients...." Cohen and Calkins (1958) and Freedman and Steinberg (1960), as well as other investigators, provided additional positive clinical findings.

Scherbel et al. (1957a) conducted the first study of hydroxychloroquine in rheumatoid arthritis and compared its efficacy with that of chloroquine. These authors pointed out in their introductory remarks that the first antimalarials used to treat rheumatoid patients—the acridine derivative, quinacrine, and the 8-aminoquinoline derivative, primaquine—although active, had exhibited very serious, even lethal, toxicities which ruled out their clinical use. Scherbel et al. (1957a) gave hydroxychloroquine to 26 patients and chloroquine to 25. These patients, all of whom had had active rheumatoid arthritis for approximately 1–2 yr, were treated for 18 mo and then evaluated. Both agents were judged to have significant, moderate, antirheumatoid activity. However, because hydroxychloroquine caused less gastrointestinal disturbance and could be administered in larger doses during the initial period of treatment, these investigators considered hydroxychloroquine "...to be the preferred antimalarial drug for treatment of disorders of connective tissue...."

Cramer (1958) used both hydroxychloroquine and chloroquine in 132 patients with rheumatoid arthritis and Marie Strümpell spondylitis. In a 6–10-mo observation period, 72% of the patients showed either remission or major improvement. The author felt that hydroxychloroquine seemed to have fewer side effects than chloroquine and might be a more practical compound, and suggested that "...this new form of antirheumatic therapy is worthy of considerably more clinical study."

Scull (1962) treated 196 poorly controlled rheumatoid arthritis patients with chloroquine, hydroxychloroquine, or placebo. In contrast to placebo treatment, 57% of the drug-treated patients showed some improvement, and the group on hydroxychloroquine reported the fewest side effects. At the same time, Mainland and Sutcliffe (1962) conducted a 6-mo, double-blind, placebo-controlled study of hydroxychloroquine in 121 patients, and Hamilton and Scott (1962) carried out a 3-mo, double-blind, placebo-controlled, crossover study with hydroxychloroquine in 41 patients. Both sets of investigators observed small, but significant, improvements with hydroxychloroquine.

Table 1 defines the critical scientific ideas and experiments leading to hydroxychloroquine and categorizes their origin.

Many reviews and books dealing with the uses and limitations of hydroxychloroquine in rheumatoid arthritis have appeared (*see*, for example, Scherbel et al., 1957a,b; Scherbel, 1961; Thompson and Werbel, 1972; Dubois, 1978; Mackenzie and Scherbel, 1980; Isaacson et al., 1982; Plaquenil Symposium, 1983; Runge, 1983; Halberg, 1984; Herxheimer, 1985; Miescher, 1986; Maksymowych and Russell, 1987).

III. Comments on Events Leading to the Use of Hydroxychloroquine in Rheumatoid Arthritis

Coatney (1963) pointed out that the crash program to develop synthetic antimalarials superior to quinacrine that took place in the USA during World War II involved the screening of some 16,000 compounds against avian models of malaria; of this large number of compounds, 400 were 4-aminoquinolines (Scherbel, 1983). Finally, after an appraisal of 80 of the most active of the 16,000 compounds in human malarias, chloroquine was judged to be the most important (Coatney, 1963).

As already described, interest in the use of antimalarial drugs, including hydroxychloroquine, for treating rheumatoid arthritis began after World War II and was based on a serendipitous clinical observation. Moreover, as Lipsky (1985) emphasized, the use of chloroquine and hydroxychloroquine, as well as other DMARDs, in the treatment of rheumatoid arthritis has been based entirely on clinical experience and not on knowledge of specific drug action.

Table 1
Profile of Observations and Ideas
Crucial to the Development of Hydroxchloroquine[a]

Sequence: Departure compound* to innovative drug**	Orient- ation	Nature of study	Research institution	National origin	Nature of discovery	Screening involved	Crucial ideas or observations
Quinacrine*							
Page (1951)	Clinical	Derma- tology	Hospi- tal	UK	Seren- dipitous	No	In 2 lupus patients, quinacrine greatly improves associated changes of rheuma- toid arthritis.
Chloroquine							
Haydu (1953)	Clinical	Rheuma- tology	Hospi- tal	USA	Orderly	No	21 of 28 rheumatoid arthritics are con- siderably improved by 6 mo of chloro- quine treatment.
Hydroxychloroquine*							
Scherbel et al. (1957a)	Clinical	Rheuma- tology	Private	USA	Orderly	No	Quinacrine con- sidered toxic; both chloroquine and hydroxychloroquine have modest anti- rheumatoid activity; hydroxychloroquine superior to chloro- quine.

*Taken from section II. Entries are those contributions without which the discovery of the agent (or additionally, in some cases, a relevant clinical application) would not have taken place or would have been materially delayed.

IV. Developments Subsequent to Hydroxychloroquine

Rheumatologists continued to study new 4-aminoquinoline antimalarials in the search for substances that would be superior to hydroxychloroquine in rheumatoid arthritis. Amodiaquin and amopyroquin (Fig. 1) were tried clinically (Bartholomew and Duff, 1963); however, neither of these antimalarials surpassed the efficacy and/or safety of hydroxychloroquine.

According to Peters (1980) the involvement of the US Army in the war in Indochina in the 1960s, coincident with the development of strains of malaria resistant to chloroquine plus the global increase in malaria transmission, led to a resurgence in the search for new antimalarials. From this most recent antimalarial effort emerged potent drugs, such as the 4-quinolinemethanol, mefloquine (Fig. 1), which have been tested in animals and humans. Rheumatologists have not reported on the use of newer antimalarials in the treatment of rheumatoid arthritis.

References

Allison, J. L., O'Brien, R. L., and Hahn, F. E.: DNA: Reaction with chloroquine. *Science* **149**: 1111–1113, 1965.

Bagnall, A. W.: The value of chloroquine in rheumatoid disease: A four-year study of continuous therapy. *Can. Med. Assoc. J.* **77**: 182–194, 1957.

Bartholomew, L. E. and Duff, I. F.: Amopyroquin (Propoquin) in rheumatoid arthritis. *Arthritis Rheum.* **6**: 356–363, 1963.

Brennecke, F. E., Alving, A. S., Arnold, J., Bergenstal, D. M., and De Wind, L.T.: A preliminary report on the effect of certain 8-aminoquinolines in the treatment of rheumatoid arthritis. *J. Lab. Clin. Med.* **38**: 795, 796, 1951.

Capell, H. A., Daymond, T. J., and Dick, W. C.: Antimalarials and other secondline drugs, in *Rheumatic Disease*, pp. 159–164, Springer-Verlag, Berlin, 1983.

Coatney, G. R.: Pitfalls in a discovery: The chronicle of chloroquine. *Am. J. Trop. Med. Hyg.* **12**: 121–128, 1963.

Cohen, A.S. and Calkins, E.: A controlled study of chloroquine as an antirheumatic agent. *Arthritis Rheum.* **1**: 297–312, 1958.

Cramer, Q.: Rheumatoid diseases. *Mo. Med.* **55**:1203–1207, 1958.

Dubois, E. L.: Antimalarials in the management of discoid and systemic lupus erythematosus. *Semin. Arthritis Rheum.* **8**: 33–51, 1978.

Dugowson, C. E. and Gilliland, B. C.: Management of rheumatoid arthritis. *DM* **32**: 1–76, 1986.

Forestier, J. and Certonciny, A.: Essai de traitement des rhumatismes inflammatoires par les antimalariques de synthése. *Rev. Rhum. Mal. Ostéoartic.* **21**: 395–398, 1954.

Freedman, A.: Chloroquine and rheumatoid arthritis: A short-term controlled trial. *Ann. Rheum. Dis.* **15**: 251–257, 1956.

Freedman, A. and Bach, F.: Mepacrine and rheumatoid arthritis. *Lancet* **2:** 321, 1952.

Freedman, A. and Steinberg, V. L.: Chloroquine in rheumatoid arthritis: A double blindfold trial of treatment for one year. *Ann. Rheum. Dis.* **19:** 243–250, 1960.

Halberg, P.: Controlled, double-blind, comparative studies of disease modifying anti-rheumatic drugs in the treatment of patients with rheumatoid arthritis. A review. *Dan. Med. Bull.* **5:** 391–402, 1984.

Hamilton, E. B. D. and Scott, J. T.: Hydroxychloroquine sulfate (Plaquenil) in treatment of rheumatoid arthritis. *Arthritis Rheum.* **5:** 502–512, 1962.

Haydu, G. G.: Rheumatoid arthritis therapy: A rationale and the use of chloroquine diphosphate. *Am. J. Med. Sci.* **225:** 71–75, 1953.

Herxheimer, A., ed.: "Disease-modifying" drugs in rheumatoid arthritis. *Drug Ther. Bull.* **23:** 101–104, 1985.

Isaacson, D., Elgart, M., and Turner, M. L.: Antimalarials in dermatology. *Int. J. Dermatol.* **21:** 379–395, 1982.

Katz, R. S.: Rheumatoid arthritis, in *Conn's Current Therapy*, R. E. Rakel, ed., pp. 789–796, W. B. Saunders, Philadelphia, 1987.

Lipsky, P. E.: Disease-modifying drugs, in *Rheumatoid Arthritis: Etiology, Diagnosis, Management,* P. D. Utsinger, N. J. Zvaifler and G. E. Ehrlich, eds., pp. 601–634, J. B. Lippincott, Philadelphia, 1985.

Mackenzie, A. H.: Antimalarial drugs for rheumatoid arthritis. *Am. J. Med.* **75(6A):** 48–58, 1983.

Mackenzie, A. H. and Scherbel, A. L.: Chloroquine and hydroxychloroquine in rheumatological therapy. *Clin. Rheum. Dis.* **6:** 545–547, 1980.

Mainland, D. and Sutcliffe, M. I.: Hydroxychloroquine sulfate in rheumatoid arthritis: A six month double blind trial. *Bull. Rheum. Dis.* **13:** 287–290, 1962.

Maksymowych, W. and Russell, A. S.: Antimalarials in rheumatology: Efficacy and safety. *Semin. Arthritis Rheum.* **16:** 206–221, 1987.

Mauss, H. and Mietzsch, F.: Atebrin, ein neues heilmittel gegen malaria. *Klin. Wochenschr.* **12:** 1276–1278, 1933.

Miescher, P. A.: Treatment of systemic lupus erythematosus. *Springer Semin. Immunopathol.* **9:** 271–282, 1986.

Page, F.: Treatment of lupus erythematosus with mepacrine. *Lancet* **2:** 755–758, 1951.

Peters, W.: Chemotherapy of malaria, in *Malaria*, vol. 1, *Epidemiology, Chemotherapy, Morphology, and Metabolism,* J. P. Kreier, ed., pp. 145–283, Academic, New York, 1980.

Plaquenil Symposium. A reassessment of Plaquenil in the treatment of rheumatoid arthritis. *Am. J. Med.* **75** (1A): 1–56, 1983.

Rollo, I. M.: Drugs used in the chemotherapy of malaria, in *The Pharmacological Basis of Therapeutics*, 4th Ed., L. S. Goodman and A. Gilman, eds., pp. 1095–1124, Macmillan, New York, 1970.

Rothermich, N. O., Whisler, R. L., Brower, A. C., and Kantor, S. M.: Antimalarials, in *Rheumatoid Arthritis*, pp. 181–189, Grune and Stratton, Orlando, FL, 1985.

Runge, L. A.: Risk/benefit analysis of hydroxychloroquine sulfate treatment in rheumatoid arthritis. *Am. J. Med.* **75** (1A): 52–56, 1983.

Rynes, R. I.: Antimalarial treatment of rheumatoid arthritis: 1985 status (editorial). *J. Rheumatol.* **4**: 657–659, 1985.

Scherbel, A. L.: Long-term maintenance therapy with 4-aminoquinoline compounds in rheumatoid arthritis, in *Inflammation and Diseases of Connective Tissues, a Hahnemann Symposium*, L. C. Mills and J. H. Moyer, eds., pp. 555–561, W. B. Saunders, Philadelphia, 1961.

Scherbel, A. L.: Use of synthetic antimalarial drugs and other agents for rheumatoid arthritis: Historic and therapeutic perspectives. *Am. J. Med.* **75** (1A): 1–4, 1983.

Scherbel, A. L., Schuchter, S. L., and Harrison, J. W.: IV. Comparison of effects of two antimalarial agents, hydroxychloroquine sulfate and chloroquine phosphate, in patients with rheumatoid arthritis. *Cleve. Clin. Q.* **24**: 98–104, 1957a.

Scherbel, A. L., Schuchter, S. L., and Harrison, J.W.: V. Chemotherapy in rheumatoid arthritis: A concept. *Cleve. Clin. Q.* **24**: 105–115, 1957b.

Schulemann, W.: Synthetic antimalarial preparations. *Proc. R. Soc. Med.* **25**: 897–905, 1932.

Schulemann, W., Schönhöfer, F., and Wingler, A.: Synthesis des Plasmochin. *Klin. Wochenschr.* **II**: 381–384, 1932.

Scull, E.: Chloroquine and hydroxychloroquine therapy in rheumatoid arthritis. *Arthritis Rheum.* **5**: 30–36, 1962.

Surrey, A. R. and Hammer, H. F.: Preparation of 7-chloro-4-[4-(N-ethyl, N-β–hydroxyethylamino)-1-methylbutylamino]-quinoline and related compounds. *J. Am. Chem. Soc.* **72**: 1814, 1815, 1950.

Thompson, P. E. and Werbel, L. M.: *Antimalarial Agents: Chemistry and Pharmacology*, Academic, New York, 1972.

Methotrexate

I. Methotrexate as an Innovative Therapeutic Agent

Methotrexate, a close structural analog of folic acid (Fig. 1), is a cell-cycle-specific, cytotoxic (cytostatic), antimetabolitic, antiproliferative agent. It acts primarily to prevent cell division during that phase of the cell cycle in which DNA synthesis is maximal (the S phase) by competitively inhibiting the enzyme dihydrofolate reductase (DHFR). DHFR catalyzes the reduction of folic acid and of dihydrofolic acid (DHF) to tetrahydrofolic acid (THF) (Fig. 1). The resultant unavailability of THF, when DHFR is inhibited, leads to cessation of the synthesis of thymidylic acid, inosinic acid, other purine metabolites, and the amino acids methionine and glycine (Letendre et al., 1985; Lampe, 1986). Inosinic acid is the precursor of purines needed for DNA and RNA syntheses, and thymidylic acid is a nucleotide that is specific to the DNA molecule (Miller et al., 1986). Methionine and glycine are important in protein synthesis.

Antiproliferative agents, such as methotrexate, have marked inhibitory effects on tissues that replicate rapidly, i.e., bone marrow cells, gastrointestinal epithelium, germinal epithelium, hair follicles, and lymphoid organs (Lampe, 1986). Although such an antiproliferative effect has untoward consequences for these normal tissues, it accounts for the extensive use of methotrexate in the treatment of neoplastic diseases and in the treatment of severe, recalcitrant, disabling psoriasis. Methotrexate is also important as a second- or third-line treatment for severe arthritic disorders.

In the application of methotrexate in cancer, cures have been reported in most cases of choriocarcinoma and related trophoblastic tumors. Methotrexate also produces some complete remissions in

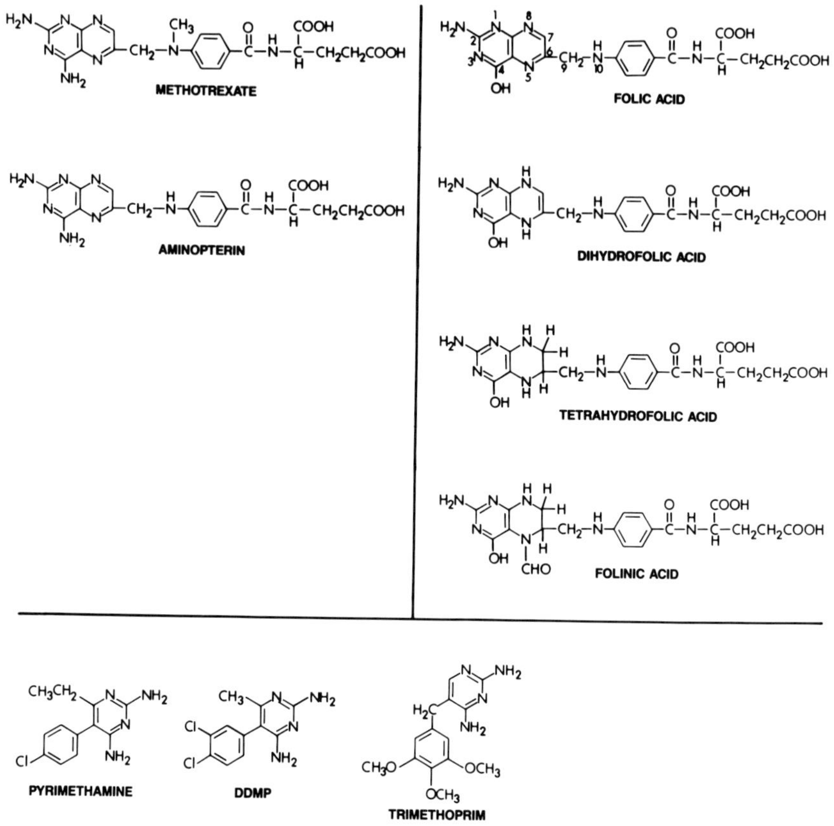

Fig. 1. The structures of methotrexate and chemically and/or pharmacologically related substances.

acute lymphocytic leukemia of childhood and, in combination with 6-mercaptopurine, is used for maintenance therapy in this indication. It is also of value alone or in combination in non-Hodgkins lymphomas; testicular cancer; head and neck, breast, lung, cervical, ovarian, and bladder carcinomas; and medulloblastoma (Calabresi and Parks, 1985; Lampe, 1986). Aggressive treatment of resistant tumors with massive (lethal) doses of methotrexate, followed by "rescue" with folinic acid, has appeared to be of value (Calvert and Turnbull, 1981a,b; Jolivet et al., 1983). Folinic acid, (N^5-formyl-THF) (Fig. 1), which is metabolized in several steps to intracellular THF, prevents the lethal consequences of the intense inhibition of DHFR.

Psoriasis is a chronic and recurrent disease characterized by dry, well-circumscribed, silvery, scaling papules and plaques commonly occurring on the scalp, elbows, knees, back, and buttocks; it is caused by an excessive epidermal cell proliferation (Berkow, 1982). The rapid turnover of epithelial cells in psoriatic skin renders them susceptible to the antiproliferative effect of methotrexate. Unfortunately, long-term, daily treatment with methotrexate frequently produces liver fibrosis and cirrhosis, especially in patients with significant alcohol intake, obesity, or diabetes (Weinstein et al., 1973). This problem is minimized, while maintaining effective action on the psoriasis, by giving a large single dose of methotrexate weekly, or by giving three oral doses weekly, administered over a 36-hour period (Kremer, 1985; Lampe, 1986).

Methotrexate has a rapid, therapeutic effect in rheumatoid arthritis, and is accepted by patients (Willkens, 1985; Tugwell et al., 1987; Wilke et al., 1987). Rheumatoid arthritis is characterized by inflammation of peripheral joints, which can result in progressive destruction of articular structures and may be generalized to all connective tissues, including vital organs (Berkow, 1982; Calabro, 1975). Methotrexate is indicated for the treatment of progressive rheumatoid arthritis that is refractory to conventional measures including salicylates, other NSAIDs, and parenteral gold (St. Clair and Polisson, 1986). Systemic administration of low doses weekly, in a pulse fashion, is effective without precipitating serious side effects (Miller et al., 1986). Its efficacy in long-term treatment, however, has not been fully established.

Methotrexate is also being studied in inflammatory conditions other than rheumatoid arthritis, namely, psoriatic arthritis, Reiter's syndrome, inflammatory myositis, vasculitis, and lupus erythematosus (Wilke et al., 1987; Nashel, 1985).

Calvert and Turnbull (1981a) pointed out that, as a cytotoxic antiproliferative agent, methotrexate has many unique features:

It is the only antimetabolite in common use that is not incorporated into nucleic acids, its action being wholly attributable to inhibition of the synthesis of essential DNA components...its cytotoxic effect may be abrogated by an antidote (FA) [folinic acid]... there are no documented carcinogenic effects of MTX [methotrexate] unlike many other cytotoxic agents...As a result of these properties, myelosuppression and gastrointestinal toxicity are wholly preventable by the appropriate use of FA. In addition, the chronic sequelae of many cytotoxic drugs (carcinogenesis and sterility) appear to be absent with MTX.

Early Clinical Research History

Cancer

In the wake of the successful clinical use of its precursor, aminopterin, in leukemic children (Farber et al., 1948) (*see* section II), methotrexate and other folate antagonists were evaluated in a variety of neoplastic disorders. Most early studies used aminopterin, methotrexate, and other antagonists interchangeably. Several of these studies confirmed Farber's finding of a beneficial action of folate antagonism in acute leukemia in children (Dameshek, 1949; Stickney et al., 1949), and others reported temporary improvement in some patients with chronic leukemias and in lymphomas such as lymphosarcoma, reticulum-cell sarcoma, and Hodgkins disease (Wright et al., 1951; Burchenal et al., 1951; Schoenbach et al., 1952).

Li et al. (1956) found that methotrexate caused unequivocal clinical improvement, along with radiological evidence of regression of pulmonary metastases, in two patients with choriocarcinoma and one patient with chorioadenoma destruens. Subsequently, marked temporary regression of mycosis fungoides was noted in three of five patients treated with methotrexate, and the drug was considered to be valuable for far-advanced cases of this disease (Wright et al., 1960). In the same year, Condit and Eliel (1960), in a preliminary study, reported that large, infrequent doses of methotrexate produced remissions in three children with acute lymphoblastic leukemia.

A huge literature has developed concerning the use of methotrexate in the treatment of cancer (*see* for references Calvert and Turnbull, 1981b; Johns and Bertino, 1982; Chabner, 1982; Jolivet et al., 1983; Calabresi and Parks, 1985).

Psoriasis

Edmundson and Guy (1958), following the successful use of aminopterin by Gubner et al. (1951) (*see* section II), were the first to use methotrexate for treating psoriasis. They administered the drug via the oral route in single doses for 6 d, withdrew it for 3 d, and then reinstituted drug for another 6 d. Seventy-five percent of their 17 patients had greater than 50% improvement of psoriatic lesions; improvement lasted for 3 mo to 1 yr after treatment. The authors felt that, although toxic effects were rarely observed in their series, considerable caution was required in the use of either methotrexate or aminopterin. Confirmatory reports of the usefulness of methotrexate in psoriasis followed (e.g., Hunter, 1962; Dobes, 1963; Strakosch, 1963). For reference to the later literature, see Weinstein (1977).

Rheumatoid Arthritis

Gubner et al. (1951) demonstrated aminopterin to be effective in rheumatoid arthritis (*see* section II). However, it was not until 1962 that sporadic preliminary reports of the use of methotrexate in rheumatoid arthritis appeared in the literature. O'Brien et al. (1962) stated that methotrexate moderately to markedly improved scores for pain on motion, tenderness, swelling, and range of motion of joints in 13 of 18 cases of psoriatic arthritis or of coexistent psoriasis and rheumatoid arthritis. It also reduced the area of the skin surface that was involved with psoriasis. This group followed up with a double-blind, placebo-controlled trial in 21 patients and found that considerable improvement in joint and skin manifestation occurred in drug-treated, but not in placebo-treated, patients (Black et al., 1964). A large literature exists concerning the use of methotrexate in arthritis (*see*, for example, Groff et al., 1983; Willkens, 1985; Letendre et al., 1985; Kremer, 1985; Miller et al., 1986; Tugwell et al., 1987; Pugh and Pugh, 1987).

II. The Scientific Departure
Leading to Methotrexate: Aminopterin

Considerable research in the early 1940s was directed toward discovering a "factor" that was essential for the growth of *Lactobacillus casei* and that stimulated hematopoiesis in animals. This growth factor was found in yeast (Snell and Peterson, 1940), spinach (Mitchell et al., 1941), and liver (Pfiffner et al., 1943), and considerable effort was expended to purify, crystallize, and characterize it (Stokstad, 1943; Hutchings et al., 1944). This search was stimulated to some extent by reports that chemically uncharacterized "folic acid" caused regression of tumors in mice (Leuchtenberger et al., 1944, 1945). These results were not confirmed.

Angier et al. (1946) determined the structure of liver *Lactobacillus casei* factor. It consisted of 2-amino-4-hydroxy pteridine linked via a 6-methylene bridge to the amino group of para-aminobenzoic acid that, in turn, formed an amide linkage to glutamic acid. This vitamin was originally named pteroylglutamic acid, but is now more commonly known as folic acid (Fig. 1).

Subsequently, colleagues of Angier synthesized several weak antimetabolites of folic acid and studied them as inhibitors of growth in microbiological and mammalian systems: "methylfolic acid" of unknown structure, pteroylaspartic acid, and a series of N^{10}-substituted derivatives of folic acid (Franklin et al., 1947; Hutchings et al., 1947; Cosulich and Smith, 1948). This group (Franklin et al., 1947) indicated that folic acid antimetabolites might be of use in the treatment of blood dyscrasias marked by erythrocytosis or by leukocytosis (leukemia). Farber et al. (1948) noted in passing that they had administered pteroylaspartic acid to a moribund leukemic child for eight days. It had not altered the clinical course of the disease, but postmortem examination revealed a very hypoplastic bone marrow—an unexpected beneficial effect.

Other groups also prepared weak antimetabolite antagonists of folic acid as a component of their research programs, but made no expression of potential medical uses for these agents (Martin et al., 1947; Mallette et al., 1947; Woolley and Pringle, 1948).

The first potent antimetabolite of folic acid, aminopterin (4 amino-folic acid) (Fig. 1) was synthesized by Seeger et al. (1947). They noted that it produced in *Streptococcus faecalis R.* an inhibition of growth that could be reversed by folic acid. The compound was lethal to mice and not readily reversed by folic acid (Franklin et al., 1948). However, Oleson et al. (1948) found aminopterin to be an antagonist for folic acid not only in *Streptococcus fecalis,* but also in chicks and weanling rats. It produced a hypoplastic bone marrow in rats. The inhibition was reversible with folic acid, but not strictly competitive. The authors speculated that a complex that was not readily dissociable might have formed between aminopterin and an enzyme that processed folic acid.

In experiments with guinea pigs, aminopterin administration led to signs of folic acid deficiency, weight loss, and death. Some animals developed normocytic anemia, all of them developed leukopenia, and half developed agranulocytosis and thrombocytopenia. Marrow hypoplasia was apparent as well. The leukopenia and thrombocytopenia, but not the anemia, were prevented by high doses of folic acid (Minnich and Moore, 1948). Swendseid et al. (1948) found that aminopterin produced anemia and leukopenia in weanling rats. Some reversal of these effects could be achieved with folic acid.

Farber et al. (1948) administered aminopterin to 16 children with acute leukemia, most of whom were moribund. Ten showed clinical, hematologic, and pathological evidence of important improvement of at least three months duration, although six did not respond well. In five of the good responders, white cell counts tended to return to normal; the percentage of immature cells fell; blast forms decreased markedly, and the relative percentages of mature leukocytes approached normal values in peripheral blood; hemoglobin, red cell count, and platelets approached normal; leukemic cells in bone marrow were decreased. However, Farber and his associates felt that the toxic effects of the drug—stomatitis with early ulceration—might limit its use.

Gubner et al. (1951) commented that, like corticosteroids and ACTH, aminopterin was known to be a potent inhibitor of connective tissue proliferation. Based on this rationale, they administered aminopterin to seven rheumatoid arthritics and to one patient with acute rheumatic fever. In all but one of the rheumatoid arthritics, significant amelioration of the arthritis occurred: symptomatic relief, subsidence of acute exudative signs of arthritic and periarthritic involvement, and functional improvement. One of these patients, who had severe psoriasis of the entire body, had a striking remission of the psoriasis. Similar striking remissions were also observed in five additional patients with psoriatic arthritis and in three patients with uncomplicated psoriasis. The authors, however, were of the opinion that "[t]he toxic effects of aminopterin place practical limitations on its use as a therapeutic agent."

Background Contributions Preceding
the Development of Aminopterin
as an Antiproliferative Agent

The search for and discovery of the folate antagonist aminopterin, and very soon thereafter methotrexate, was based on the antimetabolite concept propounded by Woods (1940) and Fildes (1940). These authors pointed out that an exogenous chemical compound, closely related in structure to an endogenous metabolite, could competitively inhibit the enzyme that normally processed the endogenous metabolite, and in this manner produce significant biological consequences.

Significant Events Following Aminopterin

Amethopterin (4 amino-N^{10}-methyl-folic acid) (Fig. 1) was synthesized by Seeger et al. (1949) and noted to have folate antagonist activity in *Streptococcus faecalis R.* It was later given the name methotrexate. In further studies this same group (Franklin et al., 1949) found that, in addition to exerting a potent competitive, reversible inhibition of folic acid in *Streptococcus faecalis R.*, methotrexate was also a potent antagonist in weanling rats and chicks. However, under the conditions of their experiments only incomplete protection could be obtained with folic acid in rats.

Table 1 defines the critical scientific ideas and experiments leading to methotrexate and categorizes their origins.

III. Comments on Events
Leading to Methotrexate

Jukes (1962), in reviewing events leading to methotrexate, stated:

In animals, a dietary deficiency of folic acid results in anaemia and leucopenia, accompanied by hypocellularity of the haemopoietic tissues in the bone marrow. These findings led to the anticipation that a substance with a biological effect antagonistic to that of folic acid would inhibit cell growth. Accordingly, in the laboratories of American Cyanamid Company, a programme was started in 1946 to synthesize chemical analogues of folic acid.

Table 1
Profile of Observations and Ideas Crucial to the Development of Methotrexate[a]

Sequence: Departure compound* to innovative drug**	Orient-ation	Nature of study	Research institution	National origin	Nature of discovery	Screening involved	Crucial ideas or observations
Aminopterin*							
Pfiffner et at. (1943)	Pre-clinical	Chem-istry/ nutrition	Univer-sity, indus-try	USA	Orderly	Targeted	An antianemia growth factor (folic acid) isolated in crystalline form from liver; authors considered it likely that the growth factors found by separate research groups in yeast, liver, and spinach were all the same substance.
Angier et al. (1946)	Pre-clinical	Chem-istry	Indus-try	USA	Orderly	No	Structure of growth factor from liver— folic acid—elucidated.
Seeger et al. (1947)	Pre-clinical	Chem-istry/ pharma-cology	Indus-try	USA	Orderly	Targeted	Aminopterin synthe-sized; first potent folate antagonist.
Gubner et al. (1951)	Clini-cal	Rheuma-tology	Univer-sity	USA	Orderly	No	Aminopterin ameliorates rheumatoid arthritis; striking remissions of psoriasis observed.
Methotrexate**							
Seeger et al. (1949)	Pre-clinical	Chem-istry/ pharma-cology	Indus-try	USA	Orderly	Targeted	Methotrexate synthe-sized; very potent folate antagonist.

[a]Taken from section II. Entries are those contributions without which the discovery of the agent (or additionally, in some cases, a relevant clinical application) would not have taken place or would have been materially delayed.

Farber and coworkers gave pteroylaspartic acid, a product of this program, to a leukemic patient in the spring of 1947 (Farber et al., 1948). This compound was the first antagonist to folic acid to be employed in Farber's studies. Johns and Bertino (1982) felt that Farber's subsequent demonstration that aminopterin was effective in producing remissions in acute leukemia (Farber et al., 1948) "...was a landmark in cancer chemotherapy: it provided the first demonstrations that an antimetabolite could be an antineoplastic agent..."

Farber (1949) commented,

> The present plan of study concerning the action of folic acid antagonists is following along the lines decided with Dr. SubbaRow [American Cyanamid Co.] in the spring of 1947. It consists essentially of the study of the action on laboratory animals and on patients with various forms of incurable cancer of related compounds in an attempt to find one which is more effective and less toxic than any we have previously employed.

In his 1966 Albert Lasker Clinical Research Award Lecture, Farber reminisced,

> Through him [Y. SubbaRow, for many years a colleague at Harvard Medical School and at the time of Farber's investigations the first director of research of the Lederle Laboratories of American Cyanamid Co.], and through his able colleagues who synthesized and made available a large series of folic acid antagonists, we were able to apply the result of our own biological studies of leukemia to the treatment of children who were dying of acute leukemia.

According to Johns and Bertino (1982), methotrexate replaced aminopterin in clinical use because it was shown to have a more favorable therapeutic index in tumor-bearing mice.

IV. Developments
Subsequent to Methotrexate

Pyrimethamine (Falco et al., 1951) (Fig. 1) showed a much greater affinity for the DHFR of plasmodia than for the mammalian enzyme, and it has become a useful treatment for malaria (Webster, 1985).

Trimethoprim (Fig. 1), a highly selective inhibitor of the DHFR of lower organisms (e.g., bacteria), is used in a synergistic combination with sulfamethoxazole in the treatment of bacterial infections.

By preventing the incorporation of para-aminobenzoic acid into folic acid, sulfamethoxazole inhibits the formation of this growth factor in those lower organisms that must make it *de novo*, and thus adds a second antifolate action to that of DHFR inhibition (Mandell and Sande, 1985).

DDMP (Fig. 1), a lipid soluble folate antagonist that more readily crosses the blood–brain barrier than does methotrexate and, therefore, should be useful against brain tumors, was developed and given extensive clinical trial (Nichol et al., 1977).

10-Deaza, 10-ethyl aminopterin is transported into some tumor cells more efficiently than into normal cells, is trapped inside the tumor cells, and is a candidate for study in humans (Sirotnak, 1983).

The aim in modern research in the folate-antagonist arena is to discover compounds that show selective toxicity for cancer cells or for infectious microorganisms as opposed to normal cells. This is to be accomplished by exploiting

1. Differences, where such exist, in the affinities of compounds for folic acid binding sites,
2. Differences in the magnitude of the cellular uptake of inhibitors or of their retention, and
3. Any other differences that may be found to exist in the pathways that lead to folic acid synthesis or utilization.

References

Angier, R. B., Boothe, J. H., Hutchings, B. L., Mowat, J. H., Semb, J., Stokstad, E. L. R., Subbarow, Y., and Waller, C. W.: The structure and synthesis of the liver *L. casei* factor. *Science* **103:** 667–669, 1946.

Berkow, R., ed.: *The Merck Manual,* 14th Ed., Merck Sharp & Dohme Research Laboratories, Rahway, NJ, 1982.

Black, R. L., O'Brien, W. M., Van Scott, E. J., Auerbach, R., Eisen, A. Z., and Bunim, J. J.: Methotrexate therapy in psoriatic arthritis: Double-blind study on 21 patients. *JAMA* **189:** 743–747, 1964.

Burchenal, J. H., Karnofsky, D. A., Kingsley-Pillers, E. M., Southam, C. M., Myers, W. P. L., Escher, G. C., Craver, L. F., Dargeon, H. W., and Rhoads, C. P.: The effect of the folic acid antagonists and 2,6-diaminopurine on neoplastic disease. *Cancer* **4:** 549–569, 1951.

Calabresi, P. and Parks, R. E., Jr.: Antiproliferative agents and drugs used for immunosuppression, in *The Pharmacological Basis of Therapeutics,* 7th

Ed., A. G. Gilman, L. S. Goodman, T. W. Rall, and F. Murad, eds., pp. 1247–1306, Macmillan, New York, 1985.

Calabro, J. J.: Long-term reappraisal of indomethacin. *Drug Ther.* **5**: 46–60, 1975.

Calvert, A. H. and Turnbull, C. P.: Proceedings of the International Symposium on Methotrexate. Introduction. *Cancer Treat. Rep.* **65** (Suppl. 1): 1,2, 1981a.

Calvert, A. H. and Turnbull, C. P., eds.: Proceedings of the International Symposium on Methotrexate. *Cancer Treat. Rep.* **65** (Suppl. 1): 1–189, 1981b.

Chabner, B. A.: Methotrexate, in *Pharmacologic Principles of Cancer Treatment*, B. A. Chabner, ed., pp. 229–255, W. B. Saunders, Philadelphia, 1982.

Condit, P. T. and Eliel, L. P.: Effects of large infrequent doses of a-methopterin on acute leukemia in children. *JAMA* **172**: 451–453, 1960.

Cosulich, D. B. and Smith, J. M., Jr.: Analogs of pteroylglutamic acid. I. N^{10}-Alkylpteroic acid and derivatives. *J. Am. Chem. Soc.* **70**: 1922–1926, 1948.

Dameshek, W.: The use of folic acid antagonists in the treatment of acute and subacute leukemia; preliminary statement. *Blood* **4**: 168–171, 1949.

Dobes, W. L.: The use of folic acid antagonists and steroids in treatment of psoriasis. *South. Med. J.* **56**: 187–192, 1963.

Edmundson, W. F. and Guy, W. B.: Treatment of psoriasis with folic acid antagonists. *Arch. Dermatol.* **78**: 200–203, 1958.

Falco, E. A., Goodwin, L. G., Hitchings, G. H., Rollo, I. M., and Russell, P. B.: 2:4-diaminopyrimidines—a new series of antimalarials. *Br. J. Pharmacol. Chemother.* **6**: 185–200, 1951.

Farber, S.: Some observations in the effect of folic acid antagonists on acute leukemia and other forms of incurable cancer. *Blood* **4**: 160–167, 1949.

Farber, S.: Chemotherapy in the treatment of leukemia and Wilms' tumor. *JAMA* **198**: 826–836, 1966.

Farber, S., Diamond, L. K., Mercer, R. D., Sylvester, R. F., and Wolff, J. A.: Temporary remissions in acute leukemia in children produced by folic acid antagonist, 4-aminopterylglutamic acid (aminopterin). *N. Engl. J. Med.* **238**: 787–793, 1948.

Fildes, P.: A rational approach to research in chemotherapy. *Lancet* **1**: 955–957, 1940.

Franklin, A. L., Stokstad, E. L. R., and Jukes, T. H.: Observations on the effect of 4-amino-pteroylglutamic acid on mice. *Proc. Soc. Exp. Biol. Med.* **67**: 398–400, 1948.

Franklin, A. L., Belt, M., Stokstad, E. L. R., and Jukes, T. H.: Biological studies with 4-amino-10-methylpteroyl-glutamic acid. *J. Biol. Chem.* **177**: 621–629, 1949.

Franklin, A. L., Stokstad, E. L. R., Belt, M., and Jukes, T. H.: Biochemical experiments with a synthetic preparation having an action antagonistic to that of pteroylglutamic acid. *J. Biol. Chem.* **169:** 427–435, 1947.

Groff, G. D., Shenberger, K. N., Wilke, W. S., and Taylor, T. H.: Low dose oral methotrexate in rheumatoid arthritis: An uncontrolled trial and review of the literature. *Semin. Arthritis Rheum.* **12:** 333–347, 1983.

Gubner, R., August, S., and Ginsberg, V.: Therapeutic suppression of tissue reactivity; Effect of aminopterin in rheumatoid arthritis and psoriasis. *Am. J. Med. Sci.* **221:** 176–182, 1951.

Hunter, G. A.: The use of methotrexate in the treatment of psoriasis. *Aust. J. Dermatol.* **6:** 248-254, 1962.

Hutchings, B. L., Stokstad, E. L. R., Bohonos, N., and Slobodkin, N. H.: Isolation of a new *Lactobacillus casei* factor. *Science* **99:** 371, 1944.

Hutchings, B. L., Mowat, J. H., Oleson, J. J., Stokstad, E. L. R., Boothe, J. H., Waller, C. W., Angier, R. B., Semb, J., and SubbaRow, Y.: Pteroylaspartic acid, an antagonist for pteroylglutamic acid. *J. Biol. Chem.* **170:** 323–328, 1947.

Johns, D. G. and Bertino, J. R.: The chemotherapeutic agents, in *Cancer Medicine*, J. F. Holland and E. Frei III, eds., pp. 775–790, Lea and Febiger, Philadelphia, 1982.

Jolivet, J., Cowan, K. H., Curt, G. A., Clendeninn, N. J., and Chabner, B. A.: The pharmacology and clinical use of methotrexate. *N. Engl. J. Med.* **309:** 1094–1104, 1983.

Jukes, T. H.: Introduction, in *Methotrexate in the Treatment of Cancer*, R. Porter and E. Wiltshaw, eds., pp. 1–10, John Wright and Sons, Bristol, UK, 1962.

Kremer, J. M.: Longterm methotrexate therapy in rheumatoid arthritis: A review. *J. Rheumatol. (Suppl.)* **12:** 25–28, 1985.

Lampe, K. F., ed.: *Drug Evaluations*, 6th Ed., American Medical Association, Chicago, 1986.

Letendre, P. W., DeJong, D. J., and Miller, D. R.: The use of methotrexate in rheumatoid arthritis. *Drug Intell. Clin. Pharm.* **19:** 349–358, 1985.

Leuchtenberger, R., Leuchtenberger, C., Laszlo, D., and Lewisohn, R.: The influence of "folic acid" on spontaneous breast cancer in mice. *Science* **101:** 46, 1945.

Leuchtenberger, C., Lewisohn, R., Laszlo, D., and Leuchtenberg, R.: "Folic acid" a tumor growth inhibitor. *Proc. Soc. Exp. Biol. Med.* **55:** 204, 205, 1944.

Li, M. C., Hertz, R., and Spencer, D. B.: Effect of methotrexate therapy upon choriocarcinoma and chorioadenoma. *Proc. Soc. Exp. Biol. Med.* **93:** 361–366, 1956.

Mallette, M. F., Taylor, E. C., Jr. and Cain, C. K.: Pyrimido [4,5-b]pyrazines. II. 2,4-diaminopyrimido [4,5-b]pyrazine and derivatives. *J. Am. Chem. Soc.* **69**: 1814–1816, 1947.

Mandell, G. L. and Sande, M. A.: Sulfonamides, trimethoprim–sulfamethoxazole, and agents for urinary tract infections, in *The Pharmacological Basis of Therapeutics*, 7th Ed., A. G. Gilman, L. S. Goodman, T. W. Rall, and F. Murad, eds., pp. 1095–1114, Macmillan, New York, 1985.

Martin, G. J., Tolman, L., and Moss, J.: *d*(-)-Methylfolic acid, displacing agent for folic acid. *Arch. Biochem* **12**: 318, 319, 1947.

Miller, D. R., Letendre, P. W., DeJong, D. J., and Fiechtner, J. J.: Methotrexate in rheumatoid arthritis: An update. *Pharmacotherapy* **6**: 170–178, 1986.

Minnich, V. and Moore, C. V.: Hypoplastic anemia induced in guinea pigs by 4-amino pteroyl glutamic acid. *Fed. Proc.* **7**: 276, 1948.

Mitchell, H. K., Snell, E. E., and Williams, R. J.: The concentration of "folic acid." *J. Am. Chem. Soc.* **63**: 2284, 1941.

Nashel, D. J.: Mechanisms of action and clinical applications of cytotoxic drugs in rheumatic disorders. *Med. Clin. North Am.* **69**: 817–840, 1985.

Nichol, C. A., Cavallito, J. C., Woolley, J. L., and Sigel, C. W.: Lipid-soluble diaminopyrimidine inhibitors of dihydrofolate reductase. *Cancer Treat. Rep.* **61**: 559–564, 1977.

O'Brien, W. M., Van Scott, E. J., Black, R. L., Eisen, A. Z., and Bunim, J. J.: Clinical Trial of amethopterin (methotrexate) in psoriatic and rheumatoid arthritis (preliminary report). *Arthritis Rheum.* **5**: 312, 1962.

Oleson, J. J. Hutchings, B. L., and SubbaRow, Y.: Studies on the inhibitory nature of 4-aminopteroylglutamic acid. *J. Biol. Chem.* **175**: 359–365, 1948.

Pfiffner, J. J., Binkley, S. B., Bloom, E. S., Brown, R. A., Bird, O. D., Emmett, A. D., Hogan, A. G. and O'Dell, B. L.: Isolation of the antianemia factor (vitamin Bc) in crystalline form from liver. *Science* **97**: 404, 405, 1943.

Pugh, M. C. and Pugh, C. B.: Current concepts in clinical therapeutics: Disease-modifying drugs for rheumatoid arthritis. *Clin. Pharm.* **6**: 475–491, 1987.

St. Clair, E. W. and Polisson, R. P.: Therapeutic approaches to the treatment of rheumatoid disease. *Med. Clin. North Am.* **70**: 285–304, 1986.

Schoenbach, E. B., Colsky, J., and Greenspan, E. M.: Observations on the effects of the folic acid antagonists, aminopterin and amethopterin, in patients with advanced neoplasms. *Cancer* **5**: 1201–1220, 1952.

Seeger, D. R., Cosulich, D. B., Smith, J. M., Jr., and Hultquist, M. E.: Analogs of pteroylglutamic acid. III. 4-amino derivatives. *J. Am. Chem. Soc.* **71**: 1753–1758, 1949.

Seeger, D. R., Smith, J. M., Jr., and Hultquist, M. E.: Antagonist for pteroylglutamic acid. *J. Am. Chem. Soc.* **69**: 2567, 1947.

Sirotnak, F. M.: Concepts in new folate analog design, in *Progress in Cancer*

Research and Therapy, vol. 28, Y.-C. Cheng, B. Goz, and M. Minikoff, eds., pp. 77–87, Raven, New York, 1983.

Snell, E. E. and Peterson, W. H.: Growth factors for bacteria. X. Additional factors required by certain lactic acid bacteria. *J. Bacteriol.* **39:** 273–285, 1940.

Stickney, J. M., Mills, S. D., Hagedorn, A. B., and Cooper, T.: The treatment of acute leukemia with folic acid antagonists. *Proc. Staff Meet. Mayo Clin.,* **24:** 525–533, 1949.

Stokstad, E. L. R.: Some properties of a growth factor for *Lactobacillus casei. J. Biol. Chem.* **149:** 573, 574, 1943.

Strakosch, E. A.: A study of the folic acid antagonists in the treatment of psoriasis (aminopterin vs. methotrexate vs. aminopterin and a corticosteroid). *Dermatologica* **126:** 259–267, 1963.

Swendseid, M. E., Wittle, E. L., Moersch, G. N., Bird, O. D., and Brown, R. A.: Studies in the rat of inhibitors of pteroylglutamic acid structurally related to this vitamin. *Fed. Proc.* **7:** 299, 1948.

Tugwell, P., Bennett, K., and Gent, M.: Methotrexate in rheumatoid arthritis. *Ann. Intern. Med.* **107:** 358–366, 1987.

Webster, L. T.: Drugs used in the chemotherapy of protozoal infections. Malaria, in *The Pharmacological Basis of Therapeutics,* 7th Ed., A. G. Gilman, L. S. Goodman, T. W. Rall, and F. Murad, eds., pp. 1029–1048, Macmillan, New York, 1985.

Weinstein, G. D.: Methotrexate. *Ann. Intern. Med.* **86:** 199–204, 1977.

Weinstein, G., Roenigk, H., Maibach, H., and Cosmides, J.: Psoriasis-liver-methotrexate interactions. *Arch. Dermatol.* **108:** 36–42, 1973.

Wilke, W. S., Biro, J. A., and Segal, A. M.: Methotrexate in the treatment of arthritis and connective tissue diseases. *Cleve. Clin. J. Med.* **54:** 327–338, 1987.

Willkens, R. F.: Short term efficacy of methotrexate in the treatment of rheumatoid arthritis. *J. Rheumatol. (Suppl.)* **12:** 21–24, 1985.

Woods, D. D.: The relation of p-aminobenzoic acid to the mechanism of the action of sulphanilamide. *Br. J. Exp. Pathol.* **21:** 74–90, 1940.

Woolley, D. W. and Pringle, A.: Some structural analogues antagonistic to pteroylglutamic acid. *J. Biol. Chem.* **174:** 327–333, 1948.

Wright, J. C., Gumport, S. L., and Golomb, F. M.: Remissions produced with use of methotrexate in patients with mycosis fungoides. *Cancer Chemother. Rep.* **9:** 11–20, 1960.

Wright, J. C., Prigot, A., Wright, B., Weintraub, S., and Wright, L. T.: An evaluation of folic acid antagonists in adults with neoplastic diseases: A study of 93 patients with incurable neoplasms. *J. Natl. Med. Assoc.* **43:** 211–240, 1951.

Cyclophosphamide

I. Cyclophosphamide
as an Innovative Therapeutic Agent

Cyclophosphamide is a cytotoxic (cytostatic), cell-cycle-non-specific, antiproliferative agent that is used in such diverse medical problems as neoplasia, tissue transplantation, and inflammatory diseases (Gershwin et al., 1974). It is an inert prodrug for a potent nitrogen mustard alkylating agent. After the metabolic activation of cyclophosphamide to the potent mustard by liver enzymes, a nonenzymatic generation of chemically reactive molecules occurs. These reactive molecules can form covalent bonds with biologically ubiquitous groups, such as amino, phosphate, hydroxyl, carboxyl, sulfhydryl and imidazole, and as a result, depending on dose, cyclophosphamide is capable of either interfering with the reproduction of cells or killing cells. This is especially true in the case of rapidly dividing cells (Golomb, 1963; Gershwin et al., 1974; Hill, 1975).

Unlike methotrexate and azathioprine, which are cell-cycle-specific antiproliferative agents (i.e., they inhibit cell function only during the S phase [the DNA-synthesizing part of the cell cycle]), cyclophosphamide can damage or kill cells whether or not they are in the process of dividing (Bertino, 1973). However, it does exert its greatest effect during the S phase (Bertino, 1973, Capell et al., 1983). Ultimately, the primary mechanism of the antiproliferative action of cyclophosphamide appears to be the covalent crosslinking of nucleic acids by the nitrogen mustard metabolites of the drug. This crosslinking results in unpaired replication of DNA and damage to DNA structure (Rothermich, et al., 1985).

Cyclophosphamide represented an innovative step beyond mechlorethamine (nitrogen mustard) and other available alkylating agents, because it was not a vesicant and did not cause tissue necrosis (Gershwin et al., 1974). Because it is chemically inert, cyclophosphamide could be administered both orally and parenterally without damage to the gastrointestinal tract or to the injection site. This yielded the notable therapeutic advantage that administration of small doses over a prolonged period of time was possible.

Cyclophosphamide was developed as an antineoplastic agent and has a broad spectrum of clinical activity. The drug is effective against a variety of malignant diseases, including carcinoma of the lung, breast, cervix, and ovary; multiple myeloma; Hodgkin's disease; and non-Hodgkin's lymphomas including Burkitt's lymphoma (Calabresi and Parks, 1985; Lampe, 1986). In combination with other agents, it is effective in the treatment of lymphoblastic leukemia of childhood and as adjuvant therapy after mastectomy in cases with axillary node involvement.

Cyclophosphamide is also used to treat nonneoplastic diseases. It is a potent immunosuppressive agent and is used as one of the primary drugs in bone marrow transplantation. It is substituted for azathioprine in patients who are undergoing organ transplantation and cannot tolerate azathioprine (Berkow, 1982). Cyclophosphamide is considered to have greater cytotoxic effect on the B-cell lymphocytes than on the T-cell lymphocytes and is a potent inhibitor of antibody production (Gershwin et al., 1974; Klein, 1982; Bennett, 1983). Some authors also hold that, as an anti-proliferative agent, cyclophosphamide may reduce the formation of immune complex that appears to initiate inflammation (Curry, 1977) and produce part of its beneficial effects by being "anti-inflammatory" as well as "immunosuppressive." According to Kaplan and Calabresi (1973), "The most impressive results [with cyclophosphamide] have been noted in the treatment of adults with progressive rheumatoid arthritis unresponsive to conventional therapy and of nephrotic syndrome in children." Rothermich et al. (1985) stated that there is general agreement that cyclophosphamide can considerably reduce the activity of rheumatoid arthritis; however, the dosage schedule remains controversial, and the potential risks for each patient are unknown.

Cyclophosphamide is also of some benefit in the treatment of patients with autoimmune blood disorders, such as idiopathic thrombocytopenia purpura, systemic lupus erythematosus, and Wegener's granulomatosis (in which it is considered the drug of choice) (Lampe, 1986).

Aside from its troublesome but not serious side effects (alopecia, nausea, and vomiting) cyclophosphamide has serious side effects including acute and long-term toxicities as well as risks of infection and neoplasia. Hemorrhagic cystitis and carcinoma of the urinary bladder are of serious concern when using this drug (Aptekar et al., 1973; Foad and Hess, 1976; Klein and Smith, 1983; Pedersen-Bjergaard et al., 1988).

Early Clinical Research History

Cancer

In two reports, one preliminary, the second somewhat more complete, Gross and Lambers (1958a,b) presented the effect of cyclophosphamide in 45 cancer patients, 28 of whom could be evaluated at the time of the reports. According to Gross and Lambers (1958a), lymphosarcomas were conspiciously susceptible, with four complete and one extensive regressions in five patients. Four of nine carcinomas showed at least partial effect, and some benefit was also seen in plasmacytoma, lymphogranulomatosis, and chronic myelosis. The authors found that the side effects that limited the extent of treatment were the subjective experiences, such as nausea and loss of appetite, and not the danger of bone marrow injury.

Coggins et al. (1959) reported a preliminary uncontrolled study of cyclophosphamide in 95 patients, 85 of whom had solid tumors. Seventy patients received an initial loading dose of 7.5 mg/kg/d for 6 d, followed by oral and intravenous injections once or twice a week. Twenty-five patients received successive massive single injections of 45–100 mg/kg of the drug given at least 18 d apart. Approximately one-third of the patients (mostly on the conservative regimen) experienced objective regression of their tumors, lasting on the average of 2 mo. Striking leukopenia was produced by both regimens and thombocytopenia only by the massive regimen. Other side effects included alopecia, nausea, vomiting, and sterile cystitis.

The authors' results suggested to them that cyclophosphamide was more effective than other available alkylating agents.

Papac et al. (1960) treated 31 carcinoma and lymphoma patients with intravenous and oral cyclophosphamide given in divided doses. Three out of seven lymphoma patients obtained significant benefit. Some positive effects were also seen in Hodgkin's disease and ovarian carcinoma.

Wall and Conrad (1961) evaluated cyclophosphamide in 130 patients who had not been responsive to other agents and noted, "The best results were obtained in lymphosarcoma, multiple myeloma, Hodgkin's disease, and chronic lymphatic leukemia." The authors concluded that cyclophosphamide may offer some advantages in selected cases.

Korst et al. (1964) reported that, of the 165 patients with multiple myeloma treated with low-dosage cyclophosphamide, 24% had mild to moderate remissions as well as an increase in survival time. A decrease in pain, improved performance, and improved blood values were most often observed. It usually took several months of treatment before positive effects occurred.

Many other clinical studies ensued and aided in characterizing the proper use of this agent: see for example, Perry et al. (1967); Samuels and Howe (1967); Bergsagel et al. (1972); Presant et al. (1976); Mouridsen et al. (1976); Santos et al. (1983); Phillips et al. (1984); and Berd et al. (1986).

Rheumatoid Arthritis

Fosdick et al. (1966), noting that cytotoxic agents, such as nitrogen mustard had had a place in the therapy of rheumatoid arthritis for years (see section II, Diaz and colleagues), took 38 patients with active disease who had deteriorated for at least 6 mo despite therapy with gold, salicylates, and other conventional methods and added oral cyclophosphamide to their previous regimen. The patients' progress was followed for 6 mo to 3 yr. Nine patients showed complete remission, 25 showed clinical improvement, and four had no improvement.

Fosdick et al. (1968) updated their report of 1966 and noted that they had treated 54 patients who were unresponsive to conventional therapy with oral cyclophosphamide. The dosage was raised until either leukopenia or clinical improvement occurred. Of 15 patients whose pain was contained at a tolerable level with corticosteroids and/or ACTH, 12 were able to stop the steroids/ACTH and three continued on reduced dosage of steroids/ACTH. Thirty-eight patients continued on the drug for 6 mo or longer and, of these, 75% showed clinical improvement. Fosdick et al. (1968) observed that, frequently, 6–12 mo of treatment with cyclophosphamide were required before improvement occurred, and that in the first few months the patient's condition might continue to deteriorate.

Fosdick et al. (1969) indicated that a total of 108 patients had received oral cyclophosphamide therapy for a period of 6 mo to 6 yr. They reported 29 complete remissions, 45 partial remissions, 21 clinical remissions and 13 "no responses." These investigators concluded, "Known risks and possible unknown effects of long-term therapy require it [cyclophosphamide] to be reserved for patients suffering from severe, active disease resistant to conventional therapy."

Additional clinical trials of cyclophosphamide in rheumatoid arthritis followed and have helped to define the limits of its usefulness: for example, *see* Cooperating Clinics Committee of the American Rheumatism Association (1970), Lidsky et al. (1973), Williams et al. (1980), McCarty and Carrera (1982), Hørslev-Petersen et al. (1983). For additional articles and books on cyclophosphamide, *see* Gershwin et al. (1974), Hill (1975), Brock (1976), Colvin (1978) and Zon (1982).

II. The Scientific Departure Leading to Cyclophosphamide: Mechlorethamine (Nitrogen Mustard)

At the end of World War II, Gilman and Philips (1946) summarized extensive, secret, wartime studies carried out with vesicant mustards. These authors noted that with the advent of the war there had been a resurgence of interest in mustard gas (used in World War I) and related agents as potential offensive weapons. There was also interest in developing antidotes to such agents.

Mustard gas (sulfur mustard) and nitrogen mustards (Fig. 1) were recognized as owing their physiological activity to the formation of reactive cyclic onium cations. When systemically administered, their outstanding action was to kill cells, and cellular susceptibility was found to be related to the rate of proliferative activity. Thus, mustards readily produced lesions in the highly proliferative tissue of intestinal tract, bone marrow, and the lymphoid system. Moreover, minimal doses were shown to interfere selectively with the mitotic activity of a variety of cells and to act directly on the structure of chromosomes.

According to Gilman and Philips (1946), the effects of the mustards on lymphoid tissue, coupled with the selective vulnerability of proliferating cells, suggested the use of mustards in neoplasms of lymphoid tissue. Since nitrogen mustards had the practical advantages that they could be made stable in solution and that the ethylenimonium ions they generated at physiological pH were measurable (whereas sulfur mustards and their ethylenesulfonium ions were both highly unstable in solution), therapeutic interest became centered in the nitrogen mustards. Methyl-*bis*(β-chloroethyl) amine, a prototype of the nitrogen mustards, became known as "nitrogen mustard" and later as mechlorethamine (Fig. 1). It was demonstrated to produce rapid dissolution of transplanted lymphosarcoma in mice, albeit at near toxic doses. Subsequently, six patients in terminal stages of various neoplastic diseases were treated. Two of these patients with lymphosarcoma, who were not responding to X-ray therapy, were injected with nitrogen mustard, and there was a rapid diminution in the size of their tumors.

Following these preliminary results, Goodman et al. (1946) gave nitrogen mustard intravenously to 67 patients suffering with lymphosarcoma, Hodgkin's disease and leukemia. In general, dramatic improvements were seen, although not all patients benefited from the therapy. The best responses were seen in patients with Hodgkin's disease; the results with lymphosarcoma were not as good (Goodman et al., 1946). The patient with lymphosarcoma went into remission for three weeks to several months; however, upon recurrence the tumors gradually became resistant to therapy. The authors suggested that the actions of nitrogen mustard "...may eventually prove of greater importance than the clinical results obtained to date."

Diaz et al. (1951) and Diaz (1951) were the first to treat rheumatoid arthritis with nitrogen mustard. Their decision was based on (1) reports of leukopenia and lympholysis being produced by mustard

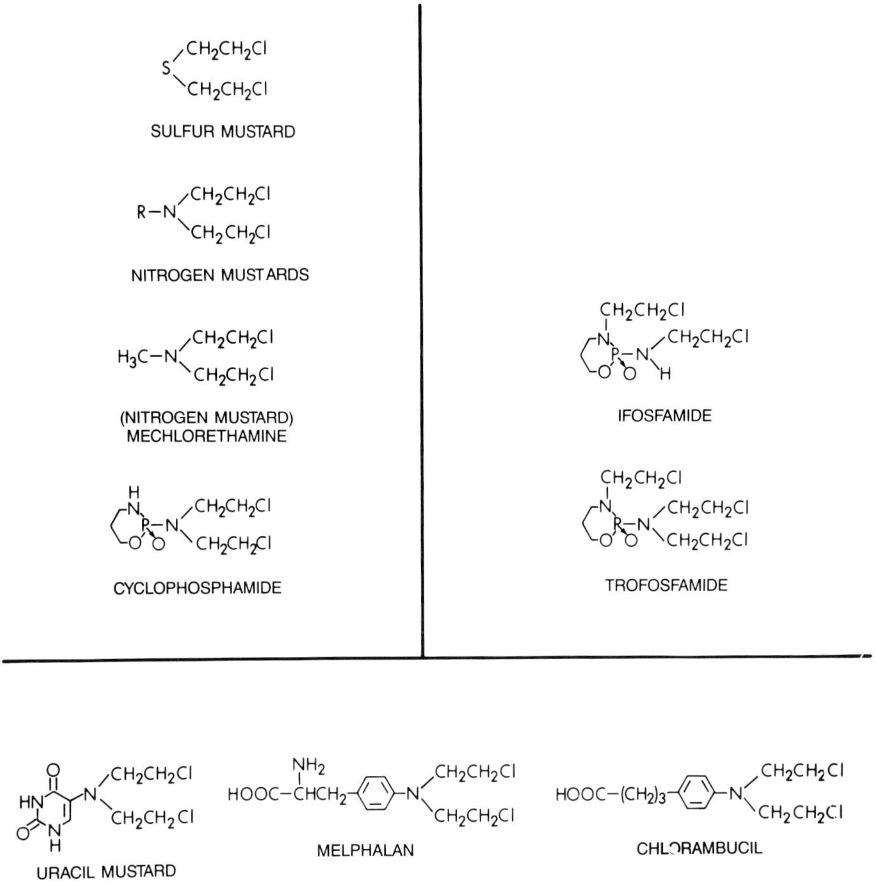

Fig. 1. The structures of cyclophosphamide and chemically and/or pharmacologically related substances.

gas and nitrogen mustard; (2) similarities among some of the effects of cortisone, ACTH, and nitrogen mustard (e.g., lympholysis and antimitotic action); and (3) the fact that Hench et al. (1949) had shown that cortisone and ACTH markedly improved the symptoms of rheumatoid arthritis. Diaz et al. (1951) reported "...remarkable results obtained with the use of nitrogen mustard in the treatment of rheumatoid arthritis. Of nine patients treated, five improved extraordinarily, with complete disappearance of the pain and swelling of the joint and recovery of normal movement." Three others showed considerable improvement. The authors stated that they had no experience with cortisone, but found it difficult to think it could be better than nitrogen mustard, the effects of which had surpassed any other therapies they had employed.

Background Contributions Preceding the Development of Mechlorethamine as an Antiproliferative Agent

According to Hektoen and Corper (1921), mustard gas was discovered by Victor Meyer in the late 1880s. It did not receive much attention until 1917, when it was used by the Germans in World War I for its poisonous effects. Meyer was credited with noting that the most severe action of mustard gas develops after its entrance into blood. Hektoen and Corper (1921) demonstrated that mustard gas prevented antibody formation in rabbits and dogs.

Krumbhaar and Krumbhaar (1919) and Krumbhaar (1919), with the US Army Medical Corps in France, studied the hematolytic changes in victims of mustard gas poisoning. The gas was found to exert direct toxicity on the bone marrow, depleting leukocytes and preventing the patient from fighting off secondary infections. Mortality was associated with severe leukopenia.

Pappenheimer and Vance (1920) injected rabbits intravenously with lethal doses of mustard gas. They reported severe lesions of bone marrow, marked reduction in circulating leukocytes, and severe lesions of intestinal tract, as well as extensive hemorrhage and edema of the lungs.

Significant Events Following Mechlorethamine

Cyclophosphamide (Fig. 1) was synthesized by Arnold et al. (1958a,b). They used the nitrogen mustard molecule as a model for the synthesis of a series of nitrogen mustard phosphamides. Their aim was to attain selective anticancer activity by making a compound that would be inert until activated by an enzyme that was found in high concentration in the body, especially in the tumor. The investigators decided to make cyclic phosphamides of nitrogen mustard since (1) the basicity of the phosphamide nitrogen and consequently the reactivity of the chlorine atoms were considerably reduced and (2) such phosphamides were subject to attack by phosphamidases that had been reported to be accumulated in tumor tissue. Two compounds, B-518-ASTA and B-485-ASTA, showed good activity, in vivo, against Yoshida ascites sarcoma of the rat, Walker carcinoma, and Jensen sarcoma. B-518 (cyclophosphamide) had less leukotoxic effects and was effective against DS carcinosarcoma, which had been particularly resistant to other forms of chemotherapy. In vitro, cyclophosphamide was inactive against tumor cells, indicating that the active form was liberated only within the body, but not by the tumors. Arnold et al. (1958a) stated, "In our opinion these results justify a clinical trial of B-518 on a wide scale."

Table 1 defines the critical scientific ideas and experiments leading to cyclophosphamide and categorizes their origins.

III. Comments on Events Leading to Cyclophosphamide

According to Golomb (1963), nitrogen mustard, known by the military code name of HN_2, was discovered when chemists working in secret during World War II found that substitution of a nitrogen atom for the sulfur atom of mustard gas greatly enhanced effectiveness.

Hill (1975) noted that modern interest in alkylating agents as anticancer agents "...must be attributed to Gilman and his colleagues who, after noting the toxicity of simple alkylating agents to lymphoid tissues and rapidly dividing cells, suggested that alkylating agents might have a therapeutic effect against tumors of lymphoid origin (Gilman and Philips, 1946)." Hill also pointed out that nitrogen mustard was the first synthetic compound clearly shown to possess antitumor activity in humans. In this regard, Gilman (1963) indicated that in the 1940s "...in the minds of most physicians the administration of drugs, other than an analgesic, in the treatment of malignant disease was the act of a charlatan."

Kaplan and Calabresi (1973) commented that "...alkylating agents and the present generation of anti-metabolites that are used to alter immune responses in man were developed in the cauldron of cytotoxicity during cancer-oriented research as part of an effort to seek methods for inhibiting the proliferation of malignant cells." In

Table 1
Profile of Observations and Ideas Crucial to the Development of Cyclophosphamide[a]

Sequence: Departure compound* to innovative drug**	Orient- ation	Nature of study	Research institution	National origin	Nature of discovery	Screening involved	Crucial ideas or observations
Nitrogen mustard*							
Gilman and Philips (1946)[b]	Pre- clinical, clinical	Chem- istry/ pharma- cology, onco- logy	Uni- versity, govern- ment	USA	Orderly	Targeted	Nitrogen mustard is lympholytic, antimi- totic; is active against lymphosarcoma in mice and humans.
Diaz (1951)	Clinical	Rheu- matol- ogy	Uni- versity	Spain	Orderly	No	Nitrogen mustard is effective in rheuma- toid arthritis.
Cyclophosphamide**							
Arnold et al. (1958a,b)	Pre- clinical	Chem- istry/ pharma- cology	Indus- try	West Germany	Orderly	Targeted	A cyclic nitrogen mustard phosphamide ester (cyclophospha- mide) is inert in vitro; a highly alkylating form is liberated in vivo; effective against animal tumors in vivo.

[a]Taken from section II. Entries are those contributions without which the discovery of the agent (or additionally, in some cases, a relevant clinical application) would not have taken place or would have been materially delayed.
[b]The classified military nature of the work covered by Gilman and Philips (1946) was reported only in summary form; it represents the work of a larger number of chemists, pharmacologists, and clinicians who are mentioned by the authors.

and around the time of the synthesis of cyclophosphamide, a feat that entailed the attachment of a cyclic phosphamide ester to *bis*-(2-chloroethyl)amine, other moeities were also being attached to this mustard in an attempt to gain specificity: for example, uracil, yielding uracil mustard (Lyttle and Petering, 1958); phenylalanine, yielding melphalan (Bergel and Stock, 1954), and an aryl group, yielding chlorambucil (Everett et al., 1953) (Fig. 1). Although these compounds, as well as other series of alkylating chemicals, have clinical utility, Calabresi and Parks (1985) stated that cyclophosphamide was the most widely used of the alkylating agents.

IV. Developments
Subsequent to Cyclophosphamide

Arnold (1967) and Brock (1967) reported the development of structural analogs of cyclophosphamide: isophosphamide (ifosfamide) and trophosophamide (trofosfamide) (Fig. 1). They are investigational drugs in cancer chemotherapy, and their spectra of activity are similar to that of cyclophosphamide (Lampe, 1986). Brock and Kuhlmann (1974) and Brock and Potel (1974) presented the pharmacology of a group of derivatives of ifosfamide wherein the chloroethyl groups were replaced, in part, by alkylsulfonyloxyalkyl groups. Of these compounds, ASTA 5122 was a more potent immunosuppressive agent than either cyclophosphamide or ifosfamide, whereas ASTA 5783 induced an unexpected stimulation of the immune system. The authors suggested clinical trials to evaluate these compounds in leukemias, autoaggressive lesions, and organ grafts.

Colvin (1978) remarked, "Although many analogues of cyclophosphamide have been synthesized and tested, only two are currently in clinical use, isophosphamide and trophosphamide."

Numerous compounds, which are either structural analogs of cyclophosphamide or precursors to its primary metabolites, continue to be synthesized and studied in the hope of providing second-generation cyclophosphamide derivatives with improved value in the treatment of cancer (Zon, 1982). This elusive goal—made difficult because the chemical complexities exhibited by cyclophosphamide metabolites present a great impediment to progress—is, nonetheless, still the goal to be achieved. Zon (1982) noted that it seemed inevitable that superior analogs will eventually be found.

References

Aptekar, R. G., Atkinson, J. P., Decker, J. L., Wolff, S. M., and Chu, E. W.: Bladder toxicity with chronic oral cyclophosphamide therapy in nonmalignant diseases. *Arthritis Rheum.* **16:** 461–467, 1973.

Arnold, H.: Ueber die Chemie neuer zytostatisch wirksamer N-Chloroaethyl-phosphorsäureesterdiamide, in *Proceedings of the Fifth International Congress Chemotherapy*, K. Spitzy and H. Haschek, eds., pp. 751–754, Verlag der Wiener Medizinischen-Akad.; Vienna, 1967.

Arnold, H., Bourseaux, F., and Brock, N.: Neuartige Krebs-Chemotherapeutika aus der Gruppe der zyklischen N-lost-phosphamidester. *Naturwissenschaften* 45: 64–66, 1958a.

Arnold, H., Bourseaux, F., and Brock, N.: Chemotherapeutic action of a cyclic nitrogen mustard phosphamide ester (B518-ASTA) in experimental tumors of the rat. *Nature* 181: 931, 1958b.

Bennett, D. R., ed.: *AMA Drug Evaluations*, 5th Ed., American Medical Association, Chicago, 1983.

Berd, D., Maguire, H. C., Jr., and Mastrangelo, M. J.: Induction of cell-mediated immunity to autologous melanoma cells and regression of metastases after treatment with a melanoma cell vaccine preceded by cyclophosphamide. *Cancer Res.* 46: 2572–2577, 1986.

Bergel, F. and Stock, J. A.: Cyto-active amino-acid and peptide derivatives. Part I. Substituted phenylalanines. *J. Chem. Soc.* II: 2409–2417, 1954.

Bergsagel, D. E., Jenkin, R. D. T., Pringle, J. F., White, D. M., Fetterly, J. C. M., Klaassen, D. J., and McDermot, R. S. R.: Lung Cancer: Clinical trial of radiotherapy alone vs. radiotherapy plus cyclophosphamide. *Cancer* 30: 621–627, 1972.

Berkow, R., ed.: *The Merck Manual*, 14th Ed., Merck Sharp & Dohme Research Laboratories, Rahway, New Jersey, 1982.

Bertino, J. R.: Chemical action and pharmacology of methotrexate, azathioprine and cyclophosphamide in man. *Arthritis Rheum.* 16: 79–83, 1973.

Brock, N.: Pharmacologische Untersuchungen mit Neuen N-Chloroathyl-phosphoraureesterdiamiden, in *Proc. Fifth Int. Congr. Chemother.*, vol. 2, K. H. Spitzy and H. Haschek, eds., pp. 155–161, Verlag der Wiener Medizinischen Akad., Vienna, 1967.

Brock, N.: Comparative pharmacologic study in vitro and in vivo with cyclophosphamide (NSC-26271), cyclophosphamide metabolites, and plain nitrogen mustard compounds. *Cancer Treat. Rep.* 60: 301–308, 1976.

Brock, N. and Kuhlmann, J.: Pharmacological studies with alkylsulfonyl-oxyalkyl substituted and chloroethyl substituted oxazaphosphorine-2-oxides. *Arzneimittelforsch.* 24: 1139–1149, 1974.

Brock, N. and Potel, J.: Pharmakologische Untersuchungen mit Alkyl-sulfonyl-oxyalkyl-bzw. Chloräthyl-substituierten Oxazaphosphorin-2-oxiden. *Arzneimittelforsch.* 24: 1149–1160, 1974.

Calabresi, P. and Parks, R. E., Jr.: Antiproliferative agents and drugs used for immunosuppression, in *The Pharmacological Basis of Therapeutics*, 7th

Ed., A. G. Gilman, L. S. Goodman, T. W. Rall, and F. Murad, eds., pp. 1247–1306, Macmillan, New York, 1985.

Capell, H. A., Daymond, T. J., Carson Dick, W.: Cytotoxic drugs, in *Rheumatic Disease*, pp. 179–186, Springer-Verlag, Berlin, 1983.

Coggins, P. R., Ravdin, R. G., and Eisman, S. H.: Clinical pharmacology and preliminary evaluation of Cytoxan (cyclophosphamide). *Cancer Chemother. Rep.* **June:** 9–11, 1959.

Colvin, M.: A review of pharmacology and clinical use of cyclophosphamide, in *Clinical Pharmacology of Anti-Neoplastic Drugs*, H. M. Pinedo, ed., pp. 245–261, Elsevier, Amsterdam, 1978.

Cooperating Clinics Committee of the American Rheumatism Association: A controlled trial of cyclophosphamide in rheumatoid arthritis. *N. Engl. J. Med.* **283:** 883–889, 1970.

Curry, H. L. F.: Immune suppression and immune enhancement, in *Rheumatoid Arthritis: Cellular Pathology and Pharmacology*, J. L. Gordon and B. L. Hazleman, eds., pp. 157–163, Elsevier, Amsterdam, 1977.

Diaz, C. J.: Treatment of dysreaction diseases with nitrogen mustards. *Ann. Rheum. Dis.* **10:** 144–151, 1951.

Diaz, C. J., Garcia, E. L., Merchante, A., and Perianes, J.: Treatment of rheumatoid arthritis with nitrogen mustard. Preliminary report. *JAMA* **147:** 1418, 1419, 1951.

Everett, J. L., Roberts, J. J., and Ross, W. C. J.: Aryl-2-halogenoalkylamines. Part XII. Some carboxylic derivatives of N N-di-2-chloroethylaniline. *J. Chem. Soc.*, **III:** 2386–2392, 1953.

Foad, B. S. I. and Hess, E. V.: Urinary bladder complications with cyclophosphamide therapy. *Arch. Intern. Med.* **136:** 616–619, 1976.

Fosdick, W. M., Parsons, J. L., and Hill, D. F.: Long-term cyclophosphamide therapy in rheumatoid arthritis: *Arthritis Rheum.* **9:** 855, 856, 1966.

Fosdick, W. M., Parsons, J. L., and Hill, D. F.: Long-term cyclophosphamide therapy in rheumatoid arthritis. *Arthritis Rheum.* **11:** 151–161, 1968.

Fosdick, W. M., Parsons, J. L., and Hill, D. F.: Long-term cyclophosphamide (CP) therapy in rheumatoid arthritis: A progress report, six years' experience. *Arthritis Rheum.* **12:** 663, 1969.

Gershwin, M. E., Goetzl, E. J., and Steinberg, A. D.: Cyclophosphamide: Use in practice. *Ann. Intern. Med.* **80:** 531–540, 1974.

Gilman, A.: The initial clinical trial of nitrogen mustard. *Am. J. Surg.* **105:** 574–578, 1963.

Gilman, A. and Philips, F. S.: The biological actions and therapeutic applications of the β-chloroethyl amines and sulphides. *Science* **103:** 409–415, 1946.

Golomb, F. M.: Agents used in cancer chemotherapy. *Am. J. Surg.* **105:** 579–590, 1963.

Goodman, L. S., Wintrobe, M. M., Dameshek, W., Goodman, M. J., Gilman, A., and McLennan, M. T.: Nitrogen mustard therapy: Use of methyl-bis (beta-chloroethyl)amine hydrochloride for Hodgkin's disease, lymphosarcoma, leukemia and certain allied and miscellaneous disorders. *JAMA* **132:** 126–132, 1946.

Gross, R. and Lambers, K.: Vorläufige klinische Beobachtungen mit einem neuen N-Lost-Phosphamidester in der Tumortherapie. *Naturwissenschaft* **45:** 66, 1958a.

Gross, R. and Lambers, K.: Erste Erfahrungen in der Behandlung maligner Tumoren mit einem neuen N-Lost-Phosphamidester. *Dtsch. Med. Wochenschr.* **83:** 458–462, 1958b.

Hektoen, L. and Corper, H. J.: The effect of mustard gas (dichlorethyl sulphid) on antibody formation. *J. Infect. Dis.* **28:** 279–285, 1921.

Hench, P. S., Kendall, E. C., Slocumb, C. H., and Polley, H. F.: The effect of a hormone of the adrenal cortex (17-hydroxy-11-dehydrocorticosterone: Compound E) and of pituitary adrenocorticotropic hormone on rheumatoid arthritis. *Proc. Staff Mtg. Mayo Clinic* **24:** 181–197, 1949.

Hill, D. L.: *A Review of Cyclophosphamide,* Charles C. Thomas, Springfield, IL, 1975.

Hørslev-Petersen, K., Beyer, J.A., and Helin, P.: Intermittent cyclophosphamide in refractory rheumatoid arthritis. *Br. Med. J.* **287:** 711, 712, 1983.

Kaplan, S. R. and Calabresi, P.: Drug therapy. Immunosuppressive agents. *N. Engl. J. Med.* **289:** 952–955, 1973.

Klein, J.: Responses dominated by T-lymphocytes, in *Immunology: The Science of Self–Nonself Discrimination,* pp. 445–574, Wiley, New York, 1982.

Klein, F. A. and Smith, M. J. V.: Urinary complications of cyclophosphamide therapy: Etiology, prevention, and management. *South. Med. J.* **76:** 1413–1416, 1983.

Korst, D. R., Clifford, G. O., Fowler, W. M., Louis, J., Will, J., and Wilson, H. E.: Multiple myeloma. II. Analysis of cyclophosphamide therapy in 165 patients. *JAMA* **189:** 758–762, 1964.

Krumbhaar, E. B.: Role of the blood and the bone marrow in certain forms of gas poisoning. I. Peripheral blood changes and their significance. *J. Am. Med. Assoc.* **72:** 39–41, 1919.

Krumbhaar, E. B. and Krumbhaar, H. D.: The blood and bone marrow in yellow cross gas (mustard gas) poisoning. *J. Med. Res.* **40:** 497–507, 1919.

Lampe, K. F., ed.: *Drug Evaluations,* 6th Ed., American Medical Association, Chicago, 1986.

Lidsky, M. D., Sharp, J. T., and Billings, S.: Double blind study of cyclophosphamide in rheumatoid arthritis. *Arthritis Rheum.* **16:** 148–153, 1973.

Lyttle, D. A. and Petering, H. G.: 5-Bis-(2-chloroethyl)-aminouracil, a new antitumor agent. *J. Am. Chem. Soc.* **80:** 6459, 6460, 1958.

McCarty, D. J., and Carrera, G. F.: Intractable rheumatoid arthritis: Treatment with combined cyclophosphamide, azathioprine, and hydroxychloroquine. *JAMA* **248:** 1718–1723, 1982.

Mouridsen, H. T., Faber, O., and Skovsted, L.: The metabolism of cyclophosphamide. Dose dependency and the effect of long-term treatment with cyclophosphamide. *Cancer* **37:** 665–670, 1976.

Papac, R., Petrakis, N. L., Amini, F., and Wood, D. A.: Comparative clinical evaluation of two alkylating agents. Mannitol mustard and cyclophosphamide (Cytoxan). *JAMA* **172:** 1387–1391, 1960.

Pappenheimer, A. M. and Vance, M.: The effects of intravenous injections of dichloroethyl sulphide in rabbits, with special reference to its leucotoxic action. *J. Exp. Med.* **31:** 71–93, 1920.

Pedersen-Bjergaard, J., Ersbøll, J., Hansen, V. L., Sørensen, B. L., Christoffersen, K., Hou-Jensen, K., Nissen, N. I., Knudsen, J. B., and Hansen, M. M.: Carcinoma of the urinary bladder after treatment with cyclophosphamide for non-Hodgkin's lymphoma. *N. Engl. J. Med.* **318:** 1028–1032, 1988.

Perry, S., Thomas, L. B., Johnson, R. E., Carbone, P. P., and Haynes, H. A.: Hodgkin's disease. Combined clinical staff conference at the National Institutes of Health. *Ann. Intern. Med.* **67:** 424–442, 1967.

Phillips, G. L., Herzig, R. H., Lazarus, H. M., Fay, J. W., Wolff, S. N., Mill, W. B., Lin, H-S., Thomas, P. R. M., Glasgow, G. P., Shina, D. C., and Herzig, G. P.: Treatment of resistant malignant lymphoma with cyclophosphamide, total body irradiation, and transplantation of cryopreserved autologous marrow. *N. Engl. J. Med.* **310:** 1557–1561, 1984.

Presant, C. A., Kolhouse, J. F., and Klahr, C.: Adriamycin, 1,3-bis(2-chloroethyl)-1-nitrosourea (BCNU-NSC 409462), and cyclophosphamide in refractory adenocarcinoma of the breast and other tumors. *Cancer* **37:** 620–628, 1976.

Rothermich, N. O., Whisler, R. L., Brower, A. C., and Kantor, S. M.: Immunosuppressive agents and other forms of treatment, in *Rheumatoid Arthritis,* pp. 226–238, Grune and Stratton, Orlando, FL, 1985.

Samuels, M. L. and Howe, C. D.: Cyclophosphamide in the management of Ewing's sarcoma. *Cancer* **20:** 961–966, 1967.

Santos, G. W., Tutschka, P. J., Brookmeyer, R., Saral, R., Beschorner, W. E., Bias, W. B., Braine, H. G., Burns, W. H., Elfenbein, G. J., Kaizer, H., Mellits, D., Sensenbrenner, L. L., Stuart, R. K., and Yeager, A. M.: Marrow transplantation for acute nonlymphocytic leukemia after treatment with busulfan and cyclophosphamide. *N. Engl. J. Med.* **309:** 1347–1353, 1983.

Wall, R. L. and Conrad, F. G.: Cyclophosphamide therapy. Its use in leu-
     kemia, lymphoma and solid tumors. *Arch. Intern. Med.* **108:** 456–482,
     1961.
Williams, H. J., Reading, J. C., Ward, J. R., and O'Brien, W. M.: Comparison
     of high and low dose cyclophosphamide therapy in rheumatoid arthritis.
     Arthritis Rheum. **23:** 521–527, 1980.
Zon, G.: Cyclophosphamide analogues, in *Progress in Medicinal Chemistry,*
     vol. 19, G. P. Ellis and G. B. West, eds., pp. 205–246, Elsevier, Amsterdam,
     1982.

Anesthesiology Group

Succinylcholine

Halothane

Fentanyl

Naloxone

Propranolol (see *Cardiovascular and Renal Group*)

Diazepam (see *Psychiatry Group*)

Succinylcholine

I. Succinylcholine as an Innovative Therapeutic Agent

Neuromuscular blocking drugs (also called muscle relaxants by anesthesiologists) are mainly used as adjuvants to surgical anesthesia (Miller and Savarese, 1981; Taylor, 1985). Once patients have been rendered insensate with an appropriate anesthetic(s), neuromuscular blocking agents provide the skeletal muscle relaxation that is needed for surgical procedures. Furthermore, in combination with an anesthetic, neuromuscular blockade is useful for other purposes (Taylor, 1985; Lampe, 1986):

1. Facilitating endotracheal intubation, laryngoscopy, bronchoscopy and esophagoscopy;
2. Various orthopedic procedures, e.g., correcting dislocations and aligning of fractures; and
3. Preventing dislocations and fractures during electroconvulsive shock therapy for affective disorders.

At the time of succinylcholine's entrance into clinical medicine in the early 1950s, the important, available neuromuscular blocking agents were d-tubocurarine, decamethonium, and gallamine. When single, effective, intravenous doses of d-tubocurarine or decamethonium were given, the onset of muscle relaxation was 3–5 min with either agent, and the durations of action were approximately 40 and 20 min, respectively; gallamine had a slightly shorter duration than d-tubocurarine (Goodman and Gilman, 1955). These durations of action were disadvantageous for brief procedures, such as endotracheal intubation, since the procedures themselves required much less time than the durations of action permitted, and the patient had then to be sustained with artificial respiration. In marked contrast to the available agents, succinylcholine in a single, effective, intravenous dose had an onset within 1 min; relaxation became maximal within 2 min and was over within 5 min (Goodman and Gilman, 1955). These time characteristics made succinylcholine ideal for most brief procedures—endotracheal intubation, laryngoscopy, endoscopy, orthopedic manipulation, and convulsive therapy.

Succinylcholine, like decamethonium, is a depolarizing neuromuscular blocking agent and stands in distinction to d-tubocurarine and gallamine, which are nondepolarizing neuromuscular blocking agents. Nondepolarizing agents act as competitive antagonists to acetylcholine at cholinergic receptors in the motor endplate. In this manner they inhibit the depolarizing action of acetylcholine (released from motor nerve endings) on this structure, and by so doing, prevent both the propagation of action potentials out onto the muscle fiber membranes and the consequent contraction. In distinction to the prevention of depolarization seen with d-tubocurarine and gallamine, succinylcholine (and decamethonium as well) acts like acetylcholine at the cholinergic receptors and depolarizes the motor endplate. However, succinylcholine persists longer than acetylcholine at these receptors and holds the endplate, and the proximate muscle membrane as well, at a potential that is below the threshold at which action potentials can be propagated—neuromuscular transmission is thereby blocked (Durant and Katz, 1982). Succinylcholine owes its very short duration of action to the fact that it is exceedingly rapidly hydrolyzed to inactive substances by pseudocholinesterase, an enzyme of plasma and liver (Miller and Savarese, 1981).

Unfortunately, both the depolarizing mechanism of action and the metabolic fate of succinylcholine entail disadvantages in the clinical application of this agent (Miller and Savarese, 1981; Durant and Katz, 1982; Taylor, 1985; Lampe, 1986). Some of the prominent problems are:

1. Muscle pains. These seem most likely to result from damage produced in muscle by the unsynchronized contractions of adjacent muscle fibers that occur during succinylcholine-induced depolarization before the onset of paralysis.

2. Decreased sensitivity of the cholinergic receptors in the muscle endplate may occur when succinylcholine is given in a single large dose, or given repeatedly or as a prolonged infusion. This desensitized state is associated with a repolarization of membranes, after which it resembles a nondepolarizing block—the endplate is not sensitive to additional succinylcholine. This prolonged desensitization (called Phase II block, dual block, or desensitization block) is best treated by maintaining artificial ventilation until it dissipates.

3. Prolonged paralysis may occur with succinylcholine if either the plasma levels or the activity of pseudocholinesterase is low because of liver disease, malnutrition, or drugs. Enzymatic activity may also be low as a result of genetically determined changes in the enzyme.

4. Although neostigmine or edrophonium—inhibitors of endplate acetylcholinesterase (true cholinesterase)—can reverse a prolonged competitive type neuromuscular blockade by elevating acetylcholine levels at the motor endplate, these agents cannot be used to reverse a prolonged depolarizing blockade. On the contrary, elevation of endplate acetylcholine reinforces a depolarizing block.

5. Depolarization releases potassium ion, and in patients with burns, trauma, or significant muscular denervation (e.g., in paraplegia) succinylcholine may elevate serum potassium to a level high enough to cause cardiac arrest.

In addition, in very rare instances, a hypersensitivity occurs to succinylcholine and/or to the anesthetic, halothane, which results in a malignant hyperthermia characterized by widespread muscular rigidity and enhanced heat production by muscles. This abberent response, which may have a genetic basis, progresses rapidly, and cardiac arrest and death occur in 30–40% of cases.

Despite these shortcomings, according to Durant and Katz (1982), "Suxamethonium [succinylcholine] has undoubtedly been the most widely used muscle relaxant during surgery and will for a while continue to have a place in the anaesthetist's armamentarium."

Early Clinical Research History

Preliminary positive reports covering the use of succinylcholine in surgery and electroshock therapy appeared in 1951 (Thesleff, 1951; Von Dardel and Thesleff, 1951; Homberg and Thesleff, 1951;

Brücke et al., 1951). Thesleff (1952), in a study of 29 patients undergoing abdominal surgery, found that intravenous injection of succinylcholine elicited a rapid and powerful muscle relaxation that was maximal within 1 min and, depending on dose, lasted for 1–12 min. Immediately preceding paralysis, brief muscle fasciculations were seen. Paralysis of the respiratory muscles required twice the dose needed for paralysis of other muscles. Muscle relaxation was the same whether barbiturate, cyclopropane, or spinal anesthesia was being used. Slow intravenous infusion of succinylcholine produced muscular relaxation that was easily controlled and could be quickly interrupted.

Von Dardel and Thesleff (1952) presented results obtained on 500 general surgical cases: in 129 patients, succinylcholine was used only for intratracheal intubation; in 206, it was used for both intubation and the operation; in 110, for the operation only; and in 55, it was given as a continuous intravenous drip. Succinylcholine was found to be suitable for short-term procedures and to be eminently suitable for lengthier operations requiring a continuous intravenous drip. No cumulative effect, tachyphylaxis, complications, or toxic actions were observed. The authors vigorously advocated the use of succinylcholine in the field of anesthesiology.

Foldes et al. (1952), in their study of 202 unselected surgical patients, found succinylcholine to be ultra-short-acting with a rapid onset. Its use was not accompanied by unwanted side effects, and the incidence of postoperative complications was low. The authors concluded, "On the basis of limited experience, succinylcholine seems to be the muscle relaxant of choice of all similar agents so far investigated."

These early, highly favorable reports of succinylcholine's lack of problems were soon tempered by others that noted prolonged action in a few patients (Harper, 1952; Love, 1952; Hewer, 1952). Evans et al. (1952) found that two patients out of more than 400 gave prolonged response to succinylcholine. In both cases the patients had very low plasma pseudocholinesterase activity. The investigators suggested that the duration of action of succinylcholine depended on the speed of its removal by the pseudocholinesterase of the plasma.

Numerous publications, chapters and books have reinforced the positive aspects that were quickly delineated for succinylcholine, but have also elaborated on its problems (*see,* for example, Goodman and Gilman, 1955; Miller and Savarese, 1981; Durant and Katz, 1982; Dorkins, 1982; Taylor, 1985; Lampe, 1986).

II. The Scientific Departure Leading to Succinylcholine: Decamethonium

The main chemical features of the active principle of curare—*d*-tubocurarine—were elucidated by King (1935), including its presumed bisquaternary nature. Ultimately, its structure was considered to have been fully delineated (King, 1948).

Barlow and Ing (1948) speculated that the extraordinary potency of tubocurarine in blocking neuromuscular transmission, when compared with the potencies of simple monoquaternary ammonium compounds, might result, in part, from the fact that tubocurarine contained two quaternary ammonium groups, and speculated further that these might be at some optimal distance apart (Fig. 1, *d*-tubocurarine, pre-1970). Barlow and Ing (1948) prepared simple molecules to test this hypothesis. Among these were a series of polymethylene *bis*-trimethylammonium dibromides of increasing chain length. Muscle relaxant activity, as judged by the rabbit head-drop assay, reached an optimum with the C_{10} member (later named decamethonium) (Fig. 1). The authors noted that, unlike tubocurarine, nearly all the compounds in this series produced contractions of the rat diaphragm in vitro at concentrations slightly lower than those needed to produce blockade.

Contemporaneous with the work of Barlow and Ing (1948), Paton and Zaimis (1948) were studying the capacity of a variety of basic substances to liberate histamine from tissues. In the course of this work, they discovered, apparently serendipitously, that C_8 *bis*-trimethyl ammonium chloride caused strong neuromuscular blockade. Following up on this lead, other homologs were made, and in the rabbit head-drop test potencies were found to increase from the

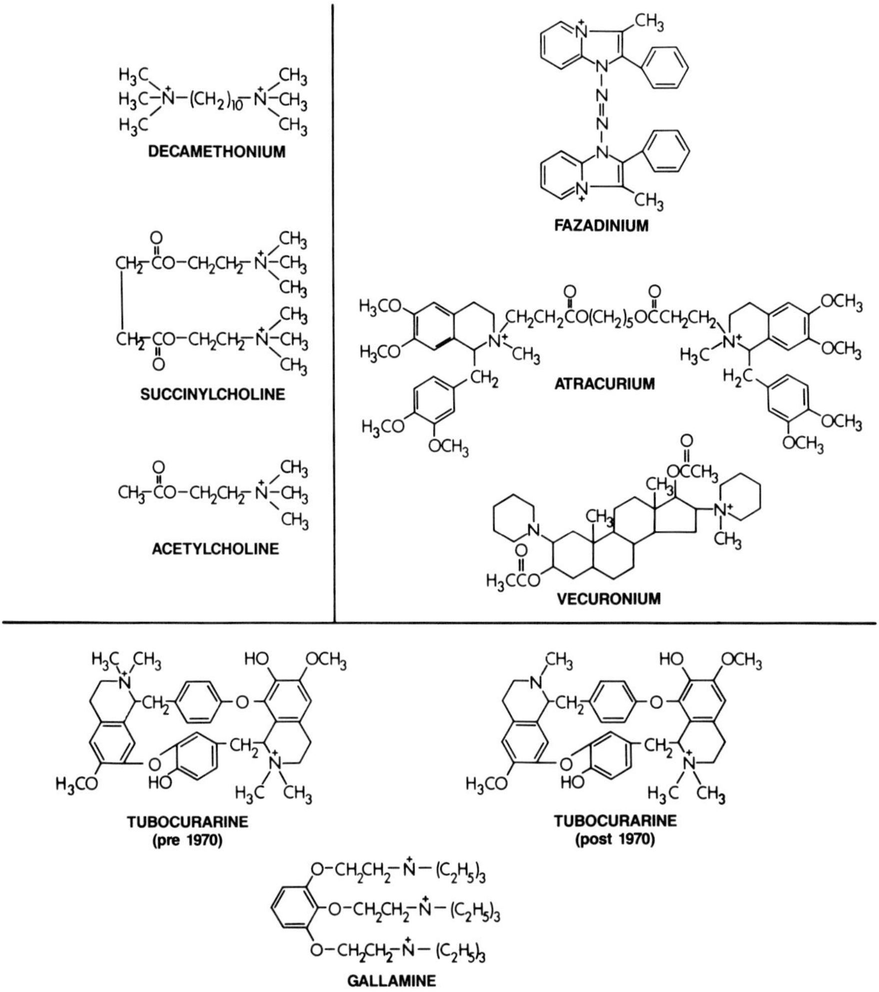

Fig. 1. The structures of succinylcholine and chemically and/or pharmacologically related substances.

C_2 to the C_8 derivative, and the C_{10} derivative (decamethonium) was even more effective. The authors carried out additional studies with the C_8 compound. Moderate intravenous doses of this molecule in the cat initially increased the response of the tibialis muscle to single maximal shocks applied to the motor nerve; the response was followed by a prolongation of the contraction and a widespread fibrillation of the musculature for 20–30 s, not unlike that resulting from the administration of anticholinesterases. Furthermore, intraarterial administration of the C_8 compound produced a twitch before blockade ensued. Paton and Zaimis (1948) were surprised to find that although the blocking action of *d*-tubocurarine was not altered when it was given after these *bis*-quaternary blocking agents, the blockade induced by the *bis*-quaternary agents was antagonized by previous administration of *d*-tubocurarine.

Background Contributions Preceding Decamethonium

Curare is a generic term for various South American arrow poisons used by aborigines for killing wild animals for food. It is an amorphous mixture of alkaloids, which comes from several plant sources and has been known for many centuries. The dramatic paralyzing actions of curare attracted the attention of early explorers and, subsequently, samples found their way back to Europe (Dorkins, 1982; Taylor, 1985). In time, Bernard (1856) described the neuromuscular blocking action of curare.

When an adequate amount of standardized, purified extract of curare became available, a number of possible clinical uses were explored, for example, treatment of tetanus (West, 1936) and spastic and dystonic states (Burman, 1939); prevention of the traumatic complications in convulsive therapy for depression (Bennett, 1940; Gray et al., 1941); adjunct use in anesthesia (Griffith and Johnson, 1942; Cullen, 1943).

Significant Work Following Decamethonium

Succinylcholine (Fig. 1) was synthesized in the late 1940s in three laboratories that were located in different countries.* Each of the three laboratories credited the development of decamethonium with being a stimulus to their own work.

---

* Succinylcholine had been synthesized earlier by Hunt and Taveau (1906), who were interested in the hypotensive effects of choline and related substances from the adrenal glands, and by Glick (1941), who made it as one of a series of choline esters of mono- and dicarboxylic acids in order to study the specificity of cholinesterase. These authors were not investigating neuromuscular blockade, and they did not discover such an effect for succinylcholine.

Bovet's group (Fusco et al., 1949) synthesized a large number of novel aliphatic double esters of dialkylethanolamine and trialkyl-ethanolammonium; included in the latter group was succinylcholine. These investigators (Bovet et al., 1949) considered succinyl-choline to be a new example of the increase that occurs in curarizing action when molecules contained two, rather than one, quaternary ammonium groups. They felt that their study of the esters of aliphatic dicarboxylic acids would complement the early knowledge regarding the weak curarizing actions of simple mono-tri-methylalkylammonium salts as well as the work of Barlow and Ing (1948) and Paton and Zaimis (1948) with the more potent polymethylene *bis*-trialkylammonium agents (the decamethonium series). Bovet et al. (1949) found that succinylcholine exerted strong curarizing effects comparable to that of *d*-tubocurarine. They fully recognized it as a "double acetylcholine" molecule (Fig. 1), and the fact that these two closely related agents, acetylcholine and suc-cinylcholine, had such totally different actions on neuromuscular transmission captured their attention. Bovet et al. (1949) expressed considerable interest in the clinical potential of this new series; however, not in succinylcholine—it produced hypertension at a high dose in the dog—but in a closely related substance that was free of this effect.

Phillips (1949), of the USA, after acknowledging the results of Bovet et al. (1949), stated, "Stimulated by the work of Barlow and Ing [1948] and Paton and Zaimis [1948]...we sought to produce compounds of similar activity by duplicating the favorable chain length, found by them to be ten atoms, between the quaternary nitrogens." This investigator prepared a series of *bis*-quaternary derivatives of aliphatic dicarboxylic acids. The first compound made was the *bis*-dimethylaminoethyl succinate *bis*-methiodide (succinylcholine), which had 10 atoms interposed between the quaternary ammonium groups. This compound was equiactive with *d*-tubocurarine, but had a much shorter duration of action. The shorter duration was tentatively attributed to the action of choline esterases because of the structural similarity between the compound and two molecules of acetylcholine coupled together.

Walker (1950), of the UK, noted that, in the work that had been carried out with decamethonium and homologs,

[t]he feature common to all the more active compounds...is that two quaternary ammonium groups are separated by a chain of between 8 and 12 atoms, indicating that the essential...requirement...may be that two such groups should occupy positions optimally separated in the same molecule. The present communication describes several extensions of this thesis...

Along with preparing a variety of compounds, this investigator commented,

As the two quaternary ammonium groups in the succinic ester of choline are separated by...10 atoms...choline succinate dibromide was prepared and examined. Shortly afterwards it was learned that Bovet...had also examined this ester..., and the appearance of a note by Phillips...is a further indication of the interest aroused in purely aliphatic compounds by the work of Paton and Zaimis [1948]. It should be noted in passing that (IX)[succinylcholine] may be considered as being derived by linking two molecules of acetylcholine...

Succinylcholine was approximately one-half as potent as decamethonium in the rabbit head-drop test.

Buttle and Zaimis (1949) noted that depolarization of muscle fibers in birds produced not only electrical inexcitability, but, in addition, contracture. They found that both decamethonium and succinylcholine, like acetylcholine, caused rigid extension of the limbs and retraction of the head in a variety of birds. On the other hand, *d*-tubocurarine and gallamine caused flaccid paralysis. The conclusion was drawn that decamethonium and succinylcholine acted essentially like acetylcholine to depolarize muscle fibers and were only superficially "curare-like" in their blocking action.

Castillo and deBeer (1950) found that succinylcholine (which they also called diacetylcholine) exhibited a strong neuromuscular blocking action of short duration in the cat, rabbit, and mouse; its action was greatly potentiated by a cholinesterase inhibitor, eserine, an agent that was known to antagonize the neuromuscular block produced by *d*-tubocurarine.

Von Dardel and Thesleff (1952), in briefly summarizing their pharmacologic work with succinylcholine, remarked, "It has been found that succinylcholine...inhibits neuromuscular transmission.

This is presumably due to the fact that succinylcholine depolarizes the muscle end-plates which thus become insensitive to the acetylcholine liberated by the neural stimulation."

Table 1 defines the critical scientific ideas and experiments leading to succinylcholine and categorizes their origin.

III. Comments on Events
Leading to Succinylcholine

Everett et al. (1970) corrected the structure that King (1935, 1948) had elaborated for *d*-tubocurarine. They showed that *d*-tubocurarine contained not two quaternary ammonium groups, but only one, with the second nitrogen bearing tertiary, not quaternary, substitution (Fig. 1, *d*-tubocurarine, post-1970). Dorkins (1982) remarked, "A group of very useful drugs was thus discovered on the premise that *d*-tubocurarine was a diquaternary salt, an assumption later found to be innaccurate." Dorkins (1982), however, further noted, "It has been pointed out that although the molecule is not diquaternary, it is likely to have two positively charged centres at normal physiological pH, because the tertiary nitrogen atom will be protonated."

IV. Developments
Subsequent to Succinylcholine

The search for a nondepolarizing, ultra-short-acting, neuromuscular blocking agent has been an ongoing endeavor during the decades since the introduction of succinylcholine. Such a molecule would be very desirable, in that it would retain the useful properties of succinylcholine while dispensing with the undesirable consequences of depolarization blockade. Entries into the field have been fazadinium, in the early 1970s, and vecuronium and atracurium, in the late 1970s and early 1980s (Fig. 1).

Fazadinium is a potent, nondepolarizing, neuromuscular blocking agent characterized in some species by a very rapid onset and a short duration of action; however, in humans it had a duration similar to that of pancuronium (Brittain and Tyers, 1973).

Table 1

Profile of Observations and Ideas Crucial to the Development of Succinylcholine[a]

Sequence: Departure compound* to innovative drug**	Orient- ation	Nature of study	Research institution	National origin	Nature of discovery	Screening involved	Crucial ideas or observations
Decamethonium*							
King (1935)	Pre- clinical	Chem- istry	Govern- ment	UK	Orderly	No	The main chemical features of d-tubo- curarine established; it is characterized as a bis-quaternary com- pound.
Barlow and Ing (1948)	Pre- clinical	Chem- istry/ pharma- cology	Uni- versity	UK	Orderly	Targeted	The potency of tubo- curarine may result from its having two separated quater- nary ammonium groups; a series of simple polymethyl- ene bis-trimethyl- ammonium com- pounds synthesized; neuromuscular blocking action is optimal with $-(CH_2)_{10}^-$ polymethylene chain length (decametho- nium).
Succinylcholine*							
Bovet et al. (1949)	Pre- clinical	Chem- istry/ pharma- cology	Govern- ment	Italy	Orderly	Targeted	Succinylcholine synthesized; like decamethonium, two quaternary groups are separated by 10 atoms; succinylcho- line is "diacetylcho- line"; it is an effect- ive neuromuscular blocking agent.

[a]Taken from section II. Entries are those contributions without which the discovery of the agent (or additionally, in some cases, a relevant clinical application) would not have taken place or would have been materially delayed.

Vecuronium is the monoquaternary homolog of the diquater- nary compound, pancuronium. One nitrogen atom of vecuronium bears tertiary rather than quaternary, substitution—a relationship reminiscent of that between the original and revised structures for *d*- tubocurarine noted in section III. Vecuronium is a potent, nondepolarizing muscle relaxant in humans. Like pancuronium, its onset time is relatively slow; its duration of action is 1/2 to 1/3 that of pancuronium (Durant et al., 1979; Fahey et al., 1981).

Atracurium is also a potent, nondepolarizing muscle relaxant. It was shown to have an onset of action in humans that permitted tracheal intubation to be performed in 1.5–2 min following administration of a low dose, but it had an intermediate duration of action (Hunt et al., 1980).

Neither vecuronium nor atracurium are truly ultra-short-acting agents comparable to succinylcholine. Atracurium and vecuronium are available in the USA; fazadinium is not.

Research at the present time continues with the same goal as in the past three decades—the discovery of a truly ultra-short-acting, nondepolarizing agent having the useful characteristics of succinylcholine, but not its problems.

References

Barlow, R. B. and Ing, H. R.: Curare-like action of polymethylene *bis*-quaternary ammonium salts. *Nature* **1:** 718, 1948.

Bennett, A. E.: Preventing traumatic complications in convulsive shock therapy by curare. *JAMA* **114:** 322–324, 1940.

Bernard, C.: Analyse physiologiques des propriétés des systémes musculaire et nerveux au moyen de curare. *Compt. Rendus Acad. Sci.* 43:825–829, 1856. Read in translation in *Readings in Pharmacology,* L. Shuster, ed., pp. 75–81, Little, Brown, Boston, 1962.

Bovet, D., Bovet-Nitti, F., Guarino, S., Longo, V. G., and Marotta, M.: Proprietá farmacodinamiche di alcuni derivati della succinilcolina dotati di azione curarica. *Rend. Ist. Super. di Sanitá* **12:** 106–137, 1949.

Brittain, R. T. and Tyers, M. B.: The pharmacology of AH 8165: A rapid-acting, short-lasting, competitive neuromuscular blocking drug. *Br. J. Anaesth.* 45: 837–843, 1973.

Brücke, H., Ginzel, K. H., Klupp, H., Pfaffenschlager, F., and Werner, G.: *Bis*-Cholinester von Dicarbonsaüren als Muskelrelaxantien in der Narkose. *Wien. Klin. Wochenschr.* 63: 464–466, 1951.

Burman, M. S.: Therapeutic use of curare and erythroidine hydrochloride for spastic and dystonic states. *Arch. Neurol. Psychiatry* **41:** 307–327, 1939.

Buttle, G. A. H. and Zaimis, E. J.: The action of decamethonium iodide in birds. *J. Pharm. Pharmacol.* **1:** 991, 992, 1949.

Castillo, J. C. and deBeer, E. J.: The neuromuscular blocking action of suc-cinylcholine(diacetylcholine). *J. Pharmacol. Exp. Ther.* **99**: 458–464, 1950.

Cullen, S. C.: The use of curare for the improvement of abdominal muscle relaxation during inhalation anesthesia; Report on 131 cases. *Surgery* **14**: 261–266, 1943.

Dorkins, H. R.: Suxamethonium—the development of a modern drug from 1906 to the present day. *Med. Hist.* **26**: 145–168, 1982.

Durant, N. N. and Katz, R. L.: Suxamethonium. *Br. J. Anaesth.* **54**: 195–208, 1982.

Durant, N. N., Marshall, I. G., Savage, D. S., Nelson, D. J., Sleigh, T., and Carlyle, I. C.: The neuromuscular and autonomic blocking activities of pancuronium, Org NC45, and other pancuronium analogues, in the cat. *J. Pharm. Pharmacol.* **31**: 831–836, 1979.

Evans, F. T., Gray, P. W. S., Lehmann, H., and Silk, E.: Sensitivity to succinyl-choline in relation to serum-cholinesterase. *Lancet* **1**: 1229, 1230, 1952.

Everett, A. J., Lowe, L. A., and Wilkinson, S.: Revision of the structures of (+)-tubocurarine chloride and (+)-chondrocurine. *J. Chem. Soc.* **13** (D): 1020, 1021, 1970.

Fahey, M. R., Morris, R. B., Miller, R. D., Sohn, Y. J., Cronnelly, R., and Gencarelli, P.: Clinical pharmacology of ORG NC45 (Norcuron): A new nondepolarizing muscle relaxant. *Anesthesiology* **55**: 6–11, 1981.

Foldes, F. F., McNall, P. G., and Borrego-Hinojosa, J. M.: Succinylcholine: A new approach to muscular relaxation in anesthesiology. *N. Engl. J. Med.* **247**: 596–600, 1952.

Fusco, R., Palazzo, G., and Knüsli, R.: Ricerche sui carari di sintesi. *Rend. Ist. Super. di Sanitá* **12**: 69–80, 1949.

Glick, D.: Some additional observations on the specificity of cholinesterase. *J. Biol. Chem.* **137**: 357–362, 1941.

Goodman, L. S. and Gilman, A.: *The Pharmacological Basis of Therapeutics*, 2nd Ed., Macmillan, New York, 1955.

Gray, R. W., Spradling, F. L., and Fechner, A. H.: The use of curare in modi-fying metrazol therapy. *Psychiatr. Q.* **15**: 159–162, 1941.

Griffith, H. R. and Johnson, E.: The use of curare in general anesthesia. *Anes-thesiology* **3**: 418–420, 1942.

Harper, J. K.: Prolonged respiratory paralysis after succinylcholine. *Br. Med. J.* **1**: 866, 1952.

Hewer, C. L.: Prolonged respiratory paralysis after succinylcholine. *Br. Med. J.* **1**: 971, 972, 1952.

Homberg, G. and Thesleff, S.: Succinylkolinjodid som muskelavslappande medel vid elektroshockbehandling. *Nord. Med.* **46**: 1567–1570, 1951.

Hunt, R. and Taveau, R.deM.: On the physiological action of certain cholin derivatives and new methods for detecting cholin. *Br. Med. J.* **II.**: 1788–1791, 1906.

Hunt, T. M., Hughes, R., and Payne, J. P.: Preliminary studies with atracurium in anaesthetized man. *Br. J. Anaesth.* **52:** 238P, 239P, 1980.

King, H.: Curare alkaloids. Part I. Tubocurarine. *J. Chem. Soc.* **2:** 1381–1389, 1935.

King, H.: Curare alkaloids. Part VII. Constitution of dextrotubocurarine chloride. *J. Chem. Soc.* **1:** 265, 266, 1948.

Lampe, K. F., ed.: *Drug Evaluations*, 6th Ed., American Medical Association, Chicago, 1986.

Love, S. H. S.: Prolonged apnoea following scoline. *Anaesthesia* **7:** 113, 114, 1952.

Miller, R. D. and Savarese, J. J.: Pharmacology of muscle relaxants, their antagonists, and monitoring of neuromuscular function, in *Anesthesia*, vol. 2, R. D. Miller, ed., pp. 487–538, Churchill Livingstone, New York, 1981.

Paton, W. D. M. and Zaimis, E. J.: Curare-like action of polymethylene *bis*-quaternary ammonium salts. *Nature* **1:** 718, 719, 1948.

Phillips, A. P.: Synthetic curare substitutes from aliphatic dicarboxylic acid aminoethyl esters. *J. Am. Chem. Soc.* **71:** 3264, 1949.

Taylor, P.: Neuromuscular blocking agents, in *The Pharmacological Basis of Therapeutics*, 7th Ed., A. G. Gilman, L. S. Goodman, T. W. Rall, and F. Murad. eds., pp. 222–235, Macmillan, New York, 1985.

Thesleff, S.: Farmakologiska och kliniska fösök med LT 1 (0.0.-succinyl-cholin-jodid. *Nord. Med.* **46:** 1045, 1951.

Thesleff, S.: An investigation of the muscle-relaxing action of succinyl-choline-iodide in man. *Acta Physiol. Scand.* **25:** 348–367, 1952.

Von Dardel, O. and Thesleff, S.: Kliniska erfarenheter med succinylkolin-jodid, ett nytt medel som ger muskelavslappning. *Nord. Med.* **46:** 1308–1311, 1951.

Von Dardel, O. and Thesleff, S.: Succinylcholine iodide as a muscular relaxant. *Acta Chir. Scandinav.* **103:** 321–336, 1952.

Walker, J.: Some new curarizing agents. *J. Chem. Soc.* **1:** 193–197, 1950.

West, R.: Intravenous curarine in the treatment of tetanus. *Lancet* **1:** 12–16, 1936.

Halothane

I. Halothane as an Innovative Therapeutic Agent

Although the obtunding of pain associated with surgery has been achievable since the nineteenth century with such agents as diethyl ether, chloroform and nitrous oxide, there was a continuing quest into the mid-twentieth century for a safe, potent, nonirritant, nonflammable, nonexplosive, volatile anesthetic. This quest culminated in the development of the halogenated hydrocarbon, halothane, in the mid-1950s.

Prior to the introduction of halothane, the most widely used inhalation anesthetics were diethyl ether and cyclopropane (Fig.1) (Dripps et al., 1961; Smith and Wollman, 1985). Diethyl ether, although a very safe anesthetic, was irritating to the respiratory tract (increasing its secretions and on occasion evoking laryngospasm), and it frequently elicited nausea and vomiting postoperatively. It also required long induction and recovery times and was flammable. Cyclopropane was employed extensively throughout the 1930s, 40s, and 50s. It was a potent gaseous anesthetic and was rapid in onset and offset. Unfortunately, it was highly flammable and explosive, and the increasing use of electronic equipment in operating rooms posed a hazard. In addition, cyclopropane often induced depression of breathing with resultant hypoxia and hypercapnia, and also elicited cardiac irregularities, such as ventricular extrasystoles and tachycardia. It both sensitized the heart to catecholamines and released these amines from adrenergic stores, which at times led to bouts of ventricular tachycardia and/or fibrillation. Furthermore, at the end of its administration, a sudden drop in CO_2 tension, and a drop in O_2 tension when a high concentration of O_2 had been used, could lead to "cyclopropane shock"—sinus tachycardia, hypotension, vasoconstriction, sweat-

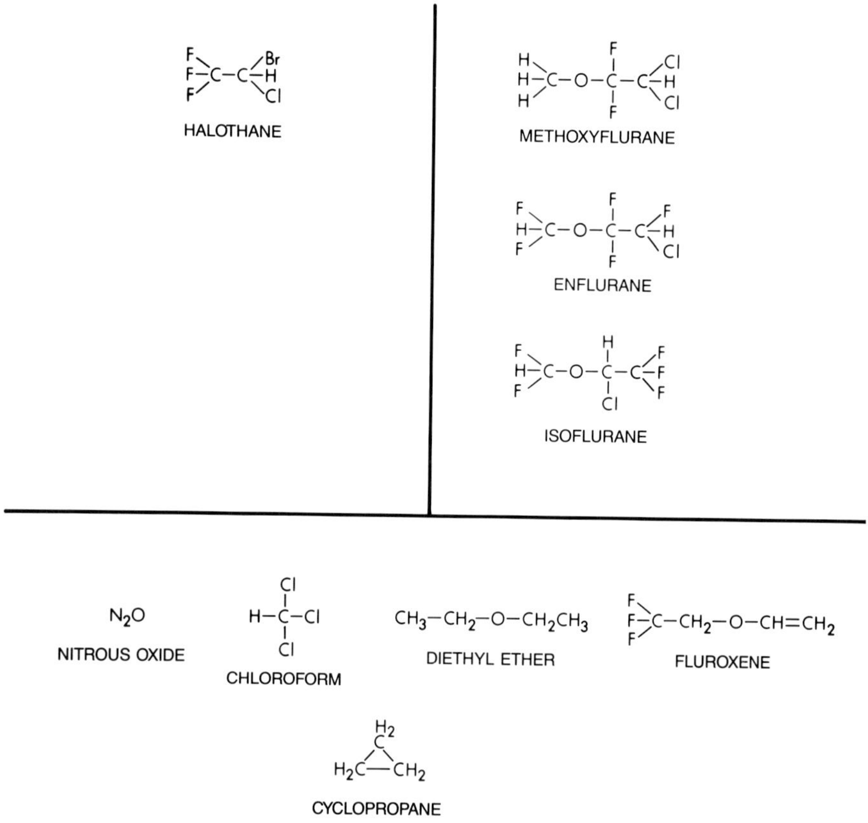

Fig. 1. The structures of halothane and chemically and/or pharmacologically related substances.

ing, and delayed recovery of consciousness. Nausea and vomiting frequently occurred after cyclopropane anesthesia (Stephen and Little, 1961; Woodbridge, 1961; Modell et al., 1976; Smith and Wollman, 1985).

Halothane represented a clear advance beyond diethyl ether, cyclopropane, and other agents available at the time. It is a potent, volatile anesthetic that gives a smooth, rapid loss of consciousness with rapid awakening when it is withdrawn. Moreover, it is neither flammable nor explosive, has a relatively low incidence of toxic effects, does not irritate the respiratory tract nor increase secretions, and is compatible with oxygen and nitrous oxide. It is used across a broad spectrum of surgical procedures (Smith, 1981;

Jones, 1984), especially in thoracic surgery, when electrocauteriza-
tion may be required. It is not used in obstetrics, however, since it
relaxes the uterus.

Halothane, in addition to its useful actions, also exerts dose-
dependent, depressant effects on left ventricular function, heart
rate, and blood pressure—all are reduced at concentrations necessary for surgical anesthesia. Severe hypotension and circulatory
failure may occur with overdosing. Halothane also produces
rapid, shallow respiration, presumably as a result of a central depressant action. These cardiovascular and respiratory effects are
manageable, however, and for most people with an undiseased
myocardium they do not pose insurmountable obstacles to the
use of halothane. Halothane does not stimulate the sympatho-
adrenal system, but sensitizes the heart to the actions of catecholamines (Modell et al., 1976; Smith, 1981; Jones, 1984; Marshall and
Wollman, 1985; Lampe, 1986). In addition, halothane may cause
both minor and, rarely, massive hepatic injury (Neuberger and
Williams, 1984).

Halothane is very effective in inducing the sleep component
of anesthesia, but is not as effective in inducing the other components. Optimal levels of analgesia require the addition of opioids
or nitrous oxide, optimal muscular relaxation requires the addition of neuromuscular blocking drugs, and control of visceral reflexes requires drugs such as atropine or local anesthetics (Modell
et al., 1976; Marshall and Wollman, 1985; Lampe, 1986). The coadministration of these adjunct agents, however, allows lower
concentrations of halothane to be used and, thus, provides a
broader margin of safety.

According to Smith and Wollman (1985), halothane "...was
introduced into clinical practice in 1956, and it revolutionized inhalational anesthesia." Marshall and Wollman (1985) noted that it
was the standard to which other volatile anesthetics are compared
and Smith (1981) commented that it was the most widely used
volatile anesthetic agent.

Early Clincial Research History

Johnstone (1956) administered halothane to 500 surgical patients. Smooth and rapidly reversible anesthesia was maintained
in all cases by continuous administration of halothane vapor along
with 50% oxygen and nitrous oxide. Brisk reflex activity returned

in two to three min after stopping the halothane. Transient post-operative nausea occurred in only 8%, and vomiting in only 4%, of patients. Halothane produced a general picture of vasodilation combined with bradycardia and hypotension and the magnitude of the hypotension was directly related to the inhaled vapor concentration of the halothane. Despite this propensity to produce hypotension, a shock syndrome similar to that observed at times with cyclopropane was completely absent with halothane usage.

In a study of 310 surgical patients, Bryce-Smith and O'Brien (1956) found halothane to have very useful anesthetic properties and the advantages of being nonflammable and nonexplosive. The hypotension it produced was not considered harmful, and the surgeons appreciated the dry operating field that was present as a consequence. However, the investigators felt that the respiratory depression they observed warranted limiting the use of halothane only to skilled anesthetists.

Hudon et al. (1957) anesthetized 1,112 surgical patients of all ages with halothane. They found that it produced smooth and easy induction and was well tolerated. A properly calibrated vaporizer and avoidance of sudden increases in concentration were necessary to avoid sudden hypotension, arrhythmias, and respiratory depression with this agent. Halothane did not elicit broncho-constriction or laryngospasm, and it diminished tracheo-bronchial secretions. The authors felt that halothane might be the equal of ether and cyclopropane as an anesthetic and that it had advantages over these agents in being nonflammable and nonexplosive, in inhibiting tracheo-bronchial secretions, and in being potent and easily reversible.

Much clinical work has confirmed and amplified the advantages and disadvantages of halothane as defined in these early studies (see, for example, Stephen and Little, 1961; Smith, 1981; Jones, 1984; Marshall and Wollman, 1985; Miller, 1986; Lampe, 1986).

II. The Scientific Work Leading to Halothane

A series of fluorinated hydrocarbons was synthesized by Suckling, of the General Chemicals Division of Imperial Chemical Industries (ICI), and examined pharmacologically by Raventós (1956). One of the agents (later named halothane) (Fig. 1), was a nonflammable, volatile liquid that exhibited potent anesthetic properties in mice, rats, dogs, cats, and monkeys. Recovery from halothane anesthesia was fast, and free from excitement, in all animal species in which it was tried. In mice and dogs, halothane proved to be approximately two times more potent than chloroform and four times more potent than diethyl ether. Halothane had a therapeutic ratio in mice of 3.3 as compared to 1.7 for diethyl ether and 1.5 for chloroform. Halothane anesthesia was accompanied by the following effects:

1. Both amplitude and frequency of respiratory movements were decreased;
2. Blood pressure fell, roughly in proportion to the concentration of the vapor;
3. Heart rate was decreased;
4. No cardiac irregularities occurred;
5. The heart was sensitized to adrenaline (injection of this amine occasionally provoked ventricular fibrillation);
6. Mouth and trachea were dry and free from secretion;
7. No vomiting occurred.

The author (Raventós, 1956) noted that halothane had already been subjected by Johnstone (1956) to initial clinical trial in surgical patients (*see* section I).

Table 1 defines the critical scientific ideas and experiments leading to halothane and categorizes their origin.

Background Contributions Preceding Halothane

According to Artusio (1962), halogenated hydrocarbons have been used almost from the beginning of the era of general inhalation anesthesia. From the mid-nineteenth century onward, chloroform, ethyl chloride, tribromethanol (with amylene hydrate), and trichloroethylene were sequentially introduced and found to be clinically useful. Unfortunately, a variety of serious toxicities or other problems curtailed their use in anesthesiology.

Since the 1930s, fluorinated hydrocarbons (originally synthesized as refrigerants) had been recognized to have CNS depressant, convulsant, and other activities in physiological systems (Booth and Bixby, 1932; Brenner, 1937; Struck and Plattner, 1940).

Robbins (1946) determined the anesthetic activity in mice of 46 hydrocarbons containing fluorine alone or in addition to other halogens. Eighteen of these compounds were given further study

Table 1
Profile of Observations and Ideas Crucial to the Development of Halothane[a]

Sequence: Route to innovative drug[**]	Orient- ation	Nature of study	Research institution	National origin	Nature of discovery	Screening involved	Crucial ideas or observations
Halothane[**] Raventós (1956)	Pre- clinical	Chem- istry/ pharma- cology	Industry	UK	Orderly	Targeted	Halothane, a volatile, fluorin- ated hydrocarbon, is a useful general anesthetic agent.

[a]Taken from section II. Entries are those contributions without which the discovery of the agent (or additionally, in some cases, a relevant clinical application) would not have taken place or would have been materially delayed.

in dogs, and the data obtained with four of them indicated that they might be useful as anesthetics. Regrettably, no further work was carried out with these molecules, one of which was CF_3CHBr_2, a close congener of halothane (Fig. 1).

Krantz et al. (1953) found trifluoroethyl vinyl ether (fluro-xene) (Fig. 1) to be a volatile inhalation anesthetic in dogs and monkeys, with a potency approximately equal to that of diethyl ether. However, it was considered to present less fire and explosion hazard than did diethyl ether. These investgators also reported on the successful use of the compound in a human volunteer. Although trifluoroethyl vinyl ether represented some improvement over diethyl ether, it was still a flammable agent, and it was readily displaced when halothane became available in 1956.

III. Comments on Events Leading to Halothane

Vitcha (1971) drew attention to the fact that, as part of the development of the atomic bomb during World War II, the need for purifying uranium isotopes prompted the development of a new fluorine chemical technology and that it was this technology that permitted the synthesis of all modern fluorinated anesthetic agents.

Suckling (1957), in reviewing the chemical program leading to halothane, noted that those properties that made compounds useful as refrigerants and aerosol propellants—volatility, low toxicity and nonflammability—were also desirable properties in an anesthetic inhalant. This author further noted that since the General Chemicals Division of ICI had considerable experience in manufacturing fluorinated refrigerants "...we decided to search among them and other fluorine containing compounds for an anesthetic." Suckling (1957) stated that several physicochemical properties were used to narrow the choice of molecules to be studied:

1. In the CF_3 and CF_2 moieties, fluorine was tightly bound and unreactive, and, in addition, these groups stabilized links between adjacent carbon atoms and halogen.
2. Keeping the percentage of hydrogen in the molecule low reduced flammability and explosiveness.
3. The significance of data on narcosis was much greater when concentrations producing narcosis were expressed as relative saturations, rather than as percentages by volume.

Suckling (1957) stated, "Some of the compounds which we chose to test were chosen because they were readily available but halothane, which was at the time an unknown compound, was selected on the basis of the considerations which I have outlined and specially made for testing as an anesthetic."

IV. Developments
Subsequent to Halothane

According to Vitcha (1971), as halothane became widely used, its shortcomings became clear, and so did the notion that it could be improved upon. These shortcomings, as noted earlier, were its respiratory and circulatory depressant actions, its sensitization of the myocardium to catecholamine-induced arrhythmias, its uterine relaxant action and propensity to increase bleeding during delivery, and occasional hepatic necrosis. Methoxyflurane, enflurane, and isoflurane, all of which are fluorinated ethers (Fig. 1), appeared as a consequence of the search for an improved halothane.

Methoxyflurane, which had originally been synthesized as part of the chemistry needed to produce the atomic bomb (Miller et al., 1948), was eventually introduced into clinical medicine as an anesthetic in the 1960s. It proved to be an effective agent, but was nephrotoxic because of metabolic liberation of significant amounts of free fluoride. As a consequence, its use became limited.

Both enflurane and its structural isomer, isoflurane, were synthesized in the mid-1960s, according to Vitcha (1971), but only reported in the early 1970s (Terrell et al., 1971, 1972). Both agents had good anesthetic properties, but shared with halothane the capacity to produce respiratory depression and hypotension. Enflurane, and particularly isoflurane, produced less sensitization of the heart to catecholamines and fewer arrhythmias than did halothane. Enflurane and isoflurane have joined halothane as widely used general anesthetics for surgery (Jones, 1984).

Stephen and Little (1961) commented that "...halothane has introduced an era of avid search for better, safe, potent, nonexplosive, volatile anesthetic drugs: in so doing, it has proven to be a real milestone in anesthesia."

References

Artusio, J. F.: General considerations of halogenated anesthetics, in *Clinical Anesthesia: Halogenated Anesthetics*, J. F. Artusio, ed., pp. 1–22, F. A. Davis, Philadelphia, 1962.

Booth, H. S. and Bixby, E. M.: Fluorine derivatives of chloroform. *Ind. Eng. Chem.* **24**: 637–641, 1932.

Brenner, C.: Note on the action of dichloro-difluoro-methane on the nervous system of the cat. *J. Pharmacol. Exp. Ther.* **59**: 176–181, 1937.

Bryce-Smith, R. and O'Brien, H. D.: Fluothane: A nonexplosive volatile anaesthetic agent. *Br. Med. J.* **2**: 969–972, 1956.

Dripps, R. D., Eckenhoff, J. E., and Vandam, L. D.: *Introduction to Anesthesia: The Principles of Safe Practice*, 2nd Ed., W. B. Saunders, Philadelphia, 1961.

Hudon, F., Jacques, A., Clavet, M., and Houde, J.: Clinical observation on fluothane anaesthesia. *Can. Anaesth. Soc. J.* **4**: 221–234, 1957.

Johnstone, M.: The human cardiovascular response to fluothane anaesthesia. *Br. J. Anaesth.* **28**: 392–410, 1956.

Jones, R. M.: Clinical comparison of inhalation anaesthetic agents. *Br. J. Anaesth.* **56**: 57S–69S, 1984.

Krantz, J. C., Jr., Carr, C. J., Lu, G., and Bell, F. K.: Anesthesia. XL. The anesthetic action of trifluoroethyl vinyl ether. *J. Pharmacol. Exp. Ther.* **108:** 488–495, 1953.

Lampe, K. F., ed.: *Drug Evaluations,* 6th Ed., American Medical Association, Chicago, 1986.

Marshall, B. E. and Wollman, H.: General anesthetics, in *The Pharmacological Basis of Therapeutics,* 7th Ed., A. G. Gilman, L. S. Goodman, T. W. Rall, and F. Murad, eds., pp. 276–301, Macmillan, New York, 1985.

Miller, R. D., ed.: *Anesthesia,* 2nd Ed., vol. 2, Churchill Livingstone, New York, 1986.

Miller, W. T., Jr., Fager, E. W., and Griswold, P. H.: The addition of methyl alcohol to fluoroethylenes. *J. Am. Chem. Soc.* **70:** 431, 432, 1948.

Modell, W., Schild, H. O., and Wilson, A.: *Applied Pharmacology,* American Ed., W. B. Saunders, Philadelphia, 1976.

Neuberger, J. and Williams, R.: Halothane anaesthesia and liver damage. *Br. Med. J.* **289:** 1136–1139, 1984.

Raventós, J.: The action of fluothane—a new volatile anaesthetic. *Br. J. Pharmacol.* **11:** 394–409, 1956.

Robbins, B. H.: Preliminary studies of the anesthetic activity of fluorinated hydrocarbons. *J. Pharmacol. Exp. Ther.* **86:** 197–204, 1946.

Smith, G.: Halothane in clinical practice. *Br. J. Anaesth.* **53:** 17S–25S, 1981.

Smith, T. C. and Wollman, H.: History and principles of anesthesiology, in *The Pharmacological Basis of Therapeutics,* 7th Ed., A. G. Gilman, L. S. Goodman, T. W. Rall, and F. Murad., eds., pp. 260–275, Macmillan, New York, 1985.

Stephen, C. R. and Little, D. M.: *Halothane,* Williams & Wilkins, Baltimore, 1961.

Struck, H. C. and Plattner, E. B.: A study of the pharmacological properties of certain saturated fluorocarbons. *J. Pharmacol. Exp. Ther.* **68:** 217–219, 1940.

Suckling, C. W.: Some chemical and physical factors in the development of fluothane. *Br. J. Anaesth.* **29:** 466–472, 1957.

Terrell, R. C., Speers, L., Szur, A. J., Treadwell, J., and Ucciardi, T. R.: General anesthetics. 1. Halogenated methyl ethyl ethers as anesthetic agents. *J. Med. Chem.* **14:** 517–519, 1971.

Terrell, R. C., Speers, L., Szur, A.J., Ucciardi, T., and Vitcha, J. F.: General anesthetics. 3. Fluorinated methyl ethyl ethers as anesthetic agents. *J. Med. Chem.* **15:** 604–606, 1972.

Vitcha, J. F.: A history of forane. *Anesthesiology* **35:** 4–7, 1971.

Woodbridge, P. D.: A technique for staying out of trouble while using cyclopropane. *Anesth. Analg.* **40:** 32–41, 1961.

Fentanyl

I. Fentanyl as an Innovative Therapeutic Agent

According to Zauder and Nichols (1971), anesthesiologists had a long-standing desire for a parenterally administered drug or combination of drugs that would produce the ideal anesthetic state. This treatment, unlike standard inhalational anesthetics, was to be easy to administer and was to provide profound analgesia, hypnosis, protection against the effects of noxious reflexes, and relaxation of skeletal musculature. Furthermore, respiration and circulation were to be unaffected, urine output was to be sustained, and the gastrointestinal tract was to maintain its normal function. Last, but not least, this ideal anesthesia was also to be rapid in onset, short in duration, and instantaneously reversible.

Two forms of combination anesthesia have become widely used as limited approximations to the ideal outlined above: balanced anesthesia and neuroleptanalgesia/anesthesia.

The term "balanced anesthesia" currently refers to the combined use of an ultra-short-acting barbiturate, an opioid analgesic, nitrous oxide, and a neuromuscular blocking agent to evoke general anesthesia (Lampe, 1986). The concept of balanced anesthesia holds that each of the compounds is given at a reasonable dose for a specific purpose (such as rapid induction of unconsciousness, analgesia, amnesia, sustained unconsciousness, muscle relaxation) with no one agent being given in troublesome excess in an attempt to achieve all of the desired effects with that agent alone (Lundy, 1926).

Neuroleptanalgesia refers to coadministration of a neuroleptic agent (usually a butyrophenone derivative) and an opiate to produce an altered state of consciousness and awareness, with consciousness not being lost during this procedure. Diagnostic procedures and minor surgery can be carried out under neuro-leptanalgesia. If 65% nitrous oxide in oxygen is added to this regimen, often along with a neuromuscular blocking agent, a state of neuroleptanesthesia is achieved. This is a state of general anes-thesia in which consciousness can rapidly be restored by stopping the nitrous oxide administration. Neuroleptanalgesia/anesthesia are both useful procedures when the cooperation of the patient may be needed (Lampe, 1986).

In recent years, the administration of high doses of an opiate alone, plus high inspired concentrations of oxygen, has been championed by some anesthesiologists as producing general an-esthesia more closely approximating the ideal (Lowenstein and Philbin, 1981; Stanley, 1987). This procedure is termed narcotic or opioid anesthesia. It has become popular because some potent nar-cotics are perceived as producing an anesthetic state while having only minor effect on most of the major organ systems, e.g., heart, liver, and kidneys (Stanley, 1982).

Morphine, meperidine, and fentanyl have all been employed in balanced anesthesia, neuroleptanalgesia/anesthesia, and nar-cotic anesthesia. Fentanyl is generally used only in anesthesia, whereas morphine is also useful in treating moderate to severe pain from a variety of causes, such as myocardial infarction and neoplasms, and meperidine is of use in obstetrics.

In its use in balanced anesthesia, fentanyl has an advantage in that it does not elicit the moderate to marked vasodilation seen with morphine and meperidine. Furthermore, fentanyl, unlike meperidine in high doses, does not tend to cause myocardial de-pression. Fentanyl has become very widely used in combination with the butyrophenone, droperidol, for inducing neuroleptan-algesia/anesthesia (Lampe, 1986).

With respect to narcotic anesthesia, Stanley (1987) noted that high doses of morphine often entail such problems as incom-plete amnesia, histamine release, lengthy postoperative respira-tory depression, marked venodilation leading to increased blood volume requirements, and hypertension. This author noted that, "In contrast [to morphine] the synthetic opioid fentanyl has be-come popular as a component of balanced...anesthesia, as a sup-plement when using an inhaled anesthetic, but also in larger doses.... as a primary or complete anesthetic." The large intravenous doses of fentanyl used in narcotic anesthesia do not depress cardiovascular function and are less prone to evoke the problems listed above for morphine. Fentanyl as a sole agent, therefore, has been found to be very useful in anesthetizing patients with diminished cardiac reserve. It is noteworthy, in this regard, that high-dose opioid analgesia, particularly with fentanyl, diminishes the hormonal "stress response" to surgery, namely, the increase in plasma concentrations of catecholamines, cortisol, ADH, growth hormone, glucose, and lactate. Increased levels of "stress hormones" are considered by some surgeons to be undesirable because they presumably promote circulatory instability and metabolic catabolism, but this concept is still a subject of some debate (Philbin et al., 1984).

Fentanyl, like other opioids, frequently produces rigidity of chest and abdominal muscles and respiratory depression. Although these are significant problems, they are not insurmountable in the use of fentanyl in anesthesia, whether as an adjunct or as a complete anesthetic (Stanley, 1987).

Early Clinical Research History

Holderness et al. (1963) noted that the combinations of neuroleptics and narcotic analgesics that had been used in the early evocations of neuroleptanalgesia—haloperidol plus phenoperidine or haloanisone plus dextromoramide—had led to problems, namely, profound hypotension, extrapyramidal disturbances, and a few instances of prolonged postoperative psychic changes. These workers studied the effects of fixed combinations (mainly 50:1 by weight) of a new butyrophenone, droperidol, and a new narcotic anesthetic, fentanyl, on 400 general surgical patients. This intravenous regimen, along with nitrous oxide/oxygen administration, produced both profound analgesia and hypnosis (i.e., a state of neuroleptanesthesia). Stability of the cardiovascular system was noteworthy—alterations in pulse rate or blood pressure were uncommon occurrences, particularly after induction was complete. Respiratory minute volume was reduced, but for a briefer period than with meperidine. In addition, intravenous fentanyl and droperidol caused a ventilatory insufficiency secondary to a catatonic rigidity of the thorax and abdominal musculature, which was of concern. This condition responded to small doses of neuromuscular blocking agents. The authors concluded that, "...this technique with nonexplosive agents...appears to merit further exploration."

Corssen et al. (1964) found that high intravenous doses of fentanyl alone, administered to seven volunteer patients, caused a slight decrease in mean pulse rate, a marked decrease in mean respiratory rate, and no consistent change in the systolic or diastolic pressure. Analgesia was very apparent; emesis occurred in only two volunteers. A total of 359 surgical patients were then treated with droperidol and fentanyl intravenously (mainly the 50:1 fixed combination), plus nitrous oxide/oxygen. The investigators found that any type of major surgery could be carried out with their regimen, provided that neuromuscular blocking agents were also used. This anesthesia produced "remarkable cardiovascular stability" and was "...of particular value for geriatric patients with minimal compensatory reserves, as well as for patients suffering from acquired or congenital heart defects." Marked, short-lived depression of respiratory function and the occurrence of muscle rigidity of the thorax and abdomen were the main problems seen with this mixture. Postoperatively, nausea and vomiting were minimal and extrapyramidal reactions did not occur. The authors concluded that, "The technic [neuroleptanesthesia] is effective, simple, safe, and nonexplosive, and appears to offer distinct advantages over conventional methods, with their high incidence of depressant and toxic effects on vital systems. The method deserves clinical attention."

Other positive clinical studies with the combination of droperidol and fentanyl followed (see, for example, Kreuscher et al., 1965; Henschel, 1966).

A fairly large clinical literature concerning the uses of fentanyl in anesthesia has appeared (see, for references, Estefanous, 1984; Stanley, 1987).

II. The Scientific Work Leading to Fentanyl

Janssen and coworkers, using meperidine (pethidine) (Fig. 1) as a starting point, prepared a large series of substituted 4-phenyl-piperidine compounds (Janssen et al., 1959a,b; Janssen and Eddy, 1960). Six compounds, bearing on the basic nitrogen of the piperi-

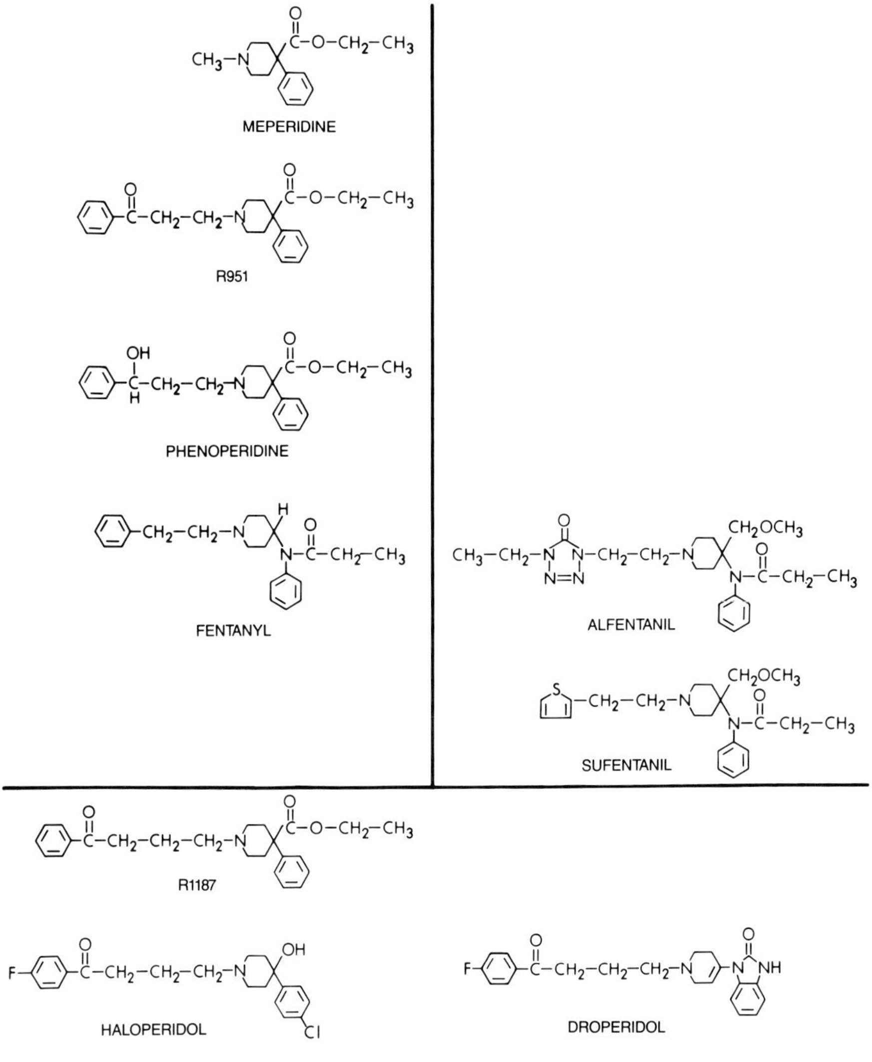

Fig. 1. The structures of fentanyl and chemically and/or pharmacologically related substances.

dine ring substitutions that were larger than the methyl group found in meperidine, were noted to have clinically useful activity. These were R951 (Fig. 1), phenoperidine (Fig. 1), pheneridine, anileridine, piminodine, and etoxeridine (Janssen, 1962). Additional results pointed to the extremely high narcotic potency of compound R 4263 (later named fentanyl). This compound, in addition to having a large substitution on the piperidine nitrogen, was an aniline derivative (Janssen, 1962) (Fig. 1).

Janssen et al. (1963a) found fentanyl to be "...the most potent morphine-like drug we have seen thus far." In the warm-water-induced tail-withdrawal reflex in rats, these investigators found fentanyl to be approximately 400 times more potent than morphine by both the subcutaneous and oral routes. It was also faster acting and shorter acting than morphine.

Gardocki and Yelnosky (1964) carried out a broad pharmacological study with fentanyl in mice, dogs, and cats. They summarized their findings as follows: fentanyl, relative to morphine, had high potency, rapid onset and short duration of action, absence of emetic activity, and minimal hypotensive activity after intravenous administration. Fentanyl, like morphine, exerted a constipating effect. It had a therapeutic ratio 25 times greater than that of morphine, by the subcutaneous route. The actions of fentanyl were readily antagonized by the narcotic antagonist nalorphine, and the bradycardia that it produced was also readily reversed by atropine.

Fentanyl plus the newly developed, short-acting butyrophenone, droperidol (Janssen et al., 1963b) (Fig. 1), were introduced for the induction of neuroleptanalgesia/anesthesia in the early 1960s as an improvement over the combination of haloperidol and phenoperidine (Shephard, 1965) (Fig. 1).

Table 1 defines the critical scientific ideas and experiments leading to fentanyl and categorizes their origin.

Background Contributions Preceding Fentanyl

Opium has been used for centuries for relieving the pain of surgery, and, in the 19th century, its active principle, morphine, began to be used in a reliable manner as a preanesthetic agent, as an adjunct to chloroform anesthesia, and, on occasion, with scopolamine as an anesthetic (Swerdlow, 1964).

Meperidine (Fig. 1), the first totally synthetic narcotic analgesic, was prepared and studied by Eisleb and Schaumann (1939) as part of a program for evaluating, as spasmolytics, structurally

Table 1
Profile of Observations and Ideas Crucial to the Development of Fentanyl[a]

Sequence: Route to innovative drug[b]	Orient- ation	Nature of study	Research institution	National origin	Nature of discovery	Screening involved	Crucial ideas or observations
Fentanyl[b]							
Janssen (1962)	Pre- clinical	Chem- istry/ pharma- cology	Industry	Belgium	Orderly	Targeted	A large series of *N*-substituted meperi-dine derivatives synthesized; several of clinical utility; the very high narcotic potency of 4-anilino-piperidines recog-nized; compound R4263 (fentanyl) is up to 5000× more po-tent than morphine.

[a]Taken from section II. Entries are those contributions without which the discovery of the agent (or additionally, in some cases, a relevant clinical application) would not have taken place or would have been materially delayed.

novel compounds related to atropine. These authors discovered that meperidine combined the spasmolytic properties of atropine and papaverine with the analgesic properties of morphine. Meperidine was found to be 7.5–10 times less potent as an analgesic than morphine, by parenteral routes in humans (Jaffe and Martin, 1985).

A decade after the discovery of meperidine, the technique of giving repeated administrations of a narcotic analgesic during the course of nitrous oxide/oxygen anesthesia was introduced as a means of ensuring adequate, sustained obtunding of pain during surgery (Neff et al., 1947; Brotman and Cullen, 1949). Subsequently, in the late 1950s, the combining of a neuroleptic state (induced initially by procaine plus hydergine, but eventually by a neuroleptic drug) along with the coadministration of an analgesic agent (originally procaine, but eventually a strong narcotic), was developed as an alternative to typical anesthetic practices. Unlike barbiturates or gases, this regimen of a neuroleptic agent plus a narcotic analgesic did not produce unconsciousness, but provided a state of passivity and indifference to pain (neuroleptanalgesia)

(De Castro and Mundeleer, 1959). Various combinations of narcotic analgesics and phenothiazine or butyrophenone neuroleptic
agents were studied; concerted interest initially settled on the combination of haloperidol with phenoperidine (De Castro and Mundeleer, 1962). Neuroleptanalgesia is generally considered to be an
outgrowth of the earlier "lytic cocktail" of Laborit (Laborit, 1949;
Laborit and Leger, 1950; *see* section II of chlorpromazine chapter).
The term "cocktail" refers to the combination of a battery of drugs,
eventually including chlorpromazine (Laborit and Huguenard,
1951), that was intended to eliminate the cellular, autonomic, and
endocrine reactions to the stress of surgery by discrete pharmacological blocking actions. Laborit referred to this procedure as
"pharmacological hibernation."

III. Comments on Events Leading to Fentanyl

Corssen et al. (1964) commented, "Since Janssen's introduction of a series of highly potent analgesic and neuroleptic agents,
an anesthetic technic has evolved, called 'neuroleptanalgesia'..."
Regarding the discovery of both of these series of compounds—
the phenyl-piperidine narcotics and the butyrophenone neuroleptics—Janssen and Tollenaere (1983) recollected, "Compound
R951 [Fig. 1] proved to be a pivotal element in our thinking because the high [narcotic] potency of R951 was contrary to the firm
belief at that time that only small chemical groups or moieties at
the nitrogen atom of the piperidine ring were compatible with high
morphinomimetic potency." In subsequently enlarging the N-
substituent of R951 by one methylene group, i.e., from a propiophenone to a butyrophenone (compound R1187) (Fig. 1), narcotic
potency dropped significantly, but was accompanied by delayed
chlorpromazine-like effects—calming, sedation and mild cata-
tonia (Janssen and Tollenaere, 1983).

Further chemical modification of R951 eventually led to
fentanyl via a series of active narcotics, as already noted; further
chemical modifications of R1187 led to haloperidol and, thence, to
the family of butyrophenones, including droperidol (Fig. 1).

IV. Developments
Subsequent to Fentanyl

The Janssen group (van Bever, et al., 1976; *see also* Janssen, 1984) prepared a series of chemical modifications of fentanyl that yielded the narcotics carfentanil, lofentanil, sufentanil, and alfentanil. The latter two agents (Fig. 1) have received significant, recent clinical attention in anesthesiology.

De Lange (1983) considered that "[b]oth alfentanil and sufentanil are attractive alternatives to fentanyl for high-dose anesthesia techniques." Alfentanil is an especially short-acting agent that has an intravenous therapeutic ratio four times greater than that of fentanyl. It is useful as an analgesic supplement to anesthesia, for anesthetic induction, and, with continuous variable rate infusion, as the major component of a general anesthetic (along with oxygen and a neuromuscular blocking agent). Alfentanil can be titrated more closely to patients' needs than can fentanyl (Reitz, 1986). It appears to be especially useful in patients undergoing short operative procedures.

Sufentanil is not as short-acting as alfentanil or fentanyl (De Lange, 1983; Janssen, 1984), but has an intravenous therapeutic ratio 100 times greater than fentanyl. It is useful for balanced anesthesia in conjunction with nitrous oxide/oxygen. It is also useful for induction and as the sole agent (along with oxygen and a neuromuscular blocking agent) in cardiovascular and neurosurgical operations (Lampe, 1986; Philbin et al., 1984; Fahmy, 1984).

Janssen (1984) expressed the view that "[t]he safe use of powerful narcotics has become possible thanks to the development of compounds with a greater dissociation between their analgesic and toxic doses...newer, more potent, and more specific opiates are no longer dangerous for patients with cardiac insufficiency..."

Philbin et al. (1984) pointed out,

Efforts to achieve an anesthetic environment that totally ablates the hormonal stress response to surgical stimulation have concentrated on high-dose narcotic anesthesia, particularly the new synthetic narcotics. This is because the high concentrations of drugs required can be administered with relative ease and side effects are easily treatable or within acceptable range. High concentrations of potent inhalation agents could also blunt these hormonal responses but at a price unacceptable in the clinical situation.

Lowenstein and Philbin (1981) felt that "[n]arcotics constitute a powerful tool in the armamentarium of anaesthetists....Whether they will provide an ideal drug remains a matter of conjecture...however, the future of narcotic 'anesthesia' looks promising indeed."

References

Brotman, M. and Cullen, S. C.: Supplementation with demerol during nitrous oxide anesthesia. *Anesthesiology* **10**: 696–705, 1949.

Corssen, G., Domino, E. F. and Sweet, R. B.: Neuroleptanalgesia and anesthesia. *Anesth. Analg.* **43**: 748–763, 1964.

De Castro, J. and Mundeleer, P.: Anesthésie sans barbiturique: La neuroleptanalgésie (R. 1406, R. 1625, hydergine, procaine). *Anesthesie, Analgesie, Reanimation* **16**: 1022–1056, 1959.

De Castro, J. and Mundeleer, P.: Die Neuroleptanalgésie. *Der Anaesthesist* **11**: 10–17, 1962.

De Lange, S.: Clinical experiences with analogues of fentanyl. *Mt. Sinai J. Med.* **50**: 312–315, 1983.

Eisleb, O. and Schaumann, O.: Dolantin, ein neuartiges Spasmolytikum und Analgetikum. *Dtsch. Med. Wochenschr.* **65**: 967, 968, 1939.

Estefanous, F. G., ed.: *Opioids in Anesthesia*, Butterworth, Boston, 1984.

Fahmy, N. R.: Sufentanil: A review, in *Opioids in Anesthesia*, F. G. Estefanous, ed., pp. 132–139, Butterworth, Boston, 1984.

Gardocki, J. F. and Yelnosky, J.: A study of some of the pharmacologic actions of fentanyl citrate. *Toxicol. Appl. Pharmacol.* **6**: 48–62, 1964.

Henschel, W. F.: Die Neuroleptanalgesie. *Landarzt* **42**: 1614–1623, 1966.

Holderness, M. C., Chase, P. E., and Dripps, R. D.: A narcotic analgesic and a butyrophenone with nitrous oxide for general anesthesia. *Anesthesiology* **24**: 336–340, 1963.

Jaffe, J. H. and Martin, W. L.: Opioid analgesics and antagonists, in *The Pharmacological Basis of Therapeutics*, 7th Ed., A. G. Gilman, L. S. Goodman, T. W. Rall, and F. Murad, eds., pp. 491–531, Macmillan, New York, 1985.

Janssen, P. A.: A review of the chemical features associated with strong morphine-like activity. *Br. J. Anaesth.* **34:** 260–268, 1962.

Janssen, P. A.: The development of new synthetic narcotics, in *Opioids in Anesthesia,* F. G. Estefanous, ed., pp. 37–44, Butterworth, Boston, 1984.

Janssen, P. A. and Eddy, N. B.: Compounds related to pethidine-IV. New general chemical methods of increasing the analgesic activity of pethidine. *J. Med. Pharm. Chem.* **2:** 31–45, 1960.

Janssen, P. A. and Tollenaere, J.: The discovery of the butyrophenone-type neuroleptics, in *Discoveries in Pharmacology,* vol. 1, M. J. Parnham and J. Bruinvels, eds., pp. 181–196, Elsevier, Amsterdam, 1983.

Janssen, P. A., Niemegeers, C. J., and Dony, J. G.: The inhibitory effect of fentanyl and other morphine-like analgesics on the warm water induced tail withdrawal reflex in rats. *Arzneimittelforsch.* **13:** 502–507, 1963a.

Janssen, P. A., Niemegeers, C. J., Schellekens, K. H., Verbruggen, F. J., and Van Neuten, J. M.: The pharmacology of dehydrobenzperidol, a new potent and short acting neuroleptic agent chemically related to haloperidol. *Arzneimittelforsch.* **13:** 205–211, 1963b.

Janssen, P. A., Jageneau, A. H., Demoen, P. J., van de Westeringh, C., Raeymaekers, A. H. M., Wouters, M. S. J., Sanczuk, S. Hermans, B. K. F., and Loomans, J. L. M.: Compounds related to pethidine-I. Mannich bases derived from norpethidine and acetophenones. *J. Med. Pharm. Chem.* **1:** 105–120, 1959a.

Janssen, P. A., Jageneau, A. H., Demoen, P. J., van de Westeringh, C., de Cannière, J. H. M., Raeymaekers, A. H. M., Wouters, M. S. J., Sanczuk, S., and Hermans, B. K. F.: Compounds related to pethidine II. Mannich bases derived from various esters of 4-carboxy-4-phenylpiperidine and acetophenones. *J. Med. Pharm. Chem.* **1:** 309–317, 1959b.

Kreuscher, H., Frey, R., and Madjidi, A.: Die "Neuroleptanalgesie." *Dtsch. Med. Wochenschr.* **90:** 721–725, 1965.

Laborit, H.: Sur l'utilization de certains agents pharmacodynamiques à action neuro-végétative en periode per- et postopératoire. *Acta Chir. Belg.* **48:** 485–492, 1949.

Laborit, H. and Huguenard, P.: Notes de technique chirurgicale. *Presse Méd.* **59:** 1329, 1951.

Laborit, H. and Leger, L.: Utilization d'un antihistaminique de synthèse en thérapeutique pré, per, et post-opératoire. *Press Méd.* **58:** 492, 1950.

Lampe, K. F., ed.: *Drug Evaluations,* 6th Ed., American Medical Association, Chicago, 1986.

Lowenstein, E. and Philbin, D. M.: Narcotic "anesthesia" in the eighties. *Anesthesiology* **55:** 195–197, 1981.

Lundy, J. S.: Balanced anesthesia. *Minn. Med.* **9**: 399–404, 1926.

Neff, W., Mayer, E. C., and de la Luz Perales, M.: Nitrous oxide and oxygen anesthesia with curare relaxation. *Calif. Med.* **66**: 67–69, 1947.

Philbin, D. M., Rosow, C. E., D'Ambra, M., Freis, E. S. , and Schneider, R. C.: Hormonal changes during narcotic anesthesia and operation, in *Opioids in Anesthesia*, F. G. Estafanous, ed., pp. 70–74, Butterworth, Boston, 1984.

Reitz, J. A.: Alfentanil in anesthesia and analgesia. *Drug Intell. Clin. Pharm.* **20**: 335–341, 1986.

Shephard, N. W., ed.: *The Application of Neuroleptanalgesia in Anesthetic and Other Practice*, Pergamon, Oxford, 1965.

Stanley, T. H.: High-dose narcotic anesthesia. *Sem. Anesthesia* **1**: 21–32, 1982.

Stanley, T. H.: Opiate anaesthesia. *Anaesth. Intensive Care* **15**: 38–59, 1987.

Swerdlow, M.: History of narcotics in anesthesia, in *Narcotics and Narcotic Antagonists*, F. Foldes, M. Swerdlow, and E. Sikes, eds., pp. 3–9, Charles C. Thomas, Springfield, IL, 1964.

van Bever, W. F. M., Niemegeers, C., Schellekens, K. H. L., and Janssen, P. A. J.: N-4-Substituted1-(2 arylethyl)-4-piperidinyl-N-phenyl-propanamides, a novel series of extremely potent analgesics with unusually high safety margin. *Arzneimittelforsch.* **26**: 1548–1551, 1976.

Zauder, H. L. and Nichols, R. J.: Intravenous anesthesia, in *A Decade of Clinical Progress*, (*Clinical Anesthesia*, vol. 7/3), L. W. Fabian, ed., pp. 318–357, F. A. Davis, Philadelphia, 1971.

Naloxone

I. Naloxone as an Innovative Therapeutic Agent

Morphine has been used effectively in medicine to suppress pain since the nineteenth century (Swerdlow, 1964). It, with other opioids, has found legitimate medical use in the treatment of moderate to severe pain, both acute and chronic, resulting from a variety of causes, such as myocardial infarction, obstetrical procedures, and neoplasms. In addition, these drugs have had wide use as adjuncts in surgical anesthesia (Lampe, 1986).

Unfortunately, the opioids that have clinical value as potent analgesics also depress respiration—their most dangerous acute manifestation—and also elicit vasodepressor actions, mood changes, drowsiness, nausea, emesis, constipation, and miosis. Moderate opioid overdosing, with consequent respiratory depression, may be encountered in medical practice as a result of an unusual response to a normal dose, to errors in calculating doses, to hypersensitivity of the elderly, or to drug interactions. In obstetrical practice, fetuses may experience respiratory depression when the mothers are given opioids during labor. Morever, severe overdosing may be encountered when there is nonmedical use (abuse) of the opioids. As is well known, chronic use of opioids can lead to physical dependence and tolerance.

Prior to the appearance of specific opioid antagonists, treatment for opioid-induced respiratory depression was largely symptomatic and supportive, and included the cautious use of such analeptic agents as pentylenetetrazol, nikethamide, or picrotoxin (Eckenhoff et al., 1952; Salomon et al., 1954). With the advent of the first important, relatively specific opioid antagonists, nalorphine and levallorphan, respiratory depression and other consequences of moderate to severe opioid overdose could be readily antagonized.

Both of these drugs, however, were not pure antagonists, but had some agonist activities. As a consequence, nalorphine and levallorphan exerted clinically significant, but limited, opioid effects in nonnarcotized people, including analgesia and depression of respiration. This respiratory depression seemed to be additive with that produced by low doses of opioids. In addition, these two agents produced dysphoric and psychotomimetic effects, such as anxiety and hallucinations, in a significant number of patients (Eckenhoff and Oech, 1960; Foldes and Torda, 1965; Modell et al., 1976; Jaffe and Martin, 1985).

Naloxone, in distinction to nalorphine and levallorphan, is essentially a pure antagonist of morphine actions, and its occupation of morphine receptors evokes essentially no agonist activities. Therefore, it displays very little, if any, opiate actions at clinically useful doses, when its high affinity for the receptors allows it readily to displace opioid agonists. Respiration and circulation are not depressed (Foldes and Torda, 1965; Foldes et al., 1969). Naloxone, in further distinction to nalorphine, does not produce physical dependence, and moreover does not produce morphine-like subjective effects, but does precipitate an abstinence syndrome in morphine-dependent people (Jasinski et al., 1967; Lampe, 1986). In addition, naloxone does not produce the dysphoric effects seen with nalorphine and levallorphan, and in fact can be used to antagonize these effects (Jaffe and Martin, 1985).

Naloxone is the drug of choice for treating opioid-induced respiratory depression (Lampe, 1986; Jaffe and Martin, 1985). The antagonism is specific and reliable enough to indicate that a respiratory depression is not opioid-induced if it is not antagonized by naloxone. Naloxone is used to reverse respiratory depression postoperatively and also in neonates when opioids have been administered to the mother during labor. It has additional utility in diagnosing physical dependence on opioids, in alleviating convulsions and coma in opioid drug abusers, and in the treatment of opioid drug abuse. Naloxone is active by parenteral routes, but is not effective following oral administration.

Early Clinical Research History

Foldes' group (Lunn et al., 1961) reported (in an abstract) that in 10 premedicated patients who were lightly anesthetized with thiopental and nitrous oxide/oxygen, naloxone completely anta-gonized the significant respiratory depression elicited by meperi-dine plus oxymorphone.

This same group (Foldes et al., 1963) found that naloxone was approximately 30 times more potent than nalorphine and six times more potent than levallorphan in antagonizing opioid-induced respiratory depression. Furthermore, the doses of naloxone that antagonized the respiratory depression caused by large doses of oxymorphone, meperidine, or alphaprodine did not cause respira-tory or circulatory depression when administered alone to pa-tients. This result was in contrast to those seen with nalorphine or levallorphan, which under the same conditions had clear respira-tory depressant actions of their own. Naloxone alone had neglible circulatory effects and had a modest effect in antagonizing the circulatory effects of oxymorphone. Foldes et al. (1963) concluded, "If further studies in conscious and anesthetized subjects confirm [these results]..., then this drug would represent a significant ad-vance in the prevention and treatment of narcotic-induced respi-ratory depression." Foldes and his group continued with careful study of naloxone vis-á-vis nalorphine and levallorphan (Foldes et al., 1964a, 1965; Foldes and Torda, 1965) and eventually concluded (Foldes et al., 1969) that naloxone "...should be considered the nar-cotic antagonist of choice for clinical use."

A considerable literature has developed concerning nalox-one, as well as other narcotic antagonists, and their uses (*see*, for references, Foldes et al., 1964b, Blumberg and Dayton, 1974; Schechter, 1980; Garrett and Way, 1983; Handal et al., 1983; McNicholas and Martin, 1984; Milne and Jhamandas, 1984; Jaffe and Martin, 1985).

II. The Scientific Departure
Leading to Naloxone: Nalorphine

McCawley et al. (1941) reported that they had synthesized *N*-allylnormorphine, the *N*-allyl derivative of morphine, (later called nalorphine) (Fig. 1). They stated that it had an antagonistic action on the depression of respiration evoked by morphine; it was considered to be stronger as an antagonist than *N*-allylnorcodeine, the *N*-allyl derivative of codeine (Fig. 1). McCawley's colleague Hart (1941) also noted, preliminarily, that *N*-allylnormorphine, as well as N-allylnorcodeine, antagonized the respiratory effects of morphine.

Weijlard and Erickson (1942), despite many efforts, were not able to repeat the preparation of nalorphine by the method outlined by McCawley et al. (1941). They described a new synthesis that they demonstrated was reliable and that yielded the product, nalorphine. This material differed in melting point by more than 100°C from the compound prepared by McCawley and coworkers. Unna (1943), an associate of Weijlard and Erickson, compared the properties of their preparation of nalorphine with those of morphine. Nalorphine was much less effective than morphine in raising the pain threshold in mice. Small doses of nalorphine, unlike morphine, did not depress respiration, but larger doses did. The compound abolished the analgesia, respiratory depression, and behavioral depression or stimulation evoked in laboratory animals by morphine. It also reduced the mortality of morphine poisoning in mice. Unna (1943) noted that he had conducted his studies as the result of a suggestion of Chauncey D. Leake of the University of California.

Hart (1943) stated that, although intravenous nalorphine caused no stimulation of respiration, it prevented the respiratory depression resulting from the subsequent administration of morphine. If given after morphine, respiration was stimulated beyond the normal level for a few minutes and then became normal.

It was pointed out by Hart and McCawley (1944) that "...the synthesis of N-allylnormorphine was undertaken with the hope that this compound might retain the analgesic and narcotic potency of morphine but lack the respiratory action." They noted the work of Weijlard and Erickson (1942) and came to the conclusion that it was highly probable that the original material prepared by them (McCawley et al., 1941) was N-allyl-O-allyl-normorphine (Fig. 1), not nalorphine. McCawley (1942), using the same method as Weijlard and Erickson (1942), "...was able to prepare N-allyl-normorphine [nalorphine] which has the same melting point as that prepared by Weijlard and Erickson." Working with proven nalorphine, Hart and McCawley (1944), unlike Unna (1943), found that it was at least as potent as morphine in raising the pain threshold and that it produced a transitory stimulation of respiration followed by a slight depression. They held the opinion that replacement of the N-methyl group of morphine by N-allyl elimi-

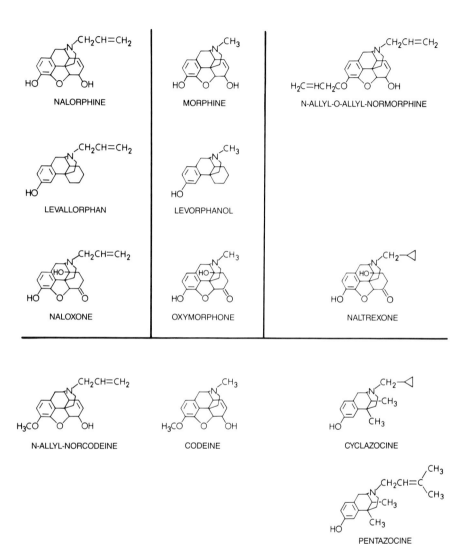

Fig. 1. The structures of naloxone and chemically and/or pharmacologically related substances.

nated the respiratory depressant action, but did not diminish the analgesic action; this opinion has not been substantiated, most workers finding both moderate analgesia and moderate respiratory depression with nalorphine.

Background Contributions Preceding Nalorphine

Von Braun (1914) devised a method for removing the N-methyl group from morphine and codeine to produce normorphine and norcodeine. Subsequently, Von Braun (1916) reacted norcodeine with allyl bromide to yield N-allylnorcodeine (Fig. 1). Pohl (1915) showed that this compound did not produce the behavioral depressant effects of codeine and that it was an antagonist of the respiratory and cerebral depressant effects of morphine. Unfortunately, this work was not followed up. McCawley et al. (1941), Hart (1941), and Hart and McCawley (1944) cited these authors for having made practical the synthesis of derivatives of morphine and codeine that differed only in the radical substituted on the nitrogen, and for demonstrating "...the very striking pharmacological properties..." of N-allylnorcodeine.

Significant Work Following Nalorphine

Schnider and Hellerbach (1950) prepared the N-allyl derivative of the opioid, levorphanol (Fig. 1). This compound, eventually named levallorphan (Fig. 1), was demonstrated by Fromherz and Pellmont (1952) to antagonize the inhibitory action of morphine on respiration in the rabbit and analgesia in the rat. The dextrorotatory N-allyl compound showed no antagonistic properties. Fromherz and Pellmont (1952) clearly recognized the earlier work of Unna (1943), and of others, with nalorphine, and also recognized that levallorphan bore the same relationship to levorphanol as did nalorphine to morphine.

Blumberg et al. (1961) reported in an abstract that the recently synthesized compound, naloxone, was a potent narcotic antagonist that, in several tests, had no analgesic properties of its own. Naloxone was the N-allyl derivative of the potent opioid oxymorphone (Fig. 1). It was seven times more potent than nalorphine in blocking oxymorphone analgesia in the hot-plate test in mice. It was 10 times more potent than nalorphine and two times more potent than levallorphan in counteracting the respiratory depression produced with oxymorphon in conscious rabbits. The compound was quickly put into clinical trial (see Lunn et al., 1961, in section I).

Table 1 defines the critical scientific ideas and experiments leading to naloxone and categorizes their origin.

III. Comments on Events Leading to Naloxone

According to Garrett and Way (1983), naloxone and other narcotic antagonists "...are the serendipitous culmination of years of research to find strong analgesics which do not have respiratory depressant properties or abuse potential."

These authors pointed out that McCawley and Hart were graduate students under Chauncey D. Leake in 1939. According to Sneader (1985), when Leake was developing vinyl ether as a volatile anesthetic he noted that ethers having an allyl group exerted respiratory stimulant properties, which suggested that an allyl function on morphine might reduce its respiratory depressant effects. Presumably, this reasoning prompted McCawley's unsuccessful initial attempt at synthesizing nalorphine. Garrett and Way (1983) also maintained that Leake, in looking for the quickest way to exploit what he thought was nalorphine, passed information on to a pharmaceutical company, Merck and Co. According to these authors, Leake and his colleagues were filled with consternation when Merck's chemists, Weijlard and Erickson (1942), published the correct synthesis for nalorphine without consulting them.

IV. Developments Subsequent to Naloxone

Blumberg et al. (1967) reported in abstract their results with three novel N-substituted derivatives of oxymorphone: the dimethylallyl, cyclobutylmethyl, and cyclopropylmethyl derivatives. The dimethylallyl compound was stated to be a moderately active analgesic and a relatively weak antagonist. The cyclobutylmethyl compound was a potent analgesic and a potent antagonist. The cyclopropylmethyl compound (later named naltrexone) (Fig.1) had little analgesic potency, but was an extremely potent

Table 1
Profile of Observations and Ideas Crucial to the Development of Naloxone[a,b]

Sequence: Departure compound* to innovative drug**	Orient- ation	Nature of study	Research institution	National origin	Nature of discovery	Screening involved	Crucial ideas or observations
Nalorphine*							
McCawley et al. (1941)	Pre- clinical	Chem- istry/ pharma- cology	Univ- ersity	USA	Orderly	Targeted	In attempting to pre- pare N-allylnormor- phine, the authors prepared N-allyl-O- allyl-normorphine; it is stated to have morphine-antagonist properties.
Weijlard and Erick- son (1942)	Pre- clinical	Chem- istry	Indus- try	USA	Orderly	No	True N-allylnormor- phine (nalorphine) synthesized.
Unna (1943)	Pre- clinical	Pharma- cology	Indus- try	USA	Orderly	Targeted	Nalorphine, a weak analgesic and respir- atory depressant, effectively antagon- izes the analgesic and respiratory- depressant effects of morphine.
Levallorphan							
Fromherz and Pellmont (1952)	Pre- clinical	Chem- istry/ pharma- cology	Indus- try	Switzer- land	Orderly	Targeted	Like nalorphine, levallorphan (the N- allyl derivative of levorphanol) effec- tively antagonizes the analgesia and respiratory-depres- sant effects of mor- phine.

(continued)

*Taken from section II. Entries are those contributions without which the discovery of the agent (or additionally, in some cases, a relevant clinical application) would not have taken place or would have been materially delayed.

[b]According to a personal communication from Blumberg, naloxone was synthesized in a pri- vate laboratory operated by M. J. Lewenstein; all original pharmacology was carried out at Endo Laboratories by Blumberg and assistants. Both Lewenstein and Blumberg were employees of the Endo Laboratories. A patent on naloxone was granted to Lewenstein and Fishman (1966).

Table 1 (continued)

Sequence: Departure compound* to innovative drug**	Orient- ation	Nature of study	Research institution	National origin	Nature of discovery	Screening involved	Crucial ideas or observations
Naloxone**							
Blumberg et al. (1961)	Pre- clinical	Chem- istry/ pharma- cology	Indus- try	USA	Orderly	Targeted	Like nalorphine and levallorphan, N-al- lylnoroxymorphone (naloxone) is a potent antagonist of morphine analgesia and respiratory de- pression; unlike these agents, nal- oxone has essentially no agonist activities at reasonable doses.

antagonist. According to Blumberg and Dayton (1974), these particular *N* substitutions were made because the same substitutions in a benzomorphan series had yielded such interesting compounds as pentazocine and cyclazocine (Fig. 1).

In humans, naltrexone, unlike naloxone, is quite active by the oral route and is relatively long-acting. Adequate oral doses, given three times a week, elicit almost continuous blockade of the subjective effects of opioids. Naltrexone is, therefore, a useful pharmacological adjunct for maintaining an opioid-free state in narcotic dependence (Martin et al., 1973; Jaffe and Martin, 1985; Lampe, 1986).

Additional opioids and opioid antagonists continue to be synthesized, especially in light of the discovery of the peptidal opioids—the enkephalins and endorphins. As pursuit of knowledge of the physiology and pathology associated with these endogenous substances (and of their interactions with mu and kappa receptors, and possibly with delta and sigma receptors as well) increases, the desire for very selective agonists and antagonists drives the drug discovery effort in this area.

Narcotic antagonists have had significant impact on opioid research. McNicholas and Martin (1984) held the opinion that, "[n]aloxone, as a prototype pure opioid antagonist ...has played a critical role in clarifying ideas about the mode of action of opioid analgesics and the physiological role of enkephalinergic and endorphinergic processes...." In a similar vein, Garrett and Way (1983) concluded that "...the great strides in the field of opiate pharmacology during the past thirty years were made possible principally by the availability of narcotic antagonists."

References

Blumberg, H. and Dayton, H. B.: Naloxone, naltrexone, and related noroxymorphones, in *Narcotic Antagonists*, M. C. Braude, L. S. Harris, E. L. May, J. P. Smith, and J. E. Villareal, eds., *Advances in Biochemical Psychopharmacology*, vol. 8, pp. 33–43, Raven, New York, 1974.

Blumberg, H., Dayton, H. B., George, M., and Rapaport, D. N.: N-Allyl-noroxymorphone: A potent narcotic antagonist. *Fed. Proc.* **20**: 311, 1961.

Blumberg, H., Dayton, H. B., and Wolf, P. S.: Analgesic and narcotic antagonist properties of noroxymorphone derivatives. *Toxicol. Appl. Pharmacol.* **10**: 406, 1967.

Eckenhoff, J. E. and Oech, S. R.: The effects of narcotics and antagonists upon respiration and circulation in man. A review. *Clin. Pharmacol. Ther.* **1**: 483–524, 1960.

Eckenhoff, J. E., Elder, J. D., and King, B. D.: N-Allylnormorphine in the treatment of morphine or Demerol narcosis. *Am. J. Med. Sci.* **223**: 191–197, 1952.

Foldes, F. F. and Torda, T. A. G.: Comparative studies with narcotics and narcotic antagonists in man. *Acta Anaesthesiol. Scand.* **9**: 121–138, 1965.

Foldes, F. F., Duncalf, D., and Kuwabara, S.: The respiratory, circulatory, and narcotic antagonistic effects of nalorphine, levallorphan, and naloxone in anaesthetized subjects. *Can. Anaesth. Soc. J.* **16**: 151–161, 1969.

Foldes, F. F., Duncalf, D., Davidson, G. M., Yun, D. S., and Shapira, M.: Comparison of the respiratory and circulatory effects of narcotic antagonists. *Anesthesiology* **25**: 95, 96, 1964a.

Foldes, F. F., Swerdlow, M., and Siker, E. S.: *Narcotics and Narcotic Antagonists*, Charles C. Thomas, Springfield, IL, 1964b.

Foldes, F. F., Lunn, J. N., Moore, J., and Brown, I.M.: N-Allylnoroxymorphone: A new potent narcotic antagonist. *Am. J. Med. Sci.*, **245**: 23–30, 1963.

Foldes, F. F., Schapira, M., Torda, T. A. G., Duncalf, D., and Shiffman, H. P.: Studies on the specificity of narcotic antagonists. *Anesthesiology*, **26**: 320–328, 1965.

Fromherz, K. and Pellmont, B.: Morphinantagonisten. *Experientia* **8**: 394, 395, 1952.

Garrett, K. M. and Way, E. L.: The history of narcotic antagonists, in *Discoveries in Pharmacology*, vol. 1, M. J. Parnham and J. Bruinvels, eds., pp. 379–393, Elsevier, Amsterdam, 1983.

Handal, K. A., Schauben, J. L., and Salamone, F. R.: Naloxone. *Ann. Emerg. Med.* **12**: 438–445, 1983.

Hart, E. R.: N-Allyl norcodeine and N-Allyl-normorphine, two antagonists to morphine. *J. Pharmacol. Exp. Ther.* **72**: 19P, 1941.

Hart, E. R.: Further observations on the antagonistic actions of N-allyl-normorphine against morphine. *Fed. Proc.* **2**: 82, 1943.

Hart, E. R. and McCawley, E. L.: The pharmacology of N-allylnormorphine as compared with morphine. *J. Pharmacol. Exp. Ther.* **82**: 339–348, 1944.

Jaffe, J. H. and Martin, W. R.: Opioid analgesics and antagonists, in *The Pharmacological Basis of Therapeutics*, 7th Ed., A. G. Gilman, L. S. Goodman, T. W. Rall, and F. Murad, eds., pp. 491–531, Macmillan, New York, 1985.

Jasinski, D. R., Martin, W. R., and Haertzen, C. A.: The human pharmacology and abuse potential of N-allylnoroxymorphone (naloxone). *J. Pharmacol. Exp. Ther.* **157**: 420–426, 1967.

Lampe, K. F., ed.: *Drug Evaluations*, 6th Ed., American Medical Association, Chicago, 1986.

Lewenstein, M. J. and Fishman, J.: Morphine derivative. US Patent 3,254,088. 1966.

Lunn, J. N., Foldes, F. F., Moore, J., and Brown, I. M.: The influence of N-allyl oxymorphone on the respiratory effects of oxymorphone in anesthetized man. *The Pharmacologist* **3**: 66, 1961.

McCawley, E. L.: The pharmacology of certain nitrogen-substituted normorphine derivatives. PhD dissertation, Graduate Division, University of California (San Francisco), 1942.

McCawley, E. L., Hart, E. R., and Marsh, D. F.: The preparation of N-allylnormorphine. *J. Am. Chem. Soc.* **63**: 314, 1941.

McNicholas, L. F. and Martin, W. R.: New and experimental therapeutic roles for naloxone and related opioid antagonists. *Drugs* **27**: 81–93, 1984.

Martin, W. R., Jasinski, D. R., and Mansky, P. A.: Naltrexone, an antagonist for the treatment of heroin dependence. Effects in man. *Arch. Gen. Psychiatry* **28**: 784–791, 1973.

Milne, B. and Jhamandas, K.: Naloxone: New therapeutic roles. *Can. Anaesth. Soc. J.* **31**: 272–278, 1984.

Modell, W., Schild, H. O., and Wilson, A.: *Applied Pharmacology*, American Ed., W. B. Saunders, Philadelphia, 1976.

Pohl, J.: Ueber das N-Allylnorcodein, einen Antagonisten des Morphins. *Z. Exper. Pathol. Ther.* **18**: 370–382, 1915.

Salomon, A., Marcus, P. S., Herschfus, J. A., and Segal, M. S.: N-Allylnormorphine (Nalline) action on narcotized and non-narcotized subjects. *Am. J. Med.* **17**: 214–222, 1954.

Schechter, A.: The role of narcotic antagonists in the rehabilitation of opiate addicts: A review of naltrexone. *Am. J. Drug Alcohol Abuse* **7**: 1–18, 1980.

Schnider, O. and Hellerbach, J.: Synthese non Morphinanen. *Helv. Chim. Acta* **33**: 1437–1448, 1950.

Sneader, W.: *Drug Discovery: The Evolution of Modern Medicine*, Wiley, New York, 1985.

Swerdlow, M.: History of narcotics in anesthesia, in *Narcotics and Narcotic Antagonists*, F. F. Foldes, M. Swerdlow, and E. S. Siker, coauthors, pp. 3–9, Charles C. Thomas, Springfield, IL, 1964.

Unna, K.: Antagonistic effect of N-allyl-normorphine upon morphine. *J. Pharmacol. Exp. Ther.* **79**: 27–31, 1943.

Von Braun, J.: Untersuchungen über Morphium-Alkaloide. I. Mitteilung. *Berichte Dtsh. Chem. Ges.* **2**: 2312–2330, 1914.

Von Braun, J.: Untersuchungen über Morphium-Alkaloide. III. Mitteilung. *Berichte Dtsch. Chem. Ges.* **1**: 977–989, 1916.

Weijlard, J. and Erickson, A.E.: N-Allylnormorphine. *J. Am. Chem. Soc.* **64**: 869, 870, 1942.

Pulmonary Group

Albuterol
Beclomethasone Dipropionate

Albuterol

I. Albuterol as an Innovative Therapeutic Agent

Bronchial asthma can be simply defined as reversible airways obstruction occurring in people with airways hypersensitivity. Since a major component of this obstruction is bronchospasm, the primary goal of asthma therapy is relief and/or prevention of bronchospasm. During the earlier part of this century, the mainstay for relief from the bronchospasm of acute severe asthmatic attacks was the endogenous adrenergic agonist, epinephrine (parenterally administered); it is still quite widely used, by subcutaneous injection, to relieve acute asthma. However, since the 1940s, the synthetic agent isoproterenol (injected and inhaled) has served as an alternative adrenergic bronchodilator for both the acute and sustained treatment of asthma, and from the 1960s onward, the synthetic adrenergic agonists metaproterenol, albuterol (salbutamol), terbutaline, and others, given by the inhalation and oral routes, have also come into wide usage.

Epinephrine, since it is a potent agonist for alpha as well as for beta receptors, produces arterial hypertension as a side effect. The hypertension is a consequence of peripheral vasoconstriction (an alpha-receptor effect) and cardiac augmentation (a beta-receptor effect), and these effects may also be associated with tachyarrhythmias and palpitations, and accompanied by headache, nervousness, and skeletal muscle tremor. Isoproterenol, on the other hand, is solely a beta agonist and has no vasoconstrictor activity; therefore, it does not evoke arterial hypertension. However, the side effects consequent on beta-induced cardiac stimulation and vasodilation—tachyarrhythmias, palpitations, hypotension—remain and can be a problem, along with the occurrence of nervousness, headache, and tremor. In addition, both epinephrine and isoproterenol are short-acting agents (Prime, 1971; Tashkin and Jenne, 1985).

Metaproterenol, albuterol, and terbutaline, at recommended clinical doses, evoke no alpha-receptor activity and elicit only a part of the array of beta-agonist actions seen with isoproterenol, the beta$_2$-receptor component. This component includes bronchodilation and vasodilation, but not cardiac stimulation (a beta$_1$ receptor component). When inhaled, these more selective beta agonists—now called beta$_2$ agonists—are virtually devoid of the side effects related to vasoconstriction and/or to cardiac stimulation that are evident with epinephrine and isoproterenol; hand tremor (a beta$_2$ action) is the primary unwanted effect that, in some patients, remains coupled to the desired bronchodilation. Beta$_2$-adrenoceptor agonists are considerably longer acting than epinephrine or isoproterenol (Lampe, 1986).

Beta$_2$-receptor stimulation is thought to be effective in asthma by increasing the levels of cyclic adenosine monophosphate in smooth muscle and in mast cells, thus inducing smooth muscle relaxation of the airways and inhibiting release of proinflammatory mediators from mast cells (Sheller and Snapper, 1987).

Albuterol is the most potent, as well as one of the most long-acting and selective, of the beta$_2$-adrenergic bronchodilators now in clinical use (Tashkin and Jenne, 1985). Delivery of this agent directly into the airways via aerosol has several advantages over oral administration: maximum relaxant effect on the bronchial smooth muscle, rapid onset of action, and minimal systemic absorption as a result of the small doses needed. When administered orally as maintenance therapy, the onset of action is slower than with inhalation therapy, and the larger dosage required often leads to undesired actions (tachycardia and considerable skeletal muscle tremor in the hands).

Theophylline, a methylxanthine bronchodilator that is active by the oral route, is frequently used with albuterol, and other beta agonists, in both the routine and emergency treatments of asthma (Berkow, 1982; Taylor et al., 1985, Lampe, 1986; Joad et al., 1987).

Sheller and Snapper (1987) held the opinion, "The use of metered dose inhalers containing bronchodilators or steroids has quietly revolutionized the treatment of asthma...," and according to Williams (1986), if beta$_2$ agonists were inhaled properly, full bronchodilation would occur without unnecessary side effects and there would be little additional need for orally administered beta$_2$ agonist or for aminophylline (theophylline plus ethylenediamine).

Gebbie (1983) also considered that the mainstay of the management of asthma in virtually all cases was the proper use of beta$_2$ agonists. When necessary, the regimen could be augmented by prophylactic measures such as sodium cromoglycate or inhaled steroids; or, in more serious cases, oral theophylline or the anticholinergic agent, ipratropium; and finally, if essential, oral steroids.

In the same vein, Dwyer (1986) was of the opinion that "[t]he major defect in the majority of asthmatic subjects involves a lack of minimal beta receptor activity allowing normal alpha and cholinergic activity to promote bronchospasm." Dwyer (1986) commented further, "We and our patients are fortunate to have available a new generation of beta$_2$ agonists, that, applied intelligently can minimize the seriousness of the incurable disease, asthma." Lampe (1986) noted that albuterol, "...is becoming the standard of this class of drugs [beta$_2$-adrenoceptor agonists] for use in asthma." Weinstein (1987), likewise, commented that albuterol "...is the most commonly prescribed inhaler in the United States today. Albuterol is currently the standard among the Adrenalinlike [epinephrine-like] medications against which new medications are compared."

Early Clinical Research History

Palmer and Diament (1969) treated 37 status asthmaticus patients with aerosol administration of albuterol. They reported that this new bronchodilator drug reduced airways obstruction without a significant fall in arterial oxygen tension. Palmer and Diament (1969) stated that a decrease in arterial oxygen saturation in patients already hypoxic from asthma was undesirable, and also that isoproterenol, because of its cardiac-stimulating properties, might evoke ventricular irritability and fatal arrhythmia in the hypoxemic myocardium. They suggested that albuterol "...because it appears to have little or no effect on the cardiovascular system may have advantages over isoprenaline [isoproterenol]." However, in order to test both drugs in the same patients before coming to a firm conclusion, Palmer and colleagues (Kelman et al., 1969) measured the effects of albuterol and isoproterenol on heart rate and circulation times in a double-blind, randomized, cross-over protocol in 10 asthmatic outpatients. Aerosol inhalation of albuterol had no significant effect on these measurements, whereas isoproterenol increased heart rate and reduced circulation times.

Choo-Kang et al. (1969), in a double-blind trial, compared inhaled isoproterenol, orciprenaline (metaproterenol) and albuterol, and placebo in 24 corticosteroid–maintained adult patients with severe chronic asthma. Albuterol had a much longer duration of action than isoproterenol; its effect on ventilatory function was slightly more intense and prolonged than that of metaproterenol. Thirteen patients selected albuterol as the most effective of the drugs. Side effects did not occur with albuterol or metaproterenol; in those patients receiving isoproterenol, a signficant increase in pulse rate was noted. These investigators concluded that, given by inhalation, albuterol could prove to be the most effective drug available for short-term treatment of asthma.

Tattersfield and McNicol (1969) and Riding et al. (1969) showed in double-blind, crossover trials that at equieffective, inhaled, bronchodilating doses, the duration of action of albuterol was longer than that of isoproterenol, and that albuterol, unlike isoproterenol, had no effect on heart rate and gave rise to no side effects.

In the next two years, many controlled clinical studies were carried out comparing the efficacy of oral, intravenous, and aerosol applications of albuterol with other agents (e.g., Choo-Kang et al., 1970, Warrell et al., 1970, Chervinsky, 1971). In addition, many books and reviews on albuterol have appeared (*see*, for example, Brittain et al., 1970, 1976; Jack, 1970; Avery, 1971; Lewis, 1971; Prime, 1971; Leifer and Wittig, 1975; Brittain and Harris, 1977; Chodosh, 1978; Tashkin and Jenne, 1985; Dwyer, 1986; Iafrate, 1986; Bronsky et al., 1987).

II. The Scientific Work Leading to Albuterol

Armstrong et al. (1957) demonstrated that a major metabolite of norepinephrine and epinephrine was 3-methoxy-4-hydroxy mandelic acid (Fig. 1) and suggested that its formation might be

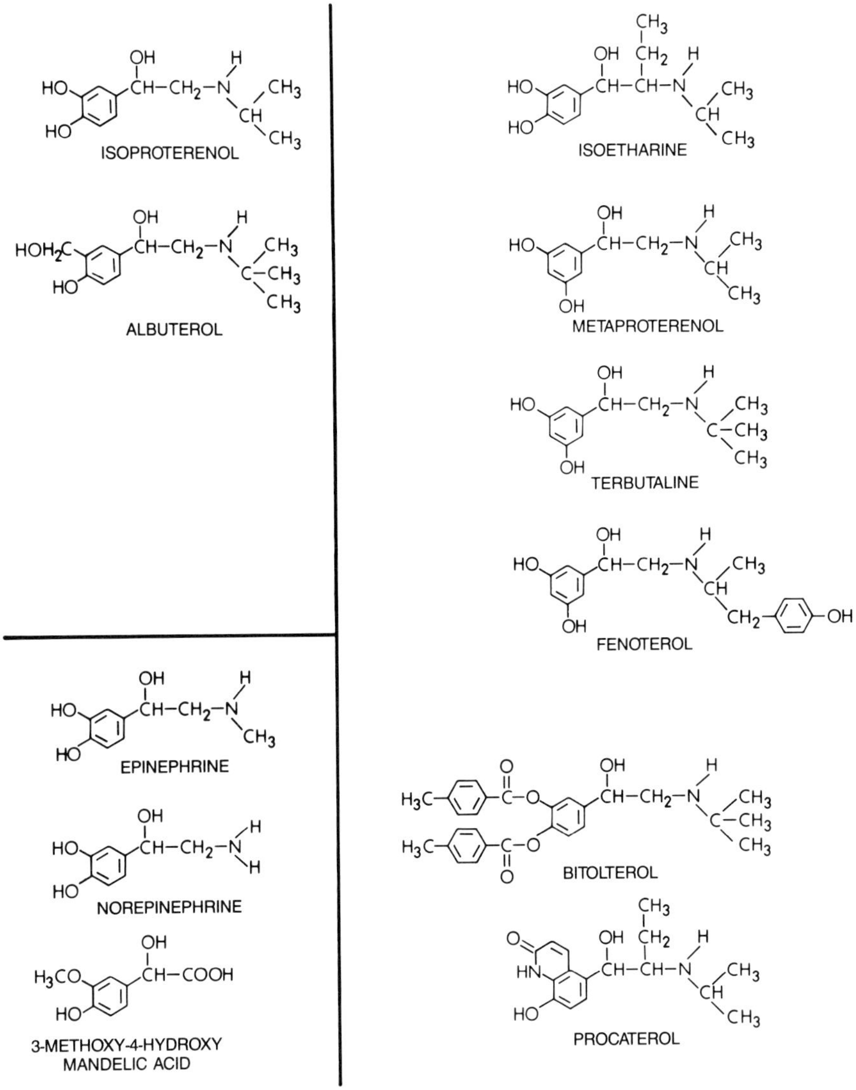

Fig. 1. The structures of albuterol and chemically and/or pharmacologically related substances.

expected from the action of amine oxidase (MAO) on norepinephrine and epinephrine, followed by methylation of the resulting 3,4-dihydroxymandelic acid.

Axelrod (1957) recognized the importance of the demonstration by Armstrong et al. (1957) that, in addition to MAO activity, another route existed for catabolizing catecholamines. He described the isolation from rat liver of an enzyme that catalyzed the O-methylation of the meta hydroxyl group of epinephrine and other catechols. This enzyme was eventually named catechol-O-methyl transferase (COMT).

Ross (1963) subsequently noted that inhibition of COMT with pyrogallol prolonged the tachycardic response of mice to isoproterenol to a much greater extent than it prolonged the tachycardic response to norepinephrine and epinephrine. It appeared to this investigator that some differences existed in the inactivation pathways for isoproterenol and for the naturally occurring catecholamines—O-methylation for the former, and uptake into tissues for the latter—and that these differences in inactivation routes could explain the difference in responses seen when COMT was inhibited.

Hartley et al. (1968) stated that the duration of the bronchodilator action of isoproterenol was known to be limited by its metabolism by COMT, and therefore they decided to try to prepare a series of compounds in which the meta phenolic group of the catechol was replaced by related functions stable to COMT. Replacement of the meta hydroxyl group by a hydroxymethyl group produced compounds exhibiting potent and long-lasting stimulation of the beta receptors in the bronchial muscle and, unlike catecholamines, these compounds were found to elicit only relatively small effects on cardiac muscle. The beta-adrenoceptor blocking agent propranolol antagonized all the actions of these agonists. AH3365, later called salbutamol or albuterol, was pointed out as a typical member of the series. It differed from isoproterenol in possessing a para hydroxyl group plus a meta hydroxymethyl group (making it a saligenin derivative instead of a catechol derivative) and in having its N-isopropyl group replaced by a tertiary butyl group (Fig. 1). Intravenous albuterol was equipotent with isoproterenol in antagonizing the bronchoconstrictor action of acetylcholine in the anesthetized guinea pig, but was 2000 times less potent than isoproterenol in increasing the contraction rate and isometric tension in isolated atria from the guinea pig.

These investigators noted,

> Our results emphasize once more the differentiation between β-adrenergic receptors in smooth and cardiac muscle [Lands and Brown, 1964] ...Further work is in progress to quantify these results and to assess their significance in the context of the concept of β-1 and β-2 receptors [of Lands et al., 1967a].

Brittain et al. (1968) gave a preliminary report of the pharmacology of albuterol. Albuterol, metaproterenol (another analog of isoproterenol), and isoproterenol were evaluated in preventing bronchospasm induced by acetylcholine in guinea pigs. At equi-effective doses, albuterol and metaproterenol had similar durations of action, and both were longer acting than isoproterenol. These workers reported, as had Hartley et al. (1968), that when tested on guinea pig atria, the stimulant effect of albuterol was 2000 times less than that of isoproterenol and half that of metaproterenol. Metabolic studies indicated that albuterol was not affected by COMT and therefore should be a longer acting drug. Brittain et al. (1968) felt that their results "...suggest that AH3365 would be an improved bronchodilator, being more selective, longer acting and safer than isoprenaline [isoproterenol], and more potent and less likely to cause side effects than orciprenaline [metaproterenol]."

Cullum et al. (1969) presented the pharmacology of albuterol in some detail, and drew the same conclusions as had their colleagues, Hartley et al. (1968) and Brittain et al. (1968), regarding its effectiveness: albuterol was much more active on bronchial smooth muscle than on cardiac muscle. They commented, "This result is compatible with the proposal of Lands [et al.] (1967a) for subdividing β receptors into β_1 receptors...and β_2 receptors...."

Table 1 defines the critical scientific ideas and experiments leading to albuterol and categorizes their origin.

Background Contributions Preceding Albuterol

Barger and Dale (1910) noted the earlier work that led to the isolation and chemical characterization of epinephrine, and went on to report the synthesis of, and structure–activity relationships for, a large series of amines related to epinephrine.

Table 1
Profile of Observations and Ideas Crucial to the Development of Albuterol[a]

Sequence: Route to innovative drug[**]	Orient-ation	Nature of study	Research institution	National origin	Nature of discovery	Screening involved	Crucial ideas or observations
Albuterol[**]							
Armstrong et al. (1957)	Clinical	Bio-chem-istry	Uni-versity	USA	Orderly	No	3 Methoxy-4-hydroxy mandelic acid is a significant urinary metabolite of norepinephrine and epinephrine; 3 O-methylation, in addition to MAO activity, is important in catabolism of norepinephrine and epinephrine.
Axelrod (1957)	Pre-clinical	Bio-chem-istry	Govern-ment	USA	Orderly	No	An enzyme (COMT) that catalyzes O-methylation of epinephrine and other catechols is isolated from rat liver.
Ross (1963)	Pre-clinical	Pharma-cology	Indus-try	Sweden	Orderly	No	The duration of action of isoproterenol, but not of norepinephrine and epinephrine, is considerably prolonged when COMT is inhibited.
Hartley et al. (1968)	Pre-clinical	Chem-istry/ pharma-cology	Indus-try	UK	Orderly	Tar-geted	Albuterol synthesized in a successful attempt to produce a beta agonist that is not a substrate for COMT; is a long-acting beta agonist; found to have greater selectivity for relaxing bronchioles than for stimulating the heart.

[a]Taken from section II. Entries are those contributions without which the discovery of the agent (or additionally, in some cases, a relevant clinical application) would not have taken place or would have been materially delayed.

Konzett (1940a,b), working with compounds supplied by C. H. Boehringer Sohn (Ingelheim, Germany), described the actions of novel analogs of epinephrine in which the N-methyl group was replaced by larger alkyl groups. Epinephrine, itself, produced bronchodilation and a biphasic action on blood pressure. However, with the larger N-substitutions, particularly the isopropyl derivative (later named isoprenaline or isoproterenol) (Fig. 1), epinephrine-like actions were modified, and bronchodilation, hypotensive effects, and vasodilation became very prominent. Isoproterenol was 10 times more effective than epinephrine as a bronchodilator. It caused a pronounced increase in heart rate.

Ahlquist (1948) suggested, as a consequence of his studies of the orders of potencies of a series of sympathomimetic amines (including isoproterenol and epinephrine) in a series of tissues and organs, that there were only two kinds of adrenergic receptors, and dubbed them alpha and beta. He concluded that alpha receptors (most readily activated by epinephrine) elicited the excitatory effects, and beta receptors (most readily activated by isoproterenol) elicited the inhibitory effects, with the controversial exception that cardiac excitation was considered to be evoked via a beta receptor.

Engelhardt et al. (1961) commented that, despite all the chemical alterations of the phenethylamine structure that had been carried out over years, placement of the two hydroxyl groups in the meta position (that is, generating resorcinol derivatives rather than catechol derivatives) had been ignored. Th152 (metaproterenol), the resorcinol analog of isoproterenol (Fig. 1), was like isoproterenol in its actions and was an agonist of beta effector sites as defined by Ahlquist, but in some respects its effect on the heart differed from isoproterenol: metaproterenol was 40 times weaker than isoproterenol in stimulating spontaneously beating cat right atrium, but approximately equipotent with it in stimulating the electrically-driven left atrium and papillary muscle; in anesthetized guinea pigs, metaproterenol did not evoke arrhythmias and did not increase myocardial vulnerability.

A sustained effort by Lands and colleagues over a period of approximately 15 years had helped to establish firmly that the molecular requirements for initiating sympathomimetic cardioacceleration and increasing the force of contraction differed from those for bronchodilator action (Lands et al., 1950; Lands and Howard, 1952; Lands and Brown, 1964; Lands et al., 1966). Lands et al. (1950) found, in anesthetized dogs, that although α-ethyl iso-proterenol (WIN 3046), later named isoetharine (Fig. 1), was only one-tenth as active as isoproterenol in preventing histamine-induced bronchoconstriction, it was 40–80 times weaker than iso-proterenol in increasing heart rate. In addition, isoetharine was more than 1000 times less potent than isoproterenol in inhibiting isolated ileum from the guinea pig, but equipotent with it in inhib-iting isolated uterus from the guinea pig. The authors related their results to those of other workers and suggested, *inter alia*, that "...the structural requirements for myocardial stimulation differ from those favorable for sympathetic excitatory or inhibitory ac-tion." Differences in the molecular requirements for optimal activ-ity in a variety of organs indicated to Lands and Brown (1964) that "...the general class of adrenotropic receptors may consist of a population with somewhat different affinities for structurally varied sympathomimetic amines." As a culmination to their years of effort, Lands et al. (1967a) reported on the effects of a series of sympathomimetic amines on fatty acid mobilization, cardiac stimulation, broncho-dilation, and vasodepression, and rapidly extended these studies to a few other organ systems (Lands et al., 1967b). They concluded, from rank ordering of potencies of the amines, that there were two beta receptor subtypes—beta$_1$ recep-tors, found in the heart, adipose tissue, and small intestine; and beta$_2$ receptors, found in the uterus, diaphragm, bronchioles, and vascular bed. They acknowledged that Ahlquist's (1948) concept, that adrenoceptors could be divided into alpha and beta receptors, had proved most useful, but felt that "...variant behavior of some compounds has acted as an annoying obstacle to the full accep-tance of this concept. The concept of two β receptor types respond-ing with different intensities to structurally varied sympath-omimetic amines provides a more satisfactory explanation..." (Lands et al., 1967b).

III. Comments on Events Leading to Albuterol

Cullum et al. (1969) stated in their introduction that meta-proterenol had been noted by Engelhardt et al. (1961) to be an ef-fective bronchodilator and that this agent "...showed that a catechol structure was not essential for β-receptor stimulant activity and that selective actions on β receptors in different organs of the body were possible."

Jack (1970) commented,

> Most of the recent successful attempts to modify isoprenaline [iso-proterenol] depend on replacing its catechol function with a grouping which is more stable in the body and which possesses some ...chemical properties of a catechol [e.g., metaproterenol, albuterol].

The comment of Jack (1970) was reinforced by Collin et al. (1970), who, in synthesizing the series of salicylic acid and sali-genin derivatives that included albuterol, stated:

> We hoped to circumvent these metabolic pathways [meaning primarily the metabolism of the catecholamines by COMT] and hence overcome some of the clinical deficiencies of isoproterenol by the preparation of compounds...which retained some of the attributes of catecholamine but which would not be subject to attack by the enzymes that inactivate the latter.

They noted, "In accord with our original hypothesis, the saligenins are not metabolized by COMT."

Brittain et al. (1970), colleagues of Jack (1970) and of Collin et al. (1970), concurred with them in commenting, "In our own laboratories attempts to improve isoprenaline [isoproterenol] concentrated on replacing the 3-hydroxyl group with metabolically stable functions to yield compounds which retained some of the properties of a catechol group."

Only later did Brittain et al. (1976) put forth the view, "Several attempts have been made during the past 15 years to make improved beta-stimulant bronchodilators and much of the credit for defining and solving the problem is due to Lands and his colleagues..." Likewise, Leifer and Wittig (1975), noting the contributions of Lands and coworkers, felt that "[t]he search for more specific beta$_2$ adrenergic agents was catalyzed by the discovery of two different beta receptors," and very much later Tashkin and Jenne (1985) concluded,

> Following the studies of Lands and Brown [1964] establishing the existence of beta$_1$ and beta$_2$ adrenergic receptors, the pharmaceuti-

cal industry increased its efforts to synthesize newer analogs of isoproterenol with a greater physiological ratio of bronchial relaxant
(beta$_2$) to cardiac stimulant (beta$_1$) effect.

IV. Developments
Subsequent to Albuterol

Terbutaline (Fig. 1), a close analog of metaproterenol in which
the isopropyl group has been replaced by a tertiary butyl group,
was reported by Bergman et al. (1969) to be a potent, beta$_2$-selective
agent. Likewise, fenoterol (Fig. 1), another close analog of metaproterenol—the isopropyl group enlarged by the addition of a
paraphenol group (Fig. 1)—was also reported to be a potent, selective beta$_2$ agonist (O'Donnell, 1970).

Attempts at making more selective, potent, and longer acting
beta$_2$ agonists continued, and many other agents have been or are
being investigated for clinical use, e.g., rimeterol, hexoprenaline,
carbuterol, quinterenol, tretoquinol, salmefenol, soterenol, zin-
terol, salmeterol, and formoterol (Csáky and Barnes, 1984).

Two of the more novel examples among the many new agents,
are bitolterol and procaterol. Bitolterol (Fig. 1) is an inactive,
diester prodrug that is administered as an aerosol and broken
down by esterase hydrolysis in the bronchial mucosa, thereby
releasing the bronchodilator, N-tertiary butyl norepinephrine.
Because the concentration of the parent diester that is achieved in
pulmonary tissue is greater than that achieved in the heart, this
drug is an effective bronchodilator with few cardiac side effects
(Minatoya, 1978; Kass and Mingo, 1980; Tashkin and Jenne, 1985;
Chervinsky, 1986). According to Chervinsky (1986), because of
slow activation, the duration of action of bitolterol extends up to
eight hours and may carry patients through the night. It may also
do away with baseline prophylactic therapy with theophyline for
the chronic asthmatic patient.

Procaterol (Fig.1) is structurally distinct from other beta agonists in that it has a carbostyril nucleus instead of an altered catechol
ring. Unlike many beta agonists, procaterol does not undergo
gastrointestinal inactivation and can be administered orally. This
agent is active in microgram quantities and may lend itself to
"bandaid" dosage formulation. It appears to be somewhat more
efficacious than other beta$_2$ agonists. Unfortunately, there is an

increase in the incidence of tremor with oral doses of the drug, but patients seem to accept this side effect (Himori and Taira, 1977; Tashkin and Jenne, 1985, and Chervinsky, 1986).

Sheller and Snapper (1987) were of the opinion that the only real difference among the many beta$_2$ agonists seems to be in the duration of their action. However, Weinstein (1987) considered that the slight structural changes in the newer asthma medications might get rid of a troublesome side effect and/or make them more potent as bronchodilators.

It should be noted that the initiation and firm establishment of the concept of beta-receptor subtypes was a direct consequence of the synthesis and screening of compounds that unexpectedly yielded selective beta$_2$ agonists, as discussed in this chapter, and of the contemporaneous, independent synthesis and screening of compounds that unexpectedly generated a group of antagonists selective for beta$_1$ and beta$_2$ adrenoceptors (*see,* for example, Levy, 1966; Lands, et al., 1967b; Dunlop and Shanks, 1968; Shanks, 1984) (*see also* section IV of the chapter on propranolol).

References

Ahlquist, R. P.: A study of the adrenotropic receptors. *Am. J. Physiol.* **153:** 586–600, 1948.

Armstrong, M. D., McMillan, A., and Shaw, K. N. F.: 3 Methoxy-4-hydroxy-D-mandelic acid, a urinary metabolite of norepinephrine. *Biochim. Biophys. Acta* **25:** 422, 423, 1957.

Avery, G. S., ed.: Salbutamol: A review. *Drugs* **1:** 274–302, 1971.

Axelrod, J.: O-Methylation of epinephrine and other catechols in vitro and in vivo. *Science* **126:** 400, 401, 1957.

Barger, G. and Dale, H. H.: Chemical structure and sympathomimetic action of amines. *J. Physiol.* **41:** 19–59, 1910.

Bergman, J., Persson, H., and Wetterlin, K.: Two new groups of selective stimulants of adrenergic β-receptors. *Experientia* **25:** 899–901, 1969.

Berkow, R., ed.: *The Merck Manual,* 14th Ed., Merck Sharp & Dohme Research Laboratories, Rahway, NJ, 1982.

Brittain, R. T. and Harris, D. M.: Albuterol, in *Pharmacological and Biochemical Properties of Drug Substances,* vol. 1, M. E. Goldberg, ed., pp. 257–276, American Pharmaceutical Association Academy of Pharmaceutical Science, Washington, DC, 1977.

Brittain, R. T., Dean, C. M., and Jack, D.: Sympathomimetic bronchodilator drugs. *Pharmacol. Ther. [B]* **2:** 423–462, 1976.

Brittain, R. T., Farmer, J. B., Jack, D., Martin, L. E., and Simpson, W. T.: α[(t-Butylamino)methyl]-4-hydroxy-*m*-xylene-a¹,a³-diol (AH. 3365): A selective β-adrenergic stimulant. *Nature* **219**: 862, 863, 1968.

Brittain, R. T., Jack, D., and Ritchie, A. C.: Recent β-adrenoreceptor stimulants, in *Advance in Research*, vol. 5, N. J. Harper and A. B. Simmonds, eds., pp. 197–253, Academic, London, 1970.

Bronsky, E., Bucholtz, G. A., Busse, W. W., Chervinsky, P., Condemi, J., Ghafouri, M. A., Hudson, L., Lakshminarayan, S., Lockey, R., Reese, M. E., Rennard, S. I., Segal, A., Smolley, L., Spector, S., Stablein, J. J., Van As, A., and Wilson, A.: Comparison of inhaled albuterol powder and aerosol in asthma. *J. Allergy Clin. Immunol.* **79**: 741–747, 1987.

Chervinsky, P.: Evaluation of a new selective beta-adrenergic receptor stimulant. *Ann. Allergy* **29**: 627–630, 1971.

Chervinsky, P.: Future drugs for the treatment of asthma, in *Current Treatment of Ambulatory Asthma*, G. A. Settipane, ed., pp. 120–122, New England and Regional Allergy Proceedings, Providence, 1986.

Choo-Kang, Y. F. J., Parker, S. S., and Grant, I. W. B.: Response of asthmatics to isoprenaline and salbutamol aerosols administered by intermittent positive-pressure ventilation. *Br. Med. J.* **4**: 465–468, 1970.

Choo-Kang, Y. F. J., Simpson, W. T., and Grant, I. W. B.: Controlled comparison of the bronchodilator effects of three β-adrenergic stimulant drugs administered by inhalation to patients with asthma. *Br. Med. J.* **2**: 287–289, 1969.

Chodosh, S.: Rational management of bronchial asthma. *Arch. Intern. Med.* **138**: 1394–1397, 1978.

Collin, D. T., Hartley, D., Jack, D., Lunts, L. H. C., Press, J. C., Ritchie A. C., and Toon, P.: Saligenin analogs of sympathomimetic catecholamines. *J. Med. Chem.* **13**: 674–680, 1970.

Csáky, T. Z. and Barnes, B. A.: *Cutting's Handbook of Pharmacology*, 7th Ed., Appleton-Century-Crofts, Norwalk, 1984.

Cullum, V. A., Farmer, J. B., Jack, D., and Levy, G. P.: Salbutamol: A new selective β-adrenoceptive receptor stimulant. *Br. J. Pharmcol.* **35**: 141–151, 1969.

Dunlop, D. and Shanks, R. G.: Selective blockade of adrenoceptive beta receptors in the heart. *Br. J. Pharmacol. Chemother.* **32**: 201–218, 1968.

Dwyer, J. M.: Beta agonists in the management of asthma, in *Current Treatment of Ambulatory Asthma*, G. A. Settipane, ed., pp. 53–58, The New England and Regional Allergy Proceedings, Providence, 1986.

Engelhardt, A., Hoefke, W., and Wick, H.: Pharmakologie des Sympathomimeticums 1-(3,5-Dihydroxyphenyl)-1-hydroxy-2-isopropylaminoäthan. *Arzneimittelforsch.* **11**: 521–525, 1961. (Read in translation in *Drugs Made in Germany* **4**: 123–131, 1961.)

Gebbie, T.: Therapeutic choices in asthma, in *Steroids in Asthma: A Re-*

appraisal in the Light of Inhalation Therapy, T. J. H. Clark, ed., pp. 83–102, Adis, Auckland, 1983.

Hartley, D., Jack, D., Lunts, L. H. C., and Ritchie, A. C.: New class of selective stimulants of beta-adrenergic receptors. *Nature* **219:** 861, 862, 1968.

Himori, N. and Taira, N.: Assessment of the selectivity of OPC-2009, a new β_2-adrenoceptor stimulant, by the use of the blood-perfused trachea *in situ* and of the isolated blood-perfused papillary muscle of the dog. *Br. J. Pharmacol.* **61:** 9–17, 1977.

Iafrate, R. P., Massey, K. L., and Hendeles, L.: Current concepts in clinical therapeutics: *Asthma. Clin. Pharm.* **5:** 206–227, 1986.

Jack, D.: Recent β-adrenoreceptor stimulants and the nature of β-adreno-receptors. *Pharm. J.* **205:** 237–240, 1970.

Joad, J. P., Ahrens, R. C., Lindgren, S. D., and Weinberger, M. M.: Relative efficacy of maintenance therapy with theophylline, inhaled albuterol, and the combination for chronic asthma. *J. Allergy Clin. Immunol.* **79:** 78–85, 1987.

Kass, I. and Mingo, T. S.: Bitolterol mesylate (WIN 32784) aerosol: A new long-acting bronchodilator with reduced chronotropic effects. *Chest* **78:** 283–287, 1980.

Kelman, G. R., Palmer, K. N. V., and Cross, M. R.: Cardiovascular effects of AH. 3365 (Salbutamol). *Nature* **221:** 1251, 1969.

Konzett, H.: Neue broncholytische hochwirksame Körper der adrenal-inreihe. *Arch. Exp. Path. Pharmak.* **197:** 27–40, 1940a.

Konzett, H.: Zur Pharmakolgie neuer adrenalinverwandter Körper. *Arch. Exp. Path. Pharmak.* **197:** 41–56, 1940b.

Lampe, K., ed. *Drug Evaluations*, 6th Ed., American Medical Association, Chicago, 1986.

Lands, A. M. and Brown, T. G., Jr.: A comparison of the cardiac stimulating and bronchodilator actions of selected sympathomimetic amines. *Proc. Soc. Exp. Biol. Med.* **116:** 331–333, 1964.

Lands, A. M. and Howard, J. W.: A comparative study of the effects of 1-arterenol, epinephrine and isopropylarterenol on the heart. *J. Pharmacol. Exper. Ther.* **106:** 65–76, 1952.

Lands, A. M., Groblewski, G. E., and Brown, T. G., Jr.: Comparison of the action of isoproterenol and several related compounds on blood pressure, heart and bronchioles. *Arch. Pharmacodyn. Ther.* **161:** 68–75, 1966.

Lands, A. M., Arnold, A., McAuliff, J. P., Luduena, F. P., and Brown, T. G., Jr.: Differentiation of receptor systems activated by sympatho-mimetic amines. *Nature* **214:** 597, 598, 1967a.

Lands, A. M., Luduena, F. P., and Buzzo, H. J.: Differentiation of receptors responsive to isoproterenol. *Life Sci.* **6:** 2241–2249, 1967b.

Lands, A. M., Luduena, F. P., Grant, J. I., and E. Ananenko: The pharmacologic action of some analogs of 1-(3,4-dihydroxyphenyl)-2-amino-1-butanol (ethylnorepinephrine). *J. Pharm. Exp. Ther.* **99**: 45–56, 1950.

Leifer, K. N. and Wittig, H. J.: The beta-2 sympathomimetic aerosols in the treatment of asthma. *Ann. Allergy* **35**: 69–80, 1975.

Levy, B.: Dimethyl isopropylmethoxamine: A selective beta-receptor blocking agent. *Br. J. Pharmacol. Chemother.* **27**: 277–285, 1966.

Lewis, A. A. G., ed.: Salbutamol. *Postgrad. Med. J.* **47** (Suppl.): 1971.

Minatoya, H.: Studies on bitolterol, di-*p*-toluate ester of *N-tert*-butylarterenol: A new long-acting bronchodilator with reduced cardiovascular effects. *J. Pharmacol. Exp. Ther.* **206**: 515–527, 1978.

O'Donnell, S. R.: A selective β-adrenoreceptor stimulant (TH1165a) related to orciprenaline. *Eur. J. Pharmacol.* **12**: 35–43, 1970.

Palmer, K. N. V. and Diament, M. L.: Effect of salbutamol on spirometry and blood-gas tensions in bronchial asthma. *Br. Med. J.* **1**: 31, 32, 1969.

Prime, F. J.: Adrenergic receptors, bronchodilators and asthma. *Drugs* **1**: 269–273, 1971.

Riding, W. D., Chatterjee, S. S., and Dinda, P.: Clinical trial of a new beta-adrenergic stimulant in asthma. *Br. J. Clin. Prac.* **23**: 217–219, 1969.

Ross, S. B.: In vivo inactivation of catecholamines in mice. *Acta Pharmacol. et Toxicol.* **20**: 267–273, 1963.

Shanks, R. G.: The discovery of beta-adrenoceptor blocking agents. *Trends Pharm. Sci.* **5**: 405–409, 1984.

Sheller, J. R. and Snapper, J. R.: Asthma in adults and adolescents, in *Conn's Current Therapy*, R. E. Rakel, ed., pp. 600–604, W. B. Saunders, Philadelphia, 1987.

Tashkin, D. P. and Jenne, J. W.: Alpha and beta adrenergic agents, in *Bronchial Asthma: Mechanisms and Therapeutics*, 2nd Ed., E. B. Weiss, M. S. Segal, and M. Stein, eds., pp. 604–639, Little Brown, Boston, 1985.

Tattersfield, A. E. and McNicol, M. W.: Salbutamol and isoproterenol: A double-blind trial to compare bronchodilator and cardiovascular activity. *N. Engl. J. Med.* **281**: 1323–1326, 1969.

Taylor, D. R., Buick, B., Kinney, C., Lowry, R. C., and McDevitt, D. G.: The efficacy of orally administered theophylline, inhaled salbutamol, and a combination of the two as chronic therapy in the management of chronic bronchitis with reversible air-flow obstruction. *Am. Rev. Respir. Dis.* **131**: 747–751, 1985.

Warrell, D. A., Robertson, D. G., Newton Howes, J., Conolly, M. E., Paterson, J. W. Beilin, L. J., and Dollery, C. T.: Comparison of cardio-respiratory effects of isoprenaline and salbutamol in patients with bronchial asthma. *Br. Med. J.* **1**: 65–70, 1970.

Weinstein, A. M.: *Asthma*, McGraw-Hill, New York, 1987.

Williams, M. H.: Inhaled versus oral bronchodilators, in *Current Treatment of Ambulatory Asthma*, E. A. Settipane, ed., pp. 75–77, New England and Regional Allergy Proceedings, Providence, 1986.

Beclomethasone Dipropionate

I. Beclomethasone Dipropionate as an Innovative Therapeutic Agent

Asthma has been defined as "[a] disease characterized by an increased responsiveness of the airways to various stimuli and manifested by slowing of forced expiration which changes in severity either spontaneously or as a result of therapy" (Joint Committee on Pulmonary Nomenclature, 1975). According to Wilson (1983a), asthma occurs in between 2 and 20% of the population in developed countries. It is a major health problem because of its disabling and disruptive nature, which often demands changes in lifestyle, and because it is associated with prolonged morbidity and some mortality.

Asthma can be either an acute or a chronic illness. Acute asthma consists of attacks of reversible bronchial obstruction brought about by contraction of bronchiolar and bronchi smooth muscle, mucosal edema, secretions in the bronchial lumen, and accumulation of mast cells in the lungs, with the chemical mediators released from the cells acting to exacerbate bronchospasm and edema (Wilson, 1983b). Attacks are characterized by wheezing, dyspnea, and respiratory distress, and they often occur at infrequent and unpredictable intervals. Asthma is generally considered to have become a chronic condition when the asthmatic has to be continuously maintained on medication to sustain a symptom-free state with adequate respiratory function between attacks (Lampe, 1986).

Glucocorticoids, administered via the intravenous route in acute asthma or by the oral route in acute and chronic asthma, have long been considered to be useful adjuncts to the bronchodilating actions of beta agonists and methylxanthines by decreasing the airways obstruction secondary to inflammation and edema. Unfortunately, the large number of serious side effects associated with systemically administered steroids has limited their use. Side effects range from those seen with acute, high-dose administration (e.g., by the intravenous route), such as electrolyte disturbances, diabetes, hypertension, mental disturbances, peptic ulcers, and many others, to those seen with long-term, oral administration, such as suppression of the hypothalamic-pituitary-adrenal axis, suppression of growth in children, osteoporosis and bone fractures, cataracts, diminished immune response, and many others (Cochrane, 1983; Siegel, 1985). Despite these toxic effects, in a small number of patients the obstructive process of asthma is sufficiently aggressive that symptoms can only be controlled by continuous glucocorticoid administration (Wilson, 1983b).

Interest in the use of glucocorticoids in chronic asthma was broadened considerably with the advent of the administration of topical steroids (beclomethasone dipropionate, betamethasone valerate) directly into the respiratory tree via inhalation (Brown, 1980). Topical steroids are those corticosteroids that are potent when applied locally (they generally bear groups that enhance their lipid solubility and penetrability into tissues) and that are more readily subject to metabolic inactivation than are the steroids that are given systemically. Thus, when taken by inhalation, the proportion of a dose of beclomethasone dipropionate that reaches the lung (<25%) is partially metabolized in the lung, and the remainder is apparently readily metabolizable by the liver as it escapes the lung. Moreover, the much larger amount (>75%) of an inhaled dose that does not go to the lung, but is swallowed, is slowly absorbed and is inactivated during its first pass through the liver (Martin et al., 1974, 1975; Brattsand et al., 1982). Little active steroid, therefore, reaches the systemic circulation, and the serious side effects common to the systemic use of steroids are avoided.

Beclomethasone dipropionate, the most intensively studied of the topical steroids used for treating asthma (Wilson, 1983b) and the standard against which other inhaled steroids are assessed (Brogden, 1983), is also the most widely used steroid for inhalation (Meltzer et al., 1985). It can be used in conjunction with bronchodilators or with cromolyn sodium. Some observers feel that it should be reserved for patients having chronic severe asthma who do not respond to these other agents (Tse and Bernstein, 1984; Siegel, 1985). It is clearly effective in treating steroid-dependent, chronic asthmatics (Brogden et al., 1984), and its use permits reduction in the dosage of oral steroids, or their elimination, in some patients (Lampe, 1986). Beclomethasone dipropionate is also effective in chronic asthma that does not require maintenance with oral steroids (Brogden et al., 1984). This drug, however, has no role in the management of acute severe asthmatic attacks, since in these conditions an inhaled substance cannot reach the site at which it needs to act (Clark and McAllister, 1983). The side actions most frequently encountered with the chronic use of inhaled beclomethasone dipropionate are oropharyngeal candidiasis (thrush), hoarseness, and sore throat (Brogden et al., 1984).

Berkow (1982) and Lampe (1986) both considered the development of beclomethasone dipropionate and related inhaled topical corticosteroids to be a "major advance" in asthma therapy. Beclomethasone dipropionate, administered intranasally, has also found use in the treatment of perennial and allergic seasonal rhinitis (Wilson, 1983b; Brogden et al., 1984).

Early Clinical Research History*

Brown et al. (1972) treated 60 patients suffering from perennial allergic asthma with inhaled beclomethasone dipropionate for up to 15 months. Of 37 steroid-dependent patients, 28 were successfully transferred to aerosol treatment; 9 were not. Of 23 patients not dependent on steroids, 19 were completely controlled with inhaled beclomethasone dipropionate. The responses of plasma cortisol (hydrocortisone) to direct stimulation of the adrenal cortex via administration of synthetic ACTH, and to indirect stimulation via administration of insulin, were not reduced during approximately one year of treatment; this indicated that adrenal suppression (a systemic effect) had not occurred during a protracted course of inhalation therapy. The best clinical results were obtained in younger, more reversible cases of asthma. Gregg (1972), in a small series of adult patients, obtained results that were very similar to those of Brown et al. (1972).

---

*In the case of beclomethasone dipropionate, the discovery of its "topical steroid" characteristics was a result of a clinical, dermatological observation (Raffle and Frain-Bell, 1967). This study is reported in section II.

Clark (1972) administered beclomethasone dipropionate via aerosol for 2–6 mo to nine asthmatic patients not taking oral steroids and to eight patients transferred from prednisolone therapy. The aerosol treatment "...provided the expected clinical benefits of corticosteroids seen in many patients with asthma." Forced expired volume in 1 s (FEV_1) was improved. Furthermore, basal cortisol levels did not fall in any of the patients and rose toward normal in those patients transferred from prednisolone. This rise in basal cortisol levels was paralleled by an increase to within normal limits (in seven out of eight cases) of the response of plasma cortisol to administered synthetic ACTH. The author concluded, "The results support the idea that inhaled beclomethasone dipropionate acts in a similar way to systemic corticosteroids in patients with asthma but seems to have less systemic effect."

On the negative side, several small studies did not attest to the effectiveness of inhaled beclomethasone dipropionate. Choo-Kang et al. (1972) measured FEV_1 and plasma cortisol levels in seven asthmatic patients. In this comparison of beclomethasone dipropionate with oral prednisolone, beclomethasone dipropionate partially relieved airways obstruction in some cases; however, its administration for 7 d sometimes depressed hypothalamic pituitary function. It was concluded that high doses of beclomethasone dipropionate by inhalation "...had no real advantage over prednisolone by mouth...in the treatment of airways obstruction...." Lower doses were considered safe but, in most cases, ineffective. Herxheimer (1972), in a note, stated that only one of 15 chronic, moderately severe asthmatics improved on inhaled beclomethasone dipropionate. He considered that his results did not warrant that controlled studies be carried out with this substance.

A double-blind, placebo-controlled, crossover comparison of oral prednisolone and aerosolized beclomethasone dipropionate was carried out in 38 steroid-dependent patients with reversible diffuse airway obstruction (Lal et al., 1972). Both treatments were found to be equieffective on the objective measurements of respiratory function that were made: FEV_1, VC (vital capacity), and PEFR (peak expiratory flow rate). Plasma cortisol levels were much higher when patients were on the aerosol than when they were on prednisolone.

Gaddie et al. (1973), in a placebo-controlled, double-blind crossover trial in 15 patients with moderately severe, chronic asthma, found significant improvement in FEV_1 with inhaled beclomethasone dipropionate, but no significant reduction in plasma cortisol levels.

A variety of reviews, symposia, and books speaks to the substantial evidence subsequently amassed to establish the usefulness of inhaled beclomethasone dipropionate and other topical steroids in asthma (*see*, for example: Brogden et al., 1975, 1984; Hoffbrand and Harris, 1975; Wilson and Marks, 1976; Abramowicz, 1976, 1985, 1987; Mygind and Clark, 1980; Williams, 1981; Wilson, 1983b; Clark, 1983; Tse and Bernstein, 1984).

II. The Scientific Work Leading to the Use of Inhaled Beclomethasone Dipropionate in Asthma

Beclomethasone dipropionate (Fig. 1) was synthesized and patented as an antiinflammatory agent by Glaxo Group Ltd. (1966).

Raffle and Frain-Bell (1967) measured plasma cortisol levels in nine dermatitis patients being effectively treated with topical beclomethasone dipropionate, and in a control group of 28 patients suffering from skin conditions other than dermatitis and not receiving topical steroid. There was no significant difference in plasma cortisol levels between the two groups and, thus, no evidence of adrenal suppression (a systemic effect) with beclomethasone dipropionate. In contrast, the authors noted that in an earlier study "...with topically applied triamcinolone acetonide there was a significant fall in plasma cortisol levels despite the progressive reduction in dosage in parallel with clinical improvement." Raffle and Frain-Bell (1968) replicated their results with beclomethasone dipropionate in a second study that employed a new ointment base for the steroid.

Two members of the Research Division of Allen and Hanburys, Ltd.—a subsidiary of Glaxo Group, Ltd.—and five hospital-based clinicians presented a précis of the chemistry and pharmacology of beclomethasone dipropionate and the results of a clinical study (Caldwell et al., 1968). It was stated that pharmacological studies in mice and dogs demonstrated beclomethasone dipropionate to be a potent antiinflammatory agent (slightly more

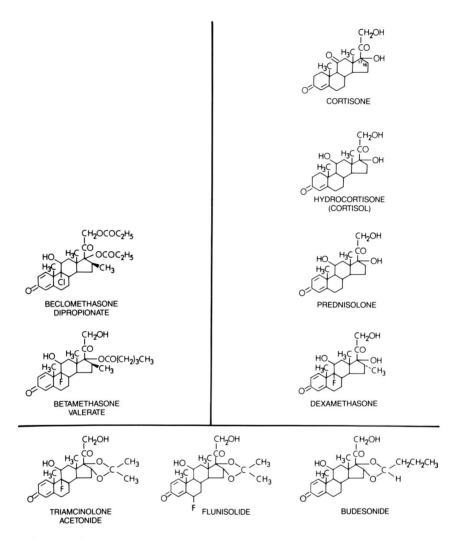

Fig. 1. The structures of beclomethasone dipropionate and chemically
and/or pharmacologically related substances.

active than betamethasone), but that it appeared almost devoid of
systemic effects in rats, having less than one-fortieth of the activity of betamethasone. In the pharmacological vasoconstrictor test
of McKenzie (1962), wherein drugs were applied topically to the
skin of humans, beclomethasone dipropionate proved to be 5000

times more potent than cortisol, 625 times more potent than beta-methasone alcohol, and 1.4 times more potent than betamethasone valerate. The clinical study concerned the effects of changes in pharmaceutical presentation on the topical potency of beclomethasone dipropionate in dermatologic patients; the drug was more active when prepared in propylene glycol and white soft paraffin than as an ointment containing a microcrystalline suspension.

Harris et al. (1973) of Allen and Hanburys, Ltd. cited (in their introductory remarks) the results of Caldwell et al. (1968), as well as those of Raffle and Frain-Bell (1967) indicating that beclomethasone dipropionate exerted topical activity on the skin without concomitant systemic activity. They went on to surmise, "Since the lungs might also be regarded as an external body surface, we thought it possible for a clinically useful, selective antiinflammatory effect to be achieved by local application of this steroid to the lungs of asthmatic patients." These authors felt that the supportive clinical findings of Brown et al. (1972), Lal et al. (1972), and Clark (1972) with inhaled beclomethasone dipropionate (supplied as pressurized aerosols by Allen and Hanburys) were encouraging. These early clinical papers are discussed in section I. Harris et al. (1973) went on to report that 2 mg/d of dexamethasone for 2 d by mouth caused clinically significant suppression of hypothalamic-pituitary-adrenal axis function in humans, whereas beclomethasone dipropionate for 2 d (up to 2 mg/d inhaled, or up to 4 mg/d by mouth) did not depress this function.

Table 1 defines the critical scientific ideas and experiments leading to the use of beclomethasone dipropionate in asthma and categorizes their origin.

Background Contributions
Preceding Beclomethasone Dipropionate

Very shortly after Hench et al. (1949) demonstrated the useful antiarthritic properties of cortisone (Fig. 1), new, more potent derivatives were synthesized, such as hydrocortisone, prednisone and prednisolone. Cortisone (Carryer et al., 1950), and these newer antiinflammatory corticosteroids, rapidly found their way into the systemic treatment of asthma, in which they were readily recognized as being very useful in the management of the disease

Table 1
Profile of Observations and Ideas
Crucial to the Development of Beclomethasone Dipropionate[a]

Sequence: Route to innovative drug[b]	Orient- ation	Nature of study	Research institution	National origin	Nature of discovery	Screening involved	Crucial ideas or observations
Beclomethasone Dipropionate[b]							
Glaxo Group Ltd. (1966)	Pre- clinical	Chem- istry/ pharma- cology	Indus- try	UK	Orderly	Targeted	Beclomethasone di- propionate, a potent antiinflammatory glucocorticoid, is synthesized.
Raffle and Frain-Bell (1967)	Clinical	Derma- tology	Hospi- tal	UK	Orderly	No	Beclomethasone di- propionate applied locally to skin is effective against dermatitis; no de- pression of plasma cortisol (i. e., no sys- temic effect) occurs.
Harris et al. (1973)	Clinical	Pharma- cology	Indus- try	UK	Orderly	No	Concept stated, preliminary support available: a clinically useful, selective anti- inflammatory effect might occur with local application of beclomethasone dipropionate to lungs of asthmatics via inhalation.

[a]Taken from section II. Entries are those contributions without which the discovery of the agent (or additionally, in some cases, a relevant clinical application) would not have taken place or would have been materially delayed.

(Clark and McAllister, 1983; Siegel, 1985). Unfortunately, as al- ready mentioned in section I, it also became very clear, very quickly, that a host of serious, even potentially lethal, side effects were associated with the heavy systemic use of the steroids.

Gelfand (1951) resorted to aerosol administration of cortisone directly into the lungs as a way of achieving localized high concen- trations where they were needed. He noted that this route of administration (for bronchodilators and antibiotics) was time-honored in the treatment of asthma. Although he had success over a two-week period in four out of five asthmatic patients, subsequent work with inhalation of several forms of hydrocortisone (Fig.1) yielded mixed opinions as to its value in asthma (*see* for example, Brockbank et al., 1956; Brockbank and Pengelly, 1958; Helm and Heyworth, 1958; Smith, 1958; Langlands and McNeill, 1960). Brattsand et al. (1982) speculated that these variable results were caused by the great dilution of inhaled drugs that occurs in the lung and to the low potency of hydrocortisone. Subsequently, inhalation of the newer, very potent, halogenated steroid, dexamethasone (Fig. 1), although clearly effective in asthma, did not result in a separation of its useful local effects from its systemic side effects (*see* for example, Linder, 1964; Siegel et al., 1964; Novey and Beall, 1965, Toogood and Lefcoe, 1965). Experience with inhalation of other potent systemic steroids was similar to that with dexamethasone and, as a consequence, glucocorticoids continued to be used in the treatment of asthma, but largely by systemic routes and only with considerable trepidation.

McKenzie (1962) developed a simple method for assaying the glucocorticoid potency of topically applied steroidal agents. The test was based on the vasoconstriction (blanching) produced in human forearm skin by alcoholic solutions of glucocorticoids. This assay quickly replaced assays based on antagonism of a variety of experimental inflammatory lesions produced on human skin. With this new assay, acetates of steroids were found to be more potent than their more water-soluble parent alcohols, whereas the very water-soluble phosphate salts were usually less effective than the parent alcohols. Thus, dexamethasone alcohol was 100 times more active than its more water-soluble phosphate salt, whereas the poorly water-soluble acetonide of triamcinolone was 1000 times more potent than its more water-soluble alcohol. Since, by intradermal injection, dexamethasone alcohol and dexamethasone phosphate, as well as triamcinolone alcohol and triamcinolone acetonide, were equiactive, the huge differences seen with these pairs of steroids when they were applied topically were considered to be in consequence of differences in their absorption through the skin. The most powerful vasoconstrictors in this test were those substances that showed the most effective topical anti-inflammatory activity in clinical use.

III. Comments on Events
Leading to Beclomethasone Dipropionate

G. H. Phillips (1976) of Glaxo Laboratories Ltd., in a review of the structure–activity relationships of locally acting corticosteroids, stated, "From our own laboratories, selecting for optimum [topical] activity as described above for the monoesters [i.e., using the human skin vasoconstrictor assay of McKenzie (1962)], beclomethasone 17,21-dipropionate emerged as a useful topical agent (Caldwell et al., 1968; Raffle and Frain-Bell, 1967 and 1968)...."

Brattsand et al. (1982) commented, "The first known GCS [glucocorticosteroid] to possess the desired 'topical' GCS action in the lung combined with only little systemic GCS activity were 17α-ester compounds beclomethasone 17α, 21-dipropionate and betamethasone 17-valerate (Fig. 1). Later on, a similar differentiation...was demonstrated also for 16α, 17α-acetonide GCS, e.g., triamcinolone acetonide and flunisolide. These GCS were originally developed for topical dermatological therapy. The potencies found in screening models intended for evaluation of the topical cutaneous anti-inflammatory activity thus seemed to be a rather good prediction also of the anti-asthmatic activity on inhalation."

Brown (1980) pointed out that the glucocorticoid betamethasone valerate was developed by Glaxo Laboratories at approximately the same time as beclomethasone dipropionate. It was a potent steroid, useful in the topical treatment of eczema, and by aerosol administration it also had shown positive results in allergic rhinitis, without adrenal suppression, as early as 1968. For no clear reason, according to the author, trials ceased, and it was not tried in asthma until 1972. Brown (1980) commented further that, because of the early, preliminary, negative results of Choo-Kang et al. (1972) (*see* section I) with beclomethasone dipropionate, by May, 1970, this drug also was almost discarded for use in asthma.

Brown (1980) felt that

The story of topical steroids for asthma is worth remembering as a cautionary tale for those involved with the development of new drugs because...one of the most important improvements in the treatment of respiratory allergy since the introduction of cortisone in 1950 was nearly discarded not once, but twice!

IV. Developments Subsequent to Beclomethasone Dipropionate

Subsequent to the demonstration of the selective topical activity of beclomethasone dipropionate and betamethasone valerate, many programs were undertaken that were aimed at synthesizing new steroids with similar properties (Phillips, 1976; Brattsand et al., 1982). These programs usually involved substituting some of the alcohol groups of potent steroids with other groups that made them less polar and, thus, better capable of penetrating into tissues. The successes resulting from this work were triamcinolone acetonide and flunisolide, both halogenated compounds, and budesonide, a nonhalogenated substance (Fig. 1). These agents have all been approved for clinical use in the United States (Tse and Bernstein, 1984; Lampe, 1986). Budesonide is of interest in that its selective topical activity appears to be determined by its nonsymmetrical acetal substitution in the 16 and 17 carbon positions (Brattsand et al., 1982). This substitution increased the spread between topical antiinflammatory potency and systemic potency when compared with the spread seen with triamcinolone acetonide, which has a symmetrical acetal substitution.

References

Abramowicz, M., ed.: Beclomethasone dipropionate (Vanceril) for asthma. *Med. Lett.* **18:** 76, 1976.

Abramowicz, M., ed.: Corticosteroid aerosols for asthma. *Med. Lett.* **27:** 5, 6, 1985.

Abramowicz, M., ed.: Drugs for asthma. *Med. Lett.* **29:** 11–16, 1987.

Berkow R., ed.: *The Merck Manual*, 14th Ed., Merck Sharp & Dohme Research Laboratories, Rahway, NJ, 1982.

Brattsand, R., Thalén, A., Roempke, K., Källström, L., and Gruvstad, E.: Development of new glucocorticosteroids with a very high ratio between topical and systemic activities. *Eur. J. Respir. Dis.* **63** (Suppl. 122): 62–73, 1982.

Brockbank, W. and Pengelly, C. D. R.: Chronic asthma treated with powder inhalations of hydrocortisone and prednisolone. *Lancet* **1:** 187, 188, 1958.

Brockbank, W., Brebner, H., and Pengelly, C. D. R.: Chronic asthma treated with aerosol hydrocortisone. *Lancet* **2:** 807, 1956.

Brogden, R. N.: Inhaled steroids: Studies in adult and childhood asthma, in *Steroids in Asthma: A Reappraisal in the Light of Inhalation Therapy*, T. J. H. Clark, ed., pp. 135–153, Adis, Auckland, 1983.

Brogden, R. N., Heel, R. C., Speight, T. M., and Avery, G. S.: Beclomethasone dipropionate. A reappraisal of its pharmacodynamic properties and therapeutic efficacy after a decade of use in asthma and rhinitis. *Drugs* 28: 99–126, 1984.

Brogden, R. N., Pinder, R. M., Sawyer, P. R., Speight, T. M., and Avery, G. S.: Beclomethasone dipropionate inhaler: A review of its pharmacology, therapeutic value and adverse effects. I: Asthma. *Drugs* 10: 166–210, 1975.

Brown, H. M.: The Introduction and early development of inhaled steroid treatment, in *Topical Steroid Treatment for Asthma and Rhinitis*, N. Mygind and T. J. H. Clark, eds., pp. 66–76, Ballière Tindall, London, 1980.

Brown, H. M., Storey, G., and George, W. H. S.: Beclomethasone dipropionate: A new steroid aerosol for the treatment of allergic asthma. *Br. Med. J.* 1: 585–590, 1972.

Caldwell, I. W., Hall-Smith, S. P., Main, R. A., Ashurst, P. J., Kirton, V., Simpson, W. T., and Williams, G. W.: Clinical evaluation of a new topical corticosteroid beclomethasone dipropionate. *Br. J. Dermatol.* 80: 111–117, 1968.

Carryer, H. M., Koelsche, G. A., Prickman, L. E., Maytum, C. K., Lake, C. F., and Williams, H. L.: The effect of cortisone on bronchial asthma and hay fever occurring in subjects sensitive to ragweed pollen. *J. Allergy* 21: 282–287, 1950.

Choo-Kang, Y. F. J., Cooper, E. J., Tribe, A. E., and Grant, I. W. B.: Beclomethasone dipropionate by inhalation in the treatment of airways obstruction. *Br. J. Dis. Chest* 66: 101–106, 1972.

Clark, T. J. H.: Effect of beclomethasone dipropionate delivered by aerosol in patients with asthma. *Lancet* 1: 1361–1364, 1972.

Clark, T. J. H., ed.: *Steroids in Asthma. A Reappraisal in the Light of Inhalation Therapy*, Adis, Auckland, 1983.

Clark, T. J. H. and McAllister, W. A. C.: Corticosteroids, in *Asthma,* 2nd Ed., T. J. H. Clark and S. Godfrey, eds., pp. 372–392, Chapman and Hall, London, 1983.

Cochrane, G. M.: Systemic steroids in asthma, in *Steroids in Asthma. A Reappraisal in the Light of Inhalation Therapy*, T. J. H. Clark, ed., pp. 103–120, Adis, Auckland, 1983.

Gaddie, J., Petrie, G. R., Reid, I. W., Sinclair, D. J. M., Skinner, C., and

Palmer, K. N. V.: Aerosol beclomethasone dipropionate in chronic bronchial asthma. *Lancet* **1:** 691–693, 1973.

Gelfand, M. L.: Administration of cortisone by the aerosol method in the treatment of bronchial asthma. *N. Engl. J. Med.* **245:** 293, 294, 1951.

Glaxo Group Ltd.: 17α,21-Diacyloxy-9α-halo-11β-hydroxy-16β-methyl-pregna-1,4-diene-3,20-diones. (Belgium Patent 649,170. Dec. 11, 1964) *Chem. Abst.* **64:** 15958c, 1966.

Gregg, I.: Treatment of asthma with beclomethasone aerosol. *Br. Med. J.* **2:** 110, 1972.

Harris, D. M., Martin, L. E., Harrison, C., and Jack, D.: The effect of oral and inhaled beclomethasone dipropionate on adrenal function. *Clin. Allergy* **3:** 243–248, 1973.

Helm, W. H. and Heyworth, F.: Bronchial asthma and chronic bronchitis treated with hydrocortisone acetate inhalations. *Br. Med. J.* **2:** 765–768, 1958.

Hench, P. S., Kendall, E. C., Slocumb, C. H., and Polley, H. F.: The effect of the hormone of the adrenal cortex (17-hydroxy-11-dehydrocorticosterone: Compound E) and of pituitary adrenocorticotropic hormone on rheumatoid arthritis; preliminary report. *Proc. Staff Mtg. Mayo Clinic* **24:** 181–197, 1949.

Herxheimer, H.: Beclomethasone aerosol in asthma. *Lancet* **2:** 91, 92, 1972.

Hoffbrand, B. I. and Harris, D. M., eds.: Beclomethasone dipropionate aerosols. *Postgrad. Med. J.* **51** (Suppl. 4): 1–113, 1975.

Joint Committee on Pulmonary Nomenclature: Pulmonary terms and symbols. *Chest* **67:** 583–593, 1975.

Lal, S., Harris, D. M., Bhalla, K. K., Singhal, S. N., and Butler, A. G.: Comparison of beclomethasone dipropionate aerosol and prednisolone in reversible airways obstruction. *Br. Med. J.* **3:** 314–317, 1972.

Lampe, K. F., ed.: *Drug Evaluations,* 6th Ed., American Medical Association, Chicago, 1986.

Langlands, J. H. M. and McNeill, R. S.: Hydrocortisone by inhalation: Effects on lung function in bronchial asthma. *Lancet* **2:** 404–406, 1960.

Linder, W. R.: Adrenal suppression by aerosol steroid inhalation. *Arch. Intern. Med.* **113:** 655, 656, 1964.

McKenzie, A. W.: Percutaneous absorption of steroids. *Arch. Dermatol.* **86:** 611–614, 1962.

Martin, L. E., Harrison, C., and Tanner, R. J. N.: Metabolism of beclomethasone dipropionate by animals and man. *Postgrad. Med. J.* **51** (Suppl. 4): 11–20, 1975.

Martin, L. E., Tanner, R. J. N., Clark, T. J. H., and Cochrane, G. M.: Absorption and metabolism of orally administered beclomethasone dipropionate. *Clin. Pharmacol. Ther.* **15:** 267–275, 1974.

Meltzer, E. O., Kemp, J. P., Welch, M. J., and Orgel, H. A.: Effect of dosing schedule on efficacy of beclomethasone dipropionate aerosol in chronic asthma. *Am. Rev. Respir. Dis.* **131:** 732–736, 1985.

Mygind, N. and Clark, T. J. H., eds.: *Topical Steroid Treatment for Asthma and Rhinitis.* Ballière Tindall, London, 1980.

Novey, H. S. and Beall, G.: Aerosolized steroids and induced Cushing's syndrome. *Arch. Intern. Med.* **115:** 602–605, 1965.

Phillips, G. H.: Locally active corticosteroids: Structure activity relationships, in *Mechanisms of Topical Corticosteroid Activity.* L. C. Wilson and R. Marks, eds., pp. 1–18, Churchill Livingstone, Edinburgh, 1976.

Raffle, E. J. and Frain-Bell, W.: The effect of topically applied beclomethasone dipropionate on adrenal function. *Br. J. Dermatol.* **79:** 487–490, 1967.

Raffle, E. J. and Frain-Bell, W.: The effect of topically applied beclomethasone. *Br. J. Dermatol.* **80:** 124, 1968.

Siegel, S. C.: Corticosteroid agents: Overview of corticosteroid therapy. *J. Allergy Clin. Immunol.* **76:** 312–320, 1985.

Siegel, S. C., Heimlich, E. M., Richards, W., and Kelley, V. C.: Adrenal function in allergy. IV. Effect of dexamethasone aerosols in asthmatic children. *Pediatrics* **33:** 245–250, 1964.

Smith, J. M.: Hydrocortisone hemisuccinate by inhalation in children with asthma. *Lancet* **2:** 1248, 1249, 1958.

Toogood, J. H. and Lefcoe, N. M.: Dexamethasone aerosol for the treatment of "steroid dependent" chronic bronchial asthmatic patients. *J. Allergy* **36:** 321–332, 1965.

Tse, C. S. T. and Bernstein, I. L.: Corticosteroid aerosols in the treatment of asthma. *Pharmacotherapy* **4:** 334–342, 1984.

Wilson, J. D.: Asthma: The dimension of the problem, in *Steroids in Asthma: A Reappraisal in the Light of Inhalation Therapy,* T. J. H. Clark, ed., pp. 1–10, Adis, Auckland, 1983a.

Wilson, J. D.: *Asthma and Allergic Diseases: A Clinician's Guide to Diagnosis and Management,* Adis Health Sci., Sydney, 1983b.

Wilson, L. and Marks, R., eds.: *Mechanisms of Topical Corticosteroid Activity,* Churchill Livingstone, Edinburgh, 1976.

Williams, M. H., Jr.: Beclomethasone dipropionate. *Ann. Intern. Med.* **95:** 464–467, 1981.

Gastrointestinal Group

Cimetidine
Chenodeoxycholic Acid
Ursodeoxycholic Acid

Cimetidine

I. Cimetidine as an Innovative Therapeutic Agent

Peptic ulcers are circumscribed lesions of the alimentary mucosa that penetrate through to its muscular layer. They occur most commonly in the proximal duodenum and also in the lesser curvature of the stomach. These ulcers are always associated with acid and pepsin secretion, and seem to result from a disturbance in the balance between the ulcerogenic potential of such secretions and the protective effects of mucus production, membrane barriers to the acid and pepsin, and the regeneration of mucosal cells (Stedman, 1982; Shearman and Finlayson, 1982; Berkow, 1982; Lampe, 1986). Venables et al. (1978) noted that 10% of the population is said to suffer peptic ulceration at some time in their lives.

Before the advent of cimetidine, the drug treatments for peptic ulcers consisted of extensive antacid therapy and/or anticholinergic drugs. Surgery was a drastic third alternative for intractable cases. Anticholinergic agents are poorly absorbed and can cause unpleasant side effects, such as dryness of the mouth, constipation, and blurring of vision. Antacids, although effective, can have side effects, such as diarrhea or constipation, that also can be unpleasant. Moreover, compliance with an antacid regimen is essential, and some patients cannot tolerate this kind of regimen.

In 1975, cimetidine, the first clinically successful histamine H_2 receptor antagonist, became available (Brimblecombe et al., 1975a). This was a significant event because, although many of the physiological actions evoked by histamine could be blocked with such known antagonists as diphenhydramine, pyrilamine, and chlorpheniramine (now called histamine H_1 receptor antagonists), these antagonists did not block all of the actions of histamine, including, significantly, its capacity to stimulate gastric acid secretion. Cimetidine, unlike the H_1 antagonists, blocked acid secretion in animals and in humans. It very quickly became the treatment of choice for peptic ulcers, and a clear and effective alternative to elective surgery. Cimetidine therapy gives relief from pain, promotes healing of ulcers, and is effective in preventing the recurrence of ulcers in many patients (Brogden et al., 1978). At reasonable clinical doses, the incidence of side effects is low.

Cimetidine also is important in the management of Zollinger-Ellison syndrome. This syndrome is characterized by peptic ulceration secondary to gastric acid hypersecretion associated with a pancreatic tumor (Fleshler, 1981). Before cimetidine, the only available treatment for this condition was total gastrectomy. Cimetidine has made gastrectomy unnecessary.

Early Clinical Research History

Wyllie and his group studied cimetidine in 18 healthy male subjects (Burland et al., 1975). It markedly inhibited histamine-induced and pentagastrin-induced gastric acid secretion in these subjects. Cimetidine appeared more active than metiamide, a precursor compound (*see* section II), and no side effects were observed.

Pounder et al. (1975) found that cimetidine reduced the 24-h intragastric acidity in six patients with duodenal ulcers to a magnitude that was compatible with successful medical treatment of the condition. This same group (Pounder et al., 1976) treated 10 patients suffering from gastric ulcers with cimetidine by the oral route for 6 wk. They found that relief of symptoms was rapid and that by the end of treatment all the ulcers had healed (as determined by endoscopy). No untoward clinical or laboratory effects were observed. The authors felt that the results of their uncontrolled pilot study should encourage controlled trials with cimetidine in gastric ulcers. Haggie et al. (1976) found similar results in an open trial in 19 patients with active duodenal ulcers. No changes in white blood cell counts and other laboratory measurements were associated with treatment. Relapses in seven of the patients occurred within 1 mo of cimetidine withdrawal.

In a double-blind, placebo-controlled trial in 44 patients with duodenal or prepyloric ulcers, Bodemar and Walan (1976) found that cimetidine by the oral route led to endoscopically determined healing in 67% and 90% of patients after 3 and 6 wk, respectively, whereas placebo elicited 17% and 36% healing at 3 and 6 wk, respectively. Basal and pentagastrin-induced acid secretion were reduced by cimetidine, but not by placebo, and consumption of antacids was reduced more by cimetidine than by placebo. Similar results were found with orally administered cimetidine in another double-blind, placebo-controlled study in 24 patients with duodenal ulcers (Blackwood et al., 1976). Many subsequent studies firmly established the effectiveness and the limitations of cimetidine in the treatment of peptic ulcers (*see* Brogden et al., 1978 for references).

Reviews and textbook treatments concerning cimetidine and H_2 receptor blockade are numerous (*see*, for example, Brimblecombe et al., 1978; Brogden et al., 1978; Misiewicz, 1978; Dyck, 1979; Hirschowitz, 1979; Black et al., 1982).

II. The Scientific Departure
Leading to Cimetidine: Burimamide

Black and his associates (1972) recounted that they started their work on the H_2 receptor in 1964 "...based on a simple analogy with catecholamine beta receptors and their antagonists and on the structure of histamine." The work took eight years and the synthesis of 700 compounds and involved the testing of these compounds as H_1 and "non-H_1" histamine agonists and antagonists in five tissue systems. The relative agonist activity of each of a series of methyl derivatives of histamine was estimated in both guinea pig ileum (H_1 receptor) and guinea pig atrium (non-H_1 receptor), and this was followed by testing in other tissues containing H_1 or non-H_1 receptors. The results all suggested that a homogeneous population of non-H_1 receptors existed. These were dubbed, provisionally, H_2 receptors. All the compounds synthesized as potential H_2 antagonists, in addition to being tested in isolated tissues, were tested for their ability to inhibit histamine stimulation of gastric acid secretion, since the authors considered it reasonable to assume that an H_2

antagonist would inhibit gastric acid secretion. Black et al. (1972) stated, "By considering the effect of structural change on activity of compounds in the screening test we progressed to N-methyl-N'-(4-(4(5)-imidazolyl)butyl)-thiourea," or burimamide (Fig. 1). Burimamide was demonstrated to be a selective, competitive inhibitor of the responses of the tissues containing H_2 receptors. It also was shown to be a surmountable, apparently competitive, inhibitor of histamine-stimulated gastric acid secretion in rats, but it did not block vagally-induced gastric acid secretion. In addition, the H_2 antagonist activities of a series of inhibitors in vitro were highly positively correlated with their capacities to inhibit histamine-stimulated gastric acid secretion in vivo. The H_2 receptor and its blockade were thus established as viable physiological and pharmacological concepts. Burimamide also inhibited the gastric acid secretion evoked by gastrin and pentagastrin in the rat and was demonstrated to reduce gastric acid secretion in response to pentagastrin in two human volunteers.

Wyllie et al. (1972) found, in human volunteers, that intravenous burimamide was considerably more effective than atropine in inhibiting gastric acid secretion and that it produced none of the side effects associated with anticholinergic therapy. However, burimamide was not adequately bioavailable by the oral route (Black et al., 1973). Clinical evaluation of this agent was discontinued.

Background Contributions Preceding Burimamide

The isolation, chemistry, and potential physiological importance of histamine captured the attention of researchers from the early twentieth century onward, and consequently histamine research has been reviewed many times (*see* for example, Code, 1965; Rocha e Silva, 1966). The development of antihistamines during and after World War II opened the door to classification of some of the actions of histamine. It became evident that the drugs that became known as the "classic" antihistamines (eventually called H_1 antagonists) could antagonize some, but not all, of the actions of histamine. For example, these antihistamines did not antagonize histamine-induced relaxation of rat uterus or histamine-induced stimulation of atria isolated from the guinea pig. Of future clinical

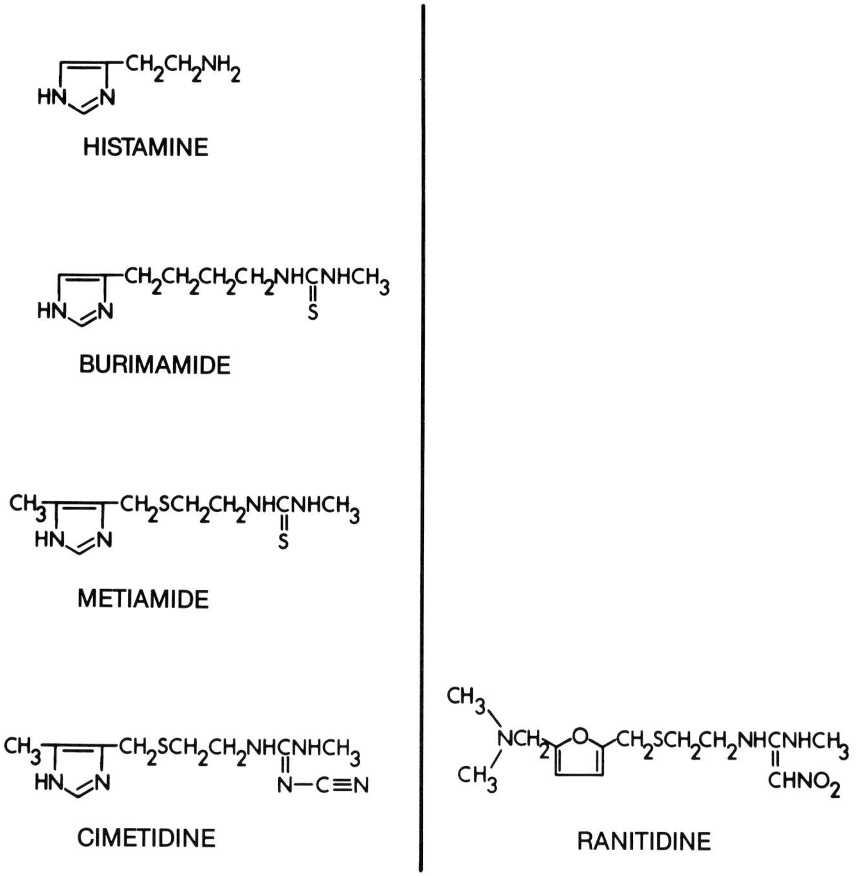

Fig. 1. The structures of cimetidine and chemically and/or pharmacologically related substances.

significance, as noted earlier, was the fact that available antihistamines also could not reduce the gastric acid secretion elicited by histamine.

Ash and Schild (1966) were the first to formalize the idea of there being more than one kind of histamine receptor. They used a series of available histamine analogs for structure–activity studies utilizing guinea pig ileum, rat uterus, and rat stomach preparations. On the basis of the relative activity of these analogs, they stated that there were at least two kinds of histamine receptors. The receptor blocked by classic antihistamines, such as mepyramine (pyrilamine), was designated H$_1$. Those actions not antagonized by classic antihistamines were mediated by histamine receptors other than H$_1$ (i.e., by non-H$_1$ receptors). Ash and Schild were hoping to find an analog of histamine that would inhibit the "other" histamine receptor. They stated, "The most satisfactory way of defining receptors is by means of antagonists...a search for this property in the compounds described...has been unproductive." Interestingly, they reported that one of their compounds, 2-mercaptohistamine, antagonized gastric acid secretion at high concentrations, but because it was also a partial agonist they did not pursue the lead.

Significant Events Following Burimamide

Black et al. (1973) studied a burimamide analog in which a methylene group had been replaced with a thio ether in the side chain and a methyl group had been added in the imidazole ring. Like burimamide, the compound was a competitive antagonist of H$_2$ receptors. It was also 10 times more potent than burimamide. Studies in volunteers showed that this compound, metiamide (Fig. 1), reduced both the volume and acidity of gastric juices. It was suggested that it should be given clinical trial. Wyllie et al. (1973) reported that intravenously administered metiamide showed marked inhibition of the gastric acid secretion induced by either histamine or pentagastrin in seven human volunteers, and Thjodleifsson and Wormsley (1975) demonstrated that pentagastrin-induced secretion of acid and pepsin in ulcer patients was reduced by intravenous doses of metiamide. These intravenous doses yielded plasma concentrations of metiamide that might be expected to occur following oral administration. Unfortunately, at the same time, Forrest et al. (1975) had to report that two patients given metiamide developed neutropenia. The neutropenia was reversed in seven to ten days after stopping metiamide, but this toxic effect was enough to cause clinical trials to be abandoned.

The search for an analog of metiamide that did not share metiamide's toxic action resulted in the development of cimetidine (Fig. 1), (Brimblecombe et al., 1975a,b). It was shown to be a competitive antagonist of the H$_2$ receptor and in vivo was two times more active than metiamide.

Table 1
Profile of Observations and Ideas Crucial to the Development of Cimetidine[a]

Sequence: Departure compound[*] to innovative drug[**]	Orient- ation	Nature of study	Research institution	National origin	Nature of discovery	Screening involved	Crucial ideas or observations
Burimamide[*]							
Black et al. (1972)	Pre- clinical	Chem- istry/ pharma- cology	Indus- try	UK	Orderly	Targeted	Burimamide discov- ed; a selective H_2 inhibitor by iv route; potential in blocking acid secretion and in treating gastric ulcers recognized.
Metiamide							
Black et al. (1973)	Pre- clinical, clinical	Chem- istry/ pharma- cology	Indus- try, univer- sity	UK	Orderly	Targeted	Burimamide analog, metiamide, devel- oped; an H_2 blocker effective via oral route (eventually shown to be toxic).
Cimetidine[**]							
Brimble- combe et al. (1975a)	Pre- clinical, clinical	Chem- istry/ pharma- cology	Indus- try	UK	Orderly	Targeted	Metiamide analog, cimetidine, devel- oped; an H_2 blocker active via oral route.

[a]Taken from section II. Entries are those contributions without which the discovery of the agent (or additionally, in some cases, a relevant clinical application) would not have taken place or would have been materially delayed.

Table 1 defines the critical scientific ideas and experiments leading to cimetidine and categorizes their origin.

III. Comments on Events Leading to Cimetidine

Ganellin (1982) commented that, at the time he and his colleagues started the 12 years of chemical effort that, in collaboration with Black and others, eventually led to cimetidine, attitudes in gastroenterology were not conducive to the use of an antagonist of histamine for controlling gastric acid secretion. Most attention at the time was directed to the newly discovered polypeptide stimulator of acid secretion, gastrin; a physiological role for histamine in the secretion of gastric acid was considered unlikely. In addition, Ganellin (1982) noted that the Eli Lilly Co. had unsuccessfully tried, during the 1950s, to find an antagonist to histamine-induced acid secretion. Because of these facts, it was generally felt that this approach was played out.

Durant et al. (1973, 1975) and Ganellin et al. (1976) discussed the extensive chemical work that was undertaken in the development of cimetidine. They used histamine as a chemical starting point and made a variety of changes in this molecule. Modifications were made in the imidazole ring, and nonpolar, lipophilic substituents were introduced at various positions, but none of these compounds antagonized the non-H_1 actions of histamine; attention was then directed to modifying the side chain. Ganellin et al. (1976) stated, "The work took several years and produced a long catalogue of nonantagonists." Ultimately, the guanidine derivative of histamine, guanylhistamine, provided a breakthrough by yielding a weakly active partial agonist (Ganellin et al., 1976). In a subsequent systematic study, the guanidinium group was replaced by a nonbasic group, the side chain was lengthened, and eventually burimamide was synthesized. Burimamide was 100 times more potent than guanylhistamine as a non-H_1 inhibitor. Unfortunately, at physiological pH, only a small portion of the drug was bioavailable. When, eventually, a methylene group was replaced with an isosteric thio ether link in the side chain and a methyl group was introduced into the imidazole ring, burimamide became metiamide. Because the thiourea group might have accounted for metiamide's toxicity, and because it was known from earlier work that guanylhistamine had exhibited partial H_2 receptor antagonism, guanidine analogs of metiamide were made. One of these analogs, the cyanoguanidine, was developed into cimetidine.

This entire chemistry story has been recounted in detail by Duncan and Parsons (1980) and Ganellin (1982). Ganellin (1982) noted, candidly, that some 200 compounds, all inactive, were prepared in the first four years and that many avenues were examined and found to be ineffective, and since in the main these are not mentioned in recountings "...the net effect may be to make the work appear to be more rational and more perceptive than is warranted."

IV. Developments
Subsequent to Cimetidine

Additional H_2-receptor blocking agents have been or are being developed, such as ranitidine, etintidine, BL 6341, and SKF 93479 (Richardson and Peterson, 1982). Ranitidine (Fig. 1) (Bradshaw et al., 1979) has been approved by the Food and Drug Administration and is marketed in the USA. This agent is more potent than cimetidine; lower dosage as well as less frequent administration are needed. It appears that there may be other advantages to ranitidine in addition to its greater potency (Brogden et al., 1978, 1982). There are several recognized side effects of cimetidine, which occur in low incidence and with high and/or prolonged doses: male breast tenderness, gynecomastia, and, possibly, impotence. These effects appear to be the result of cimetidine (which is not fully selective in binding to H_2 receptors) displacing dihydrotestosterone from androgen binding sites. Ranitidine lacks these androgenic blocking actions, since it does not readily bind to sites other than H_2 receptors (Thomas and Misiewicz, 1984). Finally, structural differences in the two molecules probably account for the fact that cimetidine, unlike ranitidine, inhibits drug metabolism through an action on cytochrome P450 enzyme systems—with the consequent problem of drug interactions if patients are taking other drugs metabolized through this system. Clinical experience will determine the position of ranitidine, or newer H_2 antagonists, vis-à-vis cimetidine as the H_2 antagonist of choice.

Hirschowitz (1979) commented that, in the wake of the work of Black et al. (1972) that led to burimamide, there followed "...the development of specific H_1 and H_2 agonists and antagonists and, by their use, the further definition of H_1 and H_2 mediated actions." For his work leading to the discoveries of cimetidine and propranolol, Black shared in the 1988 Nobel Prize in Medicine.

References

Ash, A. S. F. and Schild, H. O.: Receptors mediating some actions of histamine. *Br. J. Pharmacol. Chemother.* **27**: 427–439, 1966.

Berkow, R., ed.: *The Merck Manual*, 14th Ed., Merck Sharp & Dohme Research Laboratories, Rahway, NJ, 1982.

Black, J., Gerskowitch, V. P. , and Leff, P.: Reflections on the classification of histamine receptors, in *Pharmacology of Histamine Receptors*, C. R. Ganellin and M.E. Parsons, eds. pp. 1–9, Wright, PSG, Bristol, UK, 1982.

Black, J.W., Duncan, W. A. M., Durant, C. J., Ganellin, C. R., and Parsons, E. M.: Definition and antagonism of histamine H_2-receptors. *Nature* 236: 385–390, 1972.

Black, J.W., Duncan, W. A. M., Emmett, J. C., Ganellin, C. R., Hesselbo, T., Parsons, M. E., and Wyllie, J. H.: Metiamide: An orally active histamine H_2-receptor antagonist. *Agents Actions* 3: 133–137, 1973.

Blackwood, W. S., Maudgal, D. P., Pickard, R. G., Lawrence, D., and Northfield, T. C.: Cimetidine in duodenal ulcer: Controlled trial. *Lancet* 2: 174–176, 1976.

Bodemar, G. and Walan, A.: Cimetidine in the treatment of active duodenal and prepyloric ulcers. *Lancet* 2: 161–164, 1976.

Bradshaw, J., Brittain, R.T., Clitherow, J.W., Daly, M. J., Jack, D., Price, B. J., and Stables, R.: Ranitidine (AH 19065): A new potent, selective histamine H_2-receptor antagonist. *Br. J. Pharmacol.* 66: 464P, 1979.

Brimblecombe, R.W., Duncan, W. A. M., Durant, G.J., Emmett, J. C., Ganellin, C. R., and Parsons, M. E.: Cimetidine: A non-thiourea H_2-receptor antagonist. *J. Int. Med. Res.* 3: 86–92, 1975a.

Brimblecombe, R.W., Duncan, W. A. M., Durant, G. J., Ganellin, C. R., Parsons, M. E. and Black, J.W.: The pharmacology of cimetidine, a new histamine H_2- receptor antagonist. *Br. J. Pharmacol.* 53: 435, 436, 1975b.

Brimblecombe, R. W., Duncan, W. A. M., Durant, G. J., Emmett, J. C., Ganellin, C. R., Leslie, G. B., and Parsons, M. E.: Characterization and development of cimetidine as a histamine H_2-receptor antagonist. *Gastroenterology*, 74: 339–347, 1978.

Brogden, R. N., Heel, R. C., Speight, T. M., and Avery, G. S.: Cimetidine: A review of its pharmacological and therapeutic efficacy in peptic ulcer disease. *Drugs* 15: 93–131, 1978.

Brogden, R. N., Carmine, A. A., Heel, R. C., Speight, T. M. and Avery, G. S.: Ranitidine: A review of its pharmacology and therapeutic use in peptic ulcer disease and other allied diseases. *Drugs* 24: 267–303, 1982.

Burland, W. L., Duncan, W. A. M., Hesselbo, T., Mills, J. G., Sharpe, P. C., Haggie, S. J., and Wyllie, J. H.: Pharmacological evaluation of cimetidine, a new histamine H_2-receptor antagonist, in healthy man. *Br. J. Clin. Pharmacol.* 2: 481–486, 1975.

Code, C. F.: Histamine and gastric secretion: A later look, 1955–1965. *Fed. Proc.* 24: 1311–1321, 1965.

Duncan, W. A. M. and Parsons, M. E.: Reminiscences of the development of cimetidine. *Gastroenterology* 78: 620–625, 1980.

Durant, G. J., Emmett, J. C., and Ganellin, C. R.: Some chemical aspects of histamine H_2-receptor antagonists, in *International Symposium on Histamine H_2-Receptor Antagonists,* C. J. Wood and M. A. Simkins, ed., pp. 13–21, SKF, London, 1973.

Durant, G. J., Parsons, M. E., and Black, J.W.: Potential histamine H_2-receptor antagonists. 2. N^αguanylhistamine. *J. Med. Chem.* **18:** 830–833, 1975.

Dyck, W. P.: Cimetidine in management of peptic ulcer disease, in Symposium on New Methods of Treatment of Gastrointestinal Disease. *Surg. Clin. North Am.* **59:** 863–867, 1979.

Fleshler, B.: The impact of cimetidine on the treatment of acid-peptic disease. *Primary Care* **8:** 195–203, 1981.

Forrest, J. A. H., Shearman, D. J. C., Spence, R., and Celestin, L. R.: Neutropenia associated with metiamide. *Lancet* **1:** 392, 393, 1975.

Ganellin, C. R.: Cimetidine, in *Chronicles of Drug Discovery,* J. S. Bindra and D. Lednicer, eds., pp. 1–38, Wiley, New York, 1982.

Ganellin, C. R., Durant, G. J., and Emmett, J. C.: Some chemical aspects of histamine H_2-receptor antagonists. *Fed. Proc.* **35:** 1924–1930, 1976.

Haggie, S. J., Fermont, D. C., and Wyllie, J. H.: Treatment of duodenal ulcer with cimetidine. *Lancet* **1:** 983, 984, 1976.

Hirschowitz, B.I.: H_2 histamine receptors. *Annu. Rev. Pharmacol. Toxicol.* **19:** 203–244, 1979.

Lampe, K. F., ed.: *Drug Evaluations,* 6th Ed., American Medical Association, Chicago, 1986.

Misiewicz, J. J.: Role of cimetidine in gastrointerestinal disease: Present status and future potential. *Drugs* **15:** 89–92, 1978.

Pounder, R. E., Williams, J. G., Milton-Thompson, G. J., and Misiewicz, J. J.: 24-Hour control of intragastric acidity by cimetidine in duodenal-ulcer patients. *Lancet* **2:** 1069–1072, 1975.

Pounder, R. E., Hunt, R. H., Stekelman, M., Milton-Thompson, G. J., and Misiewicz, J. J.: Healing of gastric ulcer during treatment with cimetidine. *Lancet* **1:** 337–339, 1976.

Richardson, C. T. and Peterson, W. L.: New agents for peptic ulcer therapy. *Drug Ther.* **12:** 145–151, 1982.

Rocha e Silva, M., ed.: Histamine and antihistamines, in *Handbook of Experimental Pharmacology* , vol. 18, Part 1, pp. 991, Springer-Verlag, New York, 1966.

Shearman, D. J. C. and Finlayson, N. D. C.: *Diseases of the Gastrointestinal Tract and Liver,* Churchill Livingstone, Edinburgh, 1982.

Stedman's Medical Dictionary, 24th Ed., Williams & Wilkins, Baltimore, 1982.

Thjodleifsson, B. and Wormsley, K. G.: Aspects of the effect of metiamide on pentagastrin-stimulated and basal gastric secretion of acid and pepsin in man. *Gut* **16:** 501–508, 1975.

Thomas, J. M. and Misiewicz, G.: Histamine H_2-receptor antagonists in the short- and long-term treatment of duodenal ulcer. *Clin. Gastroenterol.* **13:** 501–542, 1984.

Venables, C. W., Stephen, J. G., Blair, E. L., Reed, J. D., and Saunders, J. D.: Cimetidine in the treatment of duodenal ulceration and the relationship of this therapy to surgical management, in *Cimetidine, The Westminster Hospital Symposium,* C. Wastell and P. Lance, eds., pp. 13–27, Churchill Livingstone, London, 1978.

Wyllie, J.H., Hesselbo, T., and Black, J.W.: Effects in man of histamine H_2-receptor blockade by burimamide. *Lancet* **2:** 1117–1120, 1972.

Wyllie, J. H., Ealding, W. D. P., Hesselbo, T. , and Black, J. W.: Inhibition of gastric secretion in man by metiamide: A new, orally active histamine H_2-receptor antagonist. *Gut* **14:** 424, 1973.

Chenodeoxycholic Acid and Ursodeoxycholic Acid

I. Chenodeoxycholic Acid and Ursodeoxycholic Acid as Innovative Therapeutic Agents

Cholelithiasis (gallstones) is a major medical and economic problem in the USA (Schoenfield, 1977; Schoenfield et al., 1981). It has been estimated to have a prevalence of 15 million women and five million men, and almost one million new cases are discovered each year (Ingelfinger, 1968; Friedman et al., 1966). Gallstones account for 5000–8000 deaths and a toll of $1 billion annually (Schoenfield et al., 1981).

Cholelithiasis and concurrent cholecystitis (inflammation of the gall bladder) are associated with disruptions of the normal metabolism of bile salts* and of their enterohepatic recycling. These disruptions frequently evoke indigestion, food intolerance, and constipation (Rains, 1964) because bile salts serve several functions critical to the absorption and solubilization of lipids:

1. A detergent, or emulsifying, action on fat particles in the intestine;
2. Micellar formation with lipid molecules in the intestine;
3. Micellar formation with lecithin and cholesterol in the bile.

In addition to gastrointestinal distress, in severe cases of stone formation, biliary colic is common (Rains, 1964; Schoenfield, 1977).

---

*Bile acids (Fig. 1) , in bile, are largely conjugated with glycine or taurine via an amide linkage at the carboxyl group. These conjugates are themselves acidic and occur as sodium salts.

377

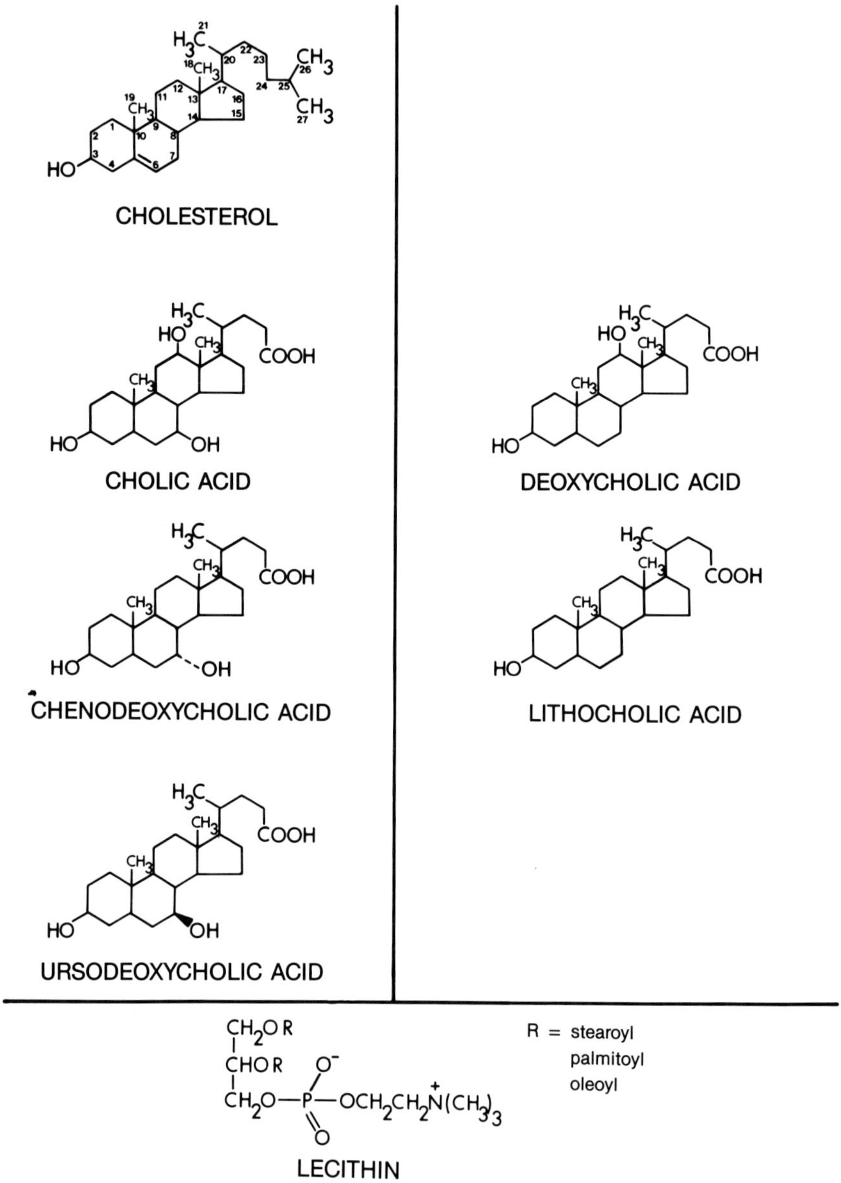

Fig. 1. The structures of chenodeoxycholic acid and ursodeoxycholic acid and chemically and/or pharmacologically related substances.

A half-million cholecystectomies (surgical removal of the gall-bladder) are performed each year (Schoenfield et al., 1981) as a therapy for gallstones. Cholecystectomy was the fifth most common therapeutic operation in the USA in 1975. This procedure generally relieves colic, but patients often continue to suffer some form of digestive discomfort. This is a result of the fact that, although the surgery can remove the mechanical effects of stones, or an infected or inflamed gallbladder, it does nothing about the disruption of bile salt metabolism (Rewbridge, 1937). In fact, cholecystectomy *per se* produces disturbances in bile salt metabolism (*see* Vernick and Kuller, 1981; Linos et al., 1981 for refs.). Some studies have suggested that cholecystectomy increases the risk of colon carcinoma (Vernick and Kuller, 1981; Linos et al., 1981; *see also* Bachrach and Hofmann, 1982).

Since the early 1970s, therapeutic experimentation with two bile acids (chenodeoxycholic acid and ursodeoxycholic acid [Fig. 1]) has been leading to a medical alternative to surgery for some patients. A definitive, placebo-controlled, multicenter study in 916 patients treated with chenodeoxycholic acid for up to two years yielded confirmed, complete dissolution of cholesterol gallstones in 13.5% of patients, and partial or complete dissolution in 40.8% (Schoenfield et al., 1981). Clinically significant, reversible hepatotoxicity (an increase in the mean level of serum aminotransferases) occurred in 3% of the drug-treated patients, and mild diarrhea occurred in 40.5% of the patients. Schoenfield et al. (1981) concluded, "Chenodiol, 750 mg/d for up to 2 years, is appropriate therapy for dissolution of gallstones in selected patients who are informed of the risks and benefits."

A multicenter, placebo-controlled, double-blind study of ursodeoxycholic acid was carried out in order to make a definitive statement regarding its efficacy (Tokyo Cooperative Gallstone Study Group, 1980). Treatment of 72 patients for six to 12 months led to the dissolution of stones, or decrease in their size and number, in 34.5% of patients. In cases with small, noncalcified stones or floating stones, 83.3% of patients were improved. Diarrhea and hepatic toxicity did not occur. The Study Group concluded that "...the results indicate that UDCA [ursodeoxycholic acid] is a safe and effective litholytic agent."

Ward et al. (1984) reviewed the literature covering ursodeoxycholic acid and concluded, "While surgery is clearly the preferred treatment in many patients with symptomatic gallstones, in a carefully selected subgroup of such patients gallstone dissolution therapy with ursodeoxycholic acid offers an important and worthwhile alternative." These authors considered ursodeoxycholic acid to be superior to chenodeoxycholic acid because it was more potent, just as effective, and better tolerated.

The Medical Letter offered the opinion, "Chenodeoxycholic acid...is a medical alternative for patients with biliary symptoms, radiolucent stones, and functioning gallbladders who are poor surgical risks or refuse to have an operation...Ursodeoxycholic acid, not yet available in the USA, is probably safer (Abramowicz, 1983)."

Early Clinical Research History

The early clinical history of chenodeoxycholic and ursodeoxycholic acids, is intimately involved in their discovery as treatments for cholesterol gallstones. This will be covered in section II.

II. The Scientific Work Leading to Chenodeoxycholic Acid and Ursodeoxycholic Acid as Treatments for Gallstones

Bile salts and lecithin (Fig. 1) had been known since the 1930s to be the two biliary constituents that, in a micellar complex, solubilize cholesterol in bile. It was also well-known that the first step in the formation of cholesterol gallstones occurred when the capacity of the bile to solubilize cholesterol (Fig. 1) was exceeded. Nonetheless, estimates of the capacity of bile from normal and cholelithiasis patients to dissolve cholesterol had been found to overlap (Isaksson, 1954a,b). Admirand and Small (1968) noted, "Consistent differences between normal bile and bile from patients with cholesterol gallstones have been difficult to demonstrate." However, by using an in vitro model system (in which the relative quantities of cholesterol, bile salts, and lecithin were plotted individually on triangular coordinates), Admirand and Small (1968) were able to make a clear distinction between normal and gallstone biles. Normal biles were less than saturated with cholesterol, whereas biles from gallstone patients were saturated. In some cases, the latter contained cholesterol microcrystals.

Subsequently, Vlahcevic et al. (1970) found that the average total bile acid pool for patients with gallstones was 1.29 g, as compared to 2.38 g in patients without gallstones. In addition, the pools of two specific bile acids, cholic acid and chenodeoxycholic acid (Fig. 1), were reduced in patients with gallstones. Vlahcevic et al. (1970) concluded "...that a diminished bile salt pool may be an important factor contributing to the production of the abnormal bile found in patients with cholesterol gallstones."

Thistle and Schoenfield (1971), over a four-month period, evaluated the effects of administering individual bile acids (*inter alia*) on the proportions of bile acids in the bile, and also on the relative concentrations of bile acids, lecithin, and cholesterol in the bile. Bile from untreated subjects with cholelithiasis was found to have a lower proportion of chenodeoxycholic acid than bile from untreated normal subjects. After the administration of chenodeoxycholic acid, this bile acid came to account for 95% of the total bile acids, and the ratio of bile acids + lecithin to cholesterol was significantly increased. On the other hand, administration of cholic acid evoked no change in this ratio. Thistle and Schoenfield (1971) suggested, as one possibility, "Chenodeoxycholic acid may be more effective than cholic acid in inhibiting cholesterol synthesis or in stimulating lecithin synthesis" and held that chenodeoxycholic acid might be of prophylactic or therapeutic value in cholelithiasis.

This same group (Danziger et al., 1972) subsequently reported complete or partial dissolution of gallstones in four of seven women given chenodeoxycholic acid for up to 22 mo. It was recognized that colonic bacteria would dehydroxylate chenodeoxycholic acid to lithocolic acid (Fig. 1), a known hepatotoxin in animals. Liver function and morphology, however, remained normal; some diarrhea was observed. These workers followed this preliminary study with a single-blind, controlled trial in 53 patients with radiolucent gallstones (Thistle and Hofmann, 1973). At 6 mo, 11 of 18 patients who were treated with chenodeoxycholic acid had a decrease in gallstone size or number. No response occurred in 17 patients treated with cholic acid or in 18 receiving a lactose placebo. Approximately 25% of those treated with chenodeoxycholic acid had transiently elevated serum glutamic oxalacetic transaminase (SGOT), but no additional liver-function changes occurred. Three patients had minor changes in liver biopsies. Thistle and Hofmann (1973) were of the opinion that chenodeoxycholic acid might eventually be of prophylactic value, especially in high-risk groups, and obviate the need for surgical treatment.

Ursodeoxycholic acid, the 7β-hydroxy epimer of chenodeoxycholic acid (Fig. 1) and the principal bile acid of bear bile, had been widely used as a cholagogue in Japanese folk medicine. Makino et al. (1975), aware of the work with chenodeoxycholic acid, carried out an open study with ursodeoxycholic acid. These authors were also aware of the work of Salen et al. (1974), which had shown that humans converted orally administered chenodeoxycholic acid to ursodeoxycholic acid, and which had raised the question of whether it was the ursodeoxycholic acid, rather than the chenodeoxycholic acid, that was responsible for the dissolution of gallstones. Makino et al., (1975) found ursodeoxycholic acid to be effective in dissolving gallstones in 4 of 11 patients treated for 4–18 mo. This same group (Nakagawa et al., 1977) conducted a 6-mo, double-blind, placebo-controlled study on 44 patients with radiolucent gallstones. Complete or partial gallstone dissolution occurred in 8 of 31 patients receiving ursodeoxycholic acid and in none of the placebo-treated group. There was no increase in the level of serum aminotransferases and no diarrhea. Ursodeoxycholic acid was approximately four times more potent than chenodeoxycholic acid.

A considerable literature has subsequently been generated concerning the relative merits of chenodeoxycholic acid and ursodeoxycholic acid. The general thrust of this literature is that both drugs are moderately effective, but that ursodeoxycholic acid is safer than chenodeoxycholic acid (for example, *see* Maton et al., 1977; Stiehl et al., 1978; Nakayama, 1980; Bachrach and Hofmann, 1982; Tint et al., 1982; Ward et al., 1984; Tint et al., 1986). The difference in safety may result from the fact that lithocolic acid, a hepatotoxin, does not increase markedly during treatment with ursodeoxycholic acid, whereas it does increase during treatment with chenodeoxycholic acid. It has been reported that the 7β-hydroxyl group of ursodeoxycholic acid is more resistant to cleavage by colon bacteria than is the 7α-hydroxyl group of chenodeoxycholic acid (Fedorowski et al., 1979; White et al., 1982).

Table 1 defines the critical scientific ideas and experiments leading to chenodeoxycholic acid and ursodeoxycholic acid in the treatment of gallstones and categorizes their origin.

Background Contributions Preceding Chenodeoxycholic Acid and Ursodeoxycholic Acid in Gallstone Therapy

Chenodeoxycholic acid was isolated from goose gall by Windhaus et al. (1924) and from human gall by Wieland and Reverey (1924). The groups agreed that the substances they had isolated from these different sources were identical. According to the Merck Index (11th edition), ursodeoxycholic acid was isolated by Shoda in 1927 and characterized by Kaziro in 1929 and 1931, and Iwasaki in 1936.

Schoenheimer and Hrdina (1931) stated, "The problem of gallstone formation is the problem of the precipitation of cholesterol out of the bile." These authors then postulated that the diseased gallbladder mucosa had a greater than normal absorptive power for bile salts (Andrews et al., 1931a). They concluded (Andrews et al., 1931b) that cholesterol stones were caused by faulty differential absorption of bile acids and cholesterol by the abnormal gallbladder wall. Andrews et al. (1932) found the bile salt:cholesterol ratio in normal bile to be 25; in bile from diseased gall bladders, the ratio was 2.5. Such a clear-cut difference apparently was not uniformly reproducible by later workers.

Spanner and Bauman (1932) noted that a 0.1% solution of lecithin plus sodium deoxycholate dissolved twice as much cholesterol as the bile salt alone. They suggested that cholesterol in bile was maintained in solution by bile salts, soaps, and phosphatides. It had been reported earlier (Hammarsten, 1905; Long and Gephart, 1908; *see also* Johnston et al., 1939) that there was a phospholipid in bile, that it was associated with bile salts, and that it was most likely lecithin. Isaksson (1951), using new methodology, showed that, contrary to current belief, human bladder bile contained a large

Table 1
Profile of Observations and Ideas Crucial to the Development
of Chenodeoxycholic Acid and Ursodeoxycholic Acid[a]

Sequence: Route to innovative drugs**	Orient- ation	Nature of study	Research institution	National origin	Nature of discovery	Screening involved	Crucial ideas or observations
Chenodeoxycholic Acid*							
Admirand and Small (1968)	Clinical	Gastro- enter- ology	Univer- sity	USA	Orderly	No	Analysis of propor- tions of cholesterol and its solubilizers, bile salts and leci- thin, show normal bile to be unsatu- rated and gallstone bile to be saturated with cholesterol.
Vlahcevic et al. (1970)	Clinical	Gastro- enter- ology	Hospital (VA), univer- sity	USA	Orderly	No	Total bile acid pool reduced in gallstone bile; cholic and chenodeoxycholic acid pools reduced.
Thistle and Schoenfield (1971)	Clinical	Gastro- enter- ology	Private	USA	Orderly	No	Chenodeoxycholic but not cholic acid increases the ratio of bile acids + lecithin to cholesterol in gallstone bile.
Danziger et al. (1972)	Clinical	Gastro- enter- ology	Private	USA	Orderly	No	Complete or partial dissolution of cho- lesterol gallstones in patients given long- term chenodeoxy- cholic acid.
Ursodeoxycholic Acid*							
Makino et al. (1975)	Clinical	Gastro- enter- ology	Univer- sity	Japan	Orderly	No	Complete or partial dissolution of cho- lesterol gallstones in patients given long- term ursodeoxy- cholic acid.

[a]Taken from section II. Entries are those contributions without which the discovery of the agent (or additionally, in some cases, a relevant clinical application) would not have taken place or would have been materially delayed.

amount of lecithin and that this was the only phospholipid present. This same author (Isaksson, 1954a) found that, in over 70% of biles from gallstone patients, the ratio of bile salts + lecithin to cholesterol was below the critical range of 11:1 for precipitation. Conversely, however, some 30% were at or over this range. In one normal patient, the ratio was below 11:1. Disconcertingly, bile salt + lecithin systems from normal biles and those from gallstone biles had the same cholesterol-dissolving capacity (Isaksson, 1954b).

Sporadic, uncontrolled studies had appeared over the years, reporting that feeding bile salts to gallstone patients had beneficial effect. Thus, Rosenak and Kohlstaedt (1936) treated 63 patients for 9 mo with a bile salt preparation containing a high percentage of deoxycholic acid. Most improvement was seen in the control of digestive symptoms and constipation. Colic pains were only somewhat attenuated. No measurement of the effects of treatment on gallstone number or size were made. Rewbridge (1937) reported the disappearance of gallstones in two of five cases in which the patients had been treated with a bile salt preparation for 9 mo. No control groups were run. In seven of nine patients receiving a bile salt preparation for 8–31 wk, "stone" shadows seen in cholangiograms of the common bile duct disappeared (Cole and Harridge, 1957). The authors were not sure if dissolution, disintegration, or passage of these "stones" had occurred in this uncontrolled study.

III. Comments on Events Leading to Chenodeoxycholic Acid and Ursodeoxycholic Acid

The impetus for the therapeutic use of chenodeoxycholic acid in cholelithiasis appears to have been the idea of supplying "replacement" therapy in what was viewed by Danziger et al. (1972) as "...a disease of decreased bile acid secretion rather than a disease of increased cholesterol secretion." Although it has subsequently been shown that chenodeoxycholic and ursodeoxycholic acids lower the lithogenic index in bile primarily by lowering cholesterol content via inhibition of synthesis and/or secretion and/or absorption of cho-lesterol, not simply by increasing a diminished bile acid pool (Tint, et al., 1986), the interim hypothesis served a useful end.

Schoenfield et al. (1981) in the introduction to the National Cooperative Gallstone Study, commented, "The pharmaceutical in-dustry probably would not have conducted a [large, multicenter] clinical trial without the protection of a patent on chenodiol."

IV. Developments
Subsequent to Chenodeoxycholic Acid
and Ursodeoxycholic Acid

As judged from the literature, there has been little or no follow-up to the bile acids in terms of the synthesis and testing of related agents for the treatment of cholelithiasis.

References

Abramowicz, M., ed.: Chenodiol for dissolving gallstones. *Medical Letter* **25:** 101, 102, 1983.

Admirand, W. H. and Small, D. M.: The physicochemical basis of cholesterol gallstone formation in man. *J. Clin. Invest.* **47:** 1043–1052, 1968.

Andrews, E., Schoenheimer, R., and Hrdina, L.: Etiology of gall stones. II. Role of the gallbladder. *Proc. Soc. Exp. Biol. Med.* **28:** 945, 946, 1931a.

Andrews, E., Schoenheimer, R., and Hrdina, L.: Etiology of gall stones. III. Bile salt-cholesterol ratio in human gall stone cases. *Proc. Soc. Exp. Biol. Med.* **28:** 945–948, 1931b.

Andrews, E., Dostal, L. E., Goff, M., and Hrdina, L.: The mechanism of cho-lesterol gallstone formation. *Ann. Surg.* **96:** 615–623, 1932.

Bachrach, W. H. and Hofmann, A. F.: Ursodeoxycholic acid in the treatment of cholesterol cholelithiasis Part I. *Dig. Dis. Sci.* **27:** 737–761, 1982.

Budavari, S., ed.: *The Merck Index*, 11th Ed., p. 1556, Merck & Co., Rahway, NJ, 1989.

Cole, W. H. and Harridge, W. H.: Disappearance of "stone" shadows in post-operative cholangiograms. *JAMA* **164:** 238–243, 1957.

Danziger, R. G., Hofmann, A. F., Schoenfield, L. J., and Thistle, J. L.: Disso-lution of cholesterol gallstones by chenodeoxycholic acid. *N. Engl. J. Med.* **286:** 1–8, 1972.

Fedorowski, T., Salen, G., Tint, G. S., and Mosbach, E.: Transformation of chenodeoxycholic acid and ursodeoxycholic acid by human intestinal bacteria. *Gastroenterology* **77**: 1068–1073, 1979.

Friedman, G. D., Kannel, W. B., and Dawber, T. R.: The epidemiology of gallbladder disease: Observations in the Framingham study. *J. Chronic Dis.* **19**: 273–292, 1966.

Hammarsten, O.: Zur Chemie der Galle. *Ergeb. Physiol.* **4**: 1–22, 1905.

Ingelfinger, F. J.: Digestive disease as a national problem. V. Gallstones. *Gastroenterology* **55**: 102–104, 1968.

Isaksson, B.: On the lipid constituents of normal bile. *Acta Soc. Med. Upsala* **56**: 177–195, 1951.

Isaksson, B.: On the lipid constituents of bile from human gallbladder containing cholesterol gallstones. A comparison with normal human bladder bile. *Acta Soc. Med. Upsala* **59**: 277–295, 1954a.

Isaksson, B.: On the dissolving power of lecithin and bile salts for cholesterol in human bladder bile. *Acta Soc. Med. Upsala* **59**: 296–306, 1954b.

Johnston, C. G., Irvin, J. L., and Walton, C.: The free choline and phospholipid of hepatic and gallbladder bile. *J. Biol. Chem.* **131**: 425–437, 1939.

Linos, D. A., Beard, C. M., O'Fallon, W. M., Dockerty, M. B., Beart, R. W. Jr., and Kurland, L. T.: Cholecystectomy and carcinoma of the colon. *Lancet* **2**: 379–381, 1981.

Long, J. H. and Gephart, F.: On the behavior of lecithin with bile salts, and the occurrence of lecithin in bile. *J. Am. Chem. Soc.* **30**: 1312–1319, 1908.

Makino, I., Shinozaki, K., Yoshino, K., and Nakagawa, S.: Dissolution of cholesterol gallstones by ursodeoxycholic acid. *Jpn. J. Gastroenterol.* **72**: 690–702, 1975.

Maton, P. N., Murphy, G. M., and Dowling, R. H.: Ursodeoxycholic acid treatment of gallstones. *Lancet* **2**: 1297–1301, 1977.

Nakagawa, S., Makino, I., Ishizaki, T., and Dohi, I.: Dissolution of cholesterol gallstones by ursodeoxycholic acid. *Lancet* **2**: 367–369, 1977.

Nakayama, F.: Oral cholelitholysis—cheno versus urso. Japanese experience. *Dig. Dis. Sci.* **25**: 129–134, 1980.

Rains, A. J. H.: *Gallstones, Causes and Treatment,* Charles C. Thomas, Springfield, IL, 1964.

Rewbridge, A. G.: The disappearance of gallstone shadows following the prolonged administration of bile salts. *Surgery* **1**: 395–400, 1937.

Rosenak, B. D. and Kohlstaedt, K. G.: Bile salt therapy in liver and gall bladder disease. *Am. J. Dig. Dis. Nutr.* **3**: 577–580, 1936.

Salen, G., Tint, G. S., Eliav, B., Deering, N., and Mosbach, E. H.: Increased formation of ursodeoxycholic acid in patients treated with chenodeoxycholic acid. *J. Clin. Invest.* **53**: 612–621, 1974.

Schoenfield, L. J.: *Diseases of the Gallbladder and Biliary System,* Wiley, New York, 1977.

Schoenfield, L. J., Lachin, J. M., The Steering Committee, and The National Cooperative Gallstone Study Group: Chenodiol (chenodeoxycholic acid) for dissolution of gallstones: The national cooperative gallstone study. *Ann. Intern. Med.* **95:** 257–282, 1981.

Schoenheimer, R. and Hrdina, L.: The etiology of gall stones. I. Chemical factors. *Proc. Soc. Exp. Biol. Med.* **28:** 944, 945, 1931.

Spanner, G. O. and Bauman, L.: The behavior of cholesterol and other bile constituents in solutions of bile salts. *J. Biol. Chem.* **98:** 181–183, 1932.

Stiehl, A., Czygan, P., Kommerell, B., Weis, H. J., and Holtermuller, K. H.: Ursodeoxycholic acid versus chenodeoxycholic acid. Comparison of their effects on bile acid and bile lipid composition in patients with cholesterol gallstones. *Gastroenterology* **75:** 1016–1020, 1978.

Thistle, J. L. and Hofmann, A. F.: Efficacy and specificity of chenodeoxycholic acid therapy for dissolving gallstones. *N. Engl. J. Med.* **289:** 655–659, 1973.

Thistle, J. L. and Schoenfield, L. J.: Induced alterations in composition of bile of persons having cholelithiasis. *Gastroenterology* **61:** 488–496, 1971.

Tint, G. S., Salen, G., and Shefer, S.: Effect of ursodeoxycholic acid and chenodeoxycholic acid on cholesterol and bile acid metabolism. *Gastroenterology* **91:** 1007–1018, 1986.

Tint, G. S., Salen, G., Colalillo, A., Graber, D., Verga, D., Speck, J., and Shefer, S.: Ursodeoxycholic acid: A safe and effective agent for dissolving cholesterol gallstones. *Ann. Intern. Med.* **97:** 351–356, 1982.

Tokyo Cooperative Gallstone Study Group: Efficacy and indications of ursodeoxycholic acid treatment for dissolving gallstones. A multicenter double-blind trial. *Gastroenterology* **78:** 542–548, 1980.

Vernick, L. J. and Kuller, L. H.: Cholecystectomy and right-sided colon cancer: An epidemiological study. *Lancet* **2:** 381–383, 1981

Vlahcevic, Z. R., Bell, C. C., Buhac, I., Farrar, J. T., and Swell, L.: Diminished bile acid pool size in patients with gallstones. *Gastroenterology* **59:** 165–173, 1970.

Ward, A., Brogden, R. N., Heel, R. C., Speight, T. M., and Avery, G. S.: Ursodeoxycholic acid. A review of its pharmacological properties and therapeutic efficacy. *Drugs* **27:** 95–131, 1984.

White, B. A., Fricke, R. J., and Hylemon, P. B.: 7β-Dehydroxylation of ursodeoxycholic acid by whole cells and cell extracts of the intestinal anaerobic bacterium, *Eubacterium* species V.P.I. 12708. *J. Lipid Res.* **23:** 145–153, 1982.

Wieland, H. and Reverey, G.: Untersuchungen über Gallensäuren. XXI. Mitteilung. Zur Kenntnis der menschlichen Galle, 1. *Z. Physiol. Chem.* **140:** 186–202, 1924.

Windhaus, A., Bohne, A., and Schwarzkopf, E.: Über die Cheno-desoxycholsäure. *Z. Physiol. Chem.* **140:** 177–185, 1924.

Analysis and Interpretation

Summaries
of the Analyses of Table 1*

In the first 28 chapters, we traced the histories of 30 lines of research that led to the discovery of 32 innovative, pharmacodynamic drugs[†]. As noted earlier, this sample of innovative drugs was not selected by the authors, but via an informal written poll of clinician-scientists who were experts in the specific therapeutic areas covered.

Using the guidelines presented in the introduction, relevant contributions from each history were placed into either the foreground or the background segment of section II of a chapter; this was followed by listing the critical contributions from each foreground segment in Table 1, column 1. The specific facts concerning each listed contribution that were then entered into the body of Table 1 were also put into a data file, and a variety of questions was asked regarding this information using SAS, a statistical analysis software package. The questions referred to the aggregate of all the drugs and in part, to each of four groups: cardiovascular and renal, psychiatry, rheumatology, anesthesiology. These four groups could be analyzed separately because they contained between 6 and 9 drugs each; the neurology, pulmonary, and gastrointestinal groups were not analyzed separately, since they contained only 2 or 3 drugs each—too small a sample size for meaningful analysis.

---

*Please see appendix for full tabulated information on which these summaries are based. Percentages have been rounded to the nearest whole number for ease of comprehension.

†For want of a better alternative, we have used the term, "pharmacodynamic drugs" to refer to agents that are useful because of their effects on mammalian systems. The term is used generically to distinguish such agents from antiinfective or chemotherapeutic drugs, which are of value not because of their effects on mammalian systems, but because they selectively inhibit or destroy microorganisms (or cancer cells) that afflict mammalian hosts.

In the aggregate analysis, two very similar, but not identical, collections of information were searched. Questions relating to the "nature of entries" (*see* IA, B, *below*) were considered to pertain to the 30 lines of research mentioned above, and the data base for this critical information (consisting of the tables from each of the chapters, including the three independent entries from the Ca antagonists chapter) was searched for answers. However, when questions were put in terms of "facts relating to the innovative drugs" (*see* II *below*), not only was this same data base searched, but also, in those cases in which two innovative drugs had been discovered sequentially from the same line of research, data for both drugs were included separately in the search; the data for the second drug of necessity contained a reprise of the data for the first drug. This was necessary for ursodeoxycholic acid (following on chenodeoxycholic acid) and for diazepam (following on chlordiazepoxide).

In addition, since three drugs (azathioprine, propranolol, and diazepam) had been voted to be innovative in more than one group, the information from their tables was included, independently, in the analyses of each of these groups: azathioprine appeared in the cardiovascular and renal group as well as in the rheumatology group; propranolol appeared in the cardiovascular and renal group as well as in the anesthesiology group; and diazepam appeared in the psychiatry, neurology, and anesthesiology groups.

The authors suggest that readers who are not interested in pursuing the highly detailed analyses of Table 1 presented in the Appendix, or in pursuing the slightly less numerical details of the summaries of the analyses of Table 1 that now commence, should skip to "Discussion of Analyses IA, IB, and II" on page 394 and "Discussion of Analysis III" on page 397.

IA. The Initiation of the 30 Lines of Research*†

Of the initial entries:

- 73% were preclinical, 23% clinical, and 3% a mixture of the two types.

---

*The terms used throughout the following summaries are defined in the chapter entitled "Definitions for Table 1."

†The information on which Summaries IA and IB are based is contained in Analysis I in the Appendix.

- 53% were industrial, 28% from universities, 13% from hospitals and 6% from government.
- 27% were serendipitous: 2 entries each from industry and universities, and 4 from hospitals. These serendipitous initial entries represented 12% of industry initiations, 22% of university initiations, and 100% of hospital initiations.

IB. The Total Number of Entries for the 30 Lines of Research

Of all entries:

- 67% were preclinical, 33% were clinical.
- 41% were from industry, 38% from university, 12% from hospital, 4% from government, 3% from private research institutions, and 1% from hospital (VA).
- 46% involved screening:
    74% of which was targeted,
    14% untargeted, and
    12% a combination of the two types.
- 40% were designated as either chemistry/pharmacology or pharmacology/chemistry (largely from industry); of this 40%, chemistry/pharmacology entries were preponderant, comprising 80% of the total.
- 17% were solely pharmacological in nature (largely from universities).
- 43% were varied in nature and reflected a relatively uniform spread across 12 other preclinical and clinical disciplines.
- The ratio *serendipitous industry entries / total industry entries* = .049; the ratio *serendipitous university entries / total university entries* = .053; and the ratio *all serendipitous nonindustry entries/all nonindustry entries* = .103.
- 47% were from the USA, 20% from the UK; 33% were spread more or less uniformly across 12 other countries.

II. The 32 Innovative Drugs

It required an average of three contributions to define the science of an innovative drug, with a range of 1–8 contributions. It took 5 yr, on average, from the initial report of a line of research to an adequate elaboration of the scientific basis for an innovative drug, with a range of 0–20 yr.

- Of the 32 drugs, 53% had only preclinical contributions, 16% only clinical, and 31% a mixture of the two types.
- Industry had at least one contribution in 75% of all the drugs discovered, whereas universities were represented in 53% and hospitals in 25%. Government and private institutions, as well as hospitals (VA), were each represented in 9% or less of the innovative drugs.
- Industry was solely responsible for 38% of the innovative drugs. Of these 12 agents, 11 were established by single contributions, and all involved screening. Hospitals alone accounted for 3%, or one agent. Other institutions, taken individually, were never solely responsible for the discovery of an innovative drug, although various combinations of university, hospital, government, and private research institutions accounted for 22%, or seven agents.
- Of the drugs, 75% had only orderly contributions; 25% had one serendipitous contribution each. All serendipitous contributions were initial contributions.
- At least one screening contribution was present in 78% of the drugs.
- When viewed by decades, serendipity was involved in 33% of the innovative drugs discovered in the 1940s, 63% in the 1950s, 8% in the 1960s, and 13% in the 1970s.
- Screening was uniformly distributed over the decades, being involved in 67% of the drugs discovered in the 1940s, 75% in the 1950s, 85% in the 1960s, and 75% in the 1970s; untargeted screening appeared in 0% of the drugs discovered in the 1940s, 25% of those discovered in the 1950s, 39% of those in the 1960s, and 50% of those in the 1970s.
- Of the drugs, 59% were developed solely in one country: 22% were discovered solely in the USA, 9% in the UK, 9% in West Germany, 6% each in Switzerland and Belgium, and 3% each in Japan and Australia. The remaining 40% required contributions from 2 or 3 countries.

Discussion of Analyses IA, IB, and II

Analyses of this sample of 32 innovative, pharmacodynamic drugs make it clear that preclinical entries were of major importance, both in initiating the 30 lines of research and throughout the development of these lines of research: in both instances, considerably more than half of the entries were preclinical. In addition, approximately half of the drugs had *only* preclinical contributions.

Industry played a strong role in the drug-discovery process. It was responsible for approximately half of the initiations of the lines of research, as well as for approximately 40% of the total number of entries and, unaided, for 12 (or nearly 40%) of the agents. In addition, industry had at least one contribution in 75% of all the drugs discovered.

Of industry entries, 90% were positive for screening; this was reflected in the fact that screening figured in nearly half of the total number of entries, as well as in the fact that nearly 80% of all the drugs discovered entailed at least one screening contribution. Interestingly, screening was uniformly distributed over the decades and appeared in an average of 75% of the drugs developed from the 1940s through the 1970s. Screening entries were predominantly targeted and chemist-driven; the latter point was judged by the fact that chemistry/pharmacology entries very clearly exceeded pharmacology/chemistry entries. Surprisingly, untargeted screening, the form of screening most heavily dependent on chance for success, increased steadily in occurrence over the decades, from none of the drugs in the 1940s to 50% of the drugs in the 1970s. Of the 12 drugs that were developed solely by industry, eight involved untargeted screening and were pharmacology/chemistry contributions, indicating the importance of this form of screening, and of the pharmacologist, in bringing about wholly industry-based pharmacotherapeutic innovations.

Although the industrial contribution (especially its unaided discovery of 12 innovative drugs) was very significant, it is also very clear that essentially half of the initiations and somewhat more than half of the total number of entries were nonindustrial entries, i.e., from universities, hospitals, private research institutions, and government. Thus, as the strongest example, universities accounted for 28% of initial entries and 38% of total entries, and had at least one contribution in half of the drugs discovered. The total of nonindustrial entries covered an array of 13 preclinical and clinical disciplines with few chemistry/pharmacology and pharmacology/chemistry entries. Without these diverse, nonindustrial contributions, approximately 60% of the drugs would not have been discovered or would have had their discoveries markedly delayed. Moreover, eight (or 25%) of the drugs were discovered solely by various combinations of nonindustrial institutions, without entries from industry.

One-quarter of the 32 innovative drugs had serendipitous initial contributions, but this type of contribution played a much greater role in the 1940s and 1950s than in the 1960s and 1970s. Serendipitous observations were involved in a higher percentage of hospital and university initiations than in industry initiations. Furthermore, as a percentage of their total entries, serendipity played an equal role for universities and for industry, but it was found to play twice as great a role when all nonindustrial contributions were looked at as a group.

III. The Innovative Drugs Taken as Groups

- Preclinical contributions were the sole type in 89% of cardiovascular and renal (CV&R) drugs, 43% of psychiatric drugs, 33% of rheumatologic drugs, and 100% of anesthesiologic drugs. On the other hand, clinical contributions were the sole type in 14% of psychiatric drugs and 33% of rheumatologic agents, but never the sole type for CV&R or anesthesiologic drugs. A mixture of both types of contributions accounted for 11, 43, 33, and 0% of CV&R, psychiatric, rheumatologic, and anesthesiologic agents, respectively.
- At least one industrial contribution was present in 100% of CV&R, 71% of psychiatric, 67% of rheumatologic, and 83% of anesthesiologic drugs.
- Universities participated in 44% of CV&R, 43% of psychiatric, 67% of rheumatologic, and 50% of anesthesiologic drugs.
- Hospitals, although not represented in the CV&R or anesthesiology categories, appeared in 57% of psychiatric and 33% of rheumatologic drugs.
- Hospitals (VA) had no representation in any of these groups, private research institutions were represented in 17% of the rheumatology group, and government was represented in 17% of both the rheumatology and the anesthesiology groups.
- Industry was solely responsible for 56% of CV&R, 43% of psychiatric, 17% of rheumatologic, and 50% of anesthesiologic drugs. Of the remaining institutions, hospitals were solely responsible for

14% of psychiatric drugs, whereas universities, government, private institutions, and hospitals (VA) were not individually responsible for any drugs in these four categories.

- Screening was a factor in the discovery of 100% of CV&R and anesthesiologic agents, and in 71% of psychiatric and 67% of rheumatologic drugs.
- Serendipitous observations aided in the discovery of 33% of CV&R, 57% of psychiatric, 17% of rheumatologic, and 17% of anesthesiologic drugs.
- The USA, unaided, was responsible for 43% and 50%, respectively, of psychiatric and rheumatologic drugs, but for only 17% of anesthesiologic and 0% of CV&R drugs. West Germany, Switzerland, and Japan accounted for 55% of CV&R drugs; Australia and Belgium for 28% of psychiatric drugs, and the UK and Belgium for 34% of anesthesiologic drugs. The remaining 44, 29, 50 and 50% of CV&R, psychiatric, rheumatologic, and anesthesiologic drugs, respectively, involved 2 or 3 countries in their discovery.

Discussion of Analysis III

When the summarized facts from the Table 1 analysis are sorted according to groups, two differing profiles emerge. All anesthesiologic drugs had only preclinical contributions, as did all but one of the CV&R drugs, which, in addition to its preclinical entries, had two clinical entries. Industry was represented in all CV&R drugs and in the bulk of anesthesiologic drugs, and, in both of these groups, industry was solely responsible for half or more of the agents. As a concomitant to industry's presence, screening appeared in all the CV&R and anesthesiologic drugs. Serendipity was a factor in only one-third or less of both groups.

In contrast to the CV&R and anesthesiology groups, the psychiatry and rheumatology groups were not so dependent on preclinical studies, with less than one-half having solely preclinical contributions and the remainder having either solely clinical or a mixture of clinical and preclinical contributions. The psychiatry and rheumatology groups, combined, contained 10 of the 12 hospital contributions that appeared in the tables; of these 10, nine were clinical in nature. Industrial contributions were contained in approximately two-thirds of psychiatric and of rheumatologic drugs, but industry was solely responsible for only somewhat less than 50% of psychiatric agents and for less than one-quarter of rheumatologic drugs (reflecting industry's reduced role relative to its role in the CV&R and anesthesiology groups). Screening, although involved in the discoveries of roughly two-thirds of the drugs in both psychiatric and rheumatologic groups, was not as important as it was in the other two groups, in which it was involved in the discovery of all the drugs; psychiatric and rheumatologic drugs were most divergent in the occurrence of serendipitous contributions, with the psychiatry group having such events in more than half of the agents and rheumatology group having them in less than one-quarter of the drugs.

In the psychiatry and rheumatology groups, innovative drugs were discovered in the 1940s, 1950s, and 1960s, but not beyond. This was also the case for the anesthesiology group. In distinction, discoveries of CV&R innovative drugs were prominent in the 1960s and 1970s.

Interpretation

The authors have worked at keeping their attitudes and opinions out of the case histories and analyses that were presented in the preceding chapters by avoiding, in large part, both the use of a narrative format and the expression of editorial comment. This was especially true for the critical parts of the chapters—the section IIs and their associated Tables. It was our intent by so doing to enable the case histories and the analyses to remain independent of our particular views.

In the present chapter, however, it is our intent to synthesize the foregoing material and to give a point of view about its meaning, both as history and as a potential guide to further discovery in the area of pharmacodynamic drugs. The authors realize that the case histories and the analyses may be subject to alternate interpretations, and we urge readers to make their own if our interpretation seems unsatisfactory.

Our primary bias is that the raison d'être for biomedical research is the alleviation of human disease and suffering, not the pursuit of knowledge as an end in itself. Our second bias is that pharmacotherapy is one of the major weapons, if not *the* major weapon, in the alleviation of suffering. Indeed, it seems to us that pharmacotherapy plays a key role in the endeavor to reduce misery and that, as a result, truly remarkable drugs have become commonplace. This is so much the case that the genesis of these agents becomes a "taken for granted" item for much of the preclinical and clinical biomedical community. This "removed status" of large segments of the biomedical community from the drug-discovery process (coupled with the anecdotal approach commonly used in describing drug discoveries, in conjunction with the seemingly innate preference of all researchers for logical constructions) is likely to lead, in the unwary onlooker, to various degrees of ignorance and error. Ignorance and error, in turn, encourage the formation of distorted ideas and attitudes about the complex process of drug discovery. Such distorted ideas can mislead all scientists—both nonindustrial and industrial—as to the nature of drug discovery and, therefore, be costly in terms of time, money, and effort spent in this pursuit. In addition, distorted attitudes can raise formidable barriers to the development of a common appreciation for each other's efforts among all scientists interested in pursuing pharmaco-therapeutic innovation. It is our hope to shed some light on what the realities of the drug discovery process may be.

The readers should already be aware that we have not defined our "study universe" in terms of new chemical entities (NCEs) approved by the FDA, although this index is considered to be a valid measure of productivity in the development of new drugs, particularly as regards the immediate contributions of the US pharmaceutical industry, and has been widely used (Wardell and Sheck, 1983; Mossinghoff, 1987). Rather, as stated in the introduction to this treatise, we were interested in the "intellectual histories" of respected innovations in pharmacotherapeutics—prime movers, so to speak—and have restricted our attention to these.

I. Actions and Interactions of the Various Research Institutions

The intellectual drive behind the discovery of innovative drugs comes predominantly from industry and universities, as shown by the fact that, together, these two institutions account for 79% (41 and 38%, respectively) of all the table entries for our sample of 32 innovative, pharmacodynamic, therapeutic agents; the remaining 21% of entries was spread among hospital, government, and private research institutions. This dominance of industry and universities is also further substantiated by the fact that industry had at least one contribution in three-quarters of all the drugs discovered and universities were represented in half of them; hospitals, government research laboratories, and private institutions, on the other hand, participated in the discovery of much lower percentages of the drugs.

Industry

The contributions of industry were predominantly chemistry-pharmacology screening collaborations; only a few purely chemical contributions (*see* methotrexate and naloxone) and a few purely pharmacological contributions (*see* naloxone, albuterol, and beclomethasone) were made by industry. In some instances, contributions from industry occurred only after significant university or other nonindustrial contributions (*see* captopril, chlorothiazide, chlorpromazine, cyclophosphamide, and albuterol); in other instances, nonindustrial and industrial contributions were interdigitated (*see* propranolol, azathioprine, imipramine, methotrexate as an antiarthritic agent, and beclomethasone dipropionate). However, the chemistry-pharmacology screening collaborations of industry played their strongest role when, as single-contribution lines of research, they produced innovative drugs (*see* verapamil, nifedipine, diltiazem, furosemide, cyclosporine, haloperidol, chlordiazepoxide, carbamazepine, indomethacin, halothane, and fentanyl) or when, in a series of contributions, they led to a discovery (*see* diazepam), or essentially did so (*see* naloxone and cimetidine).

University

University contributions, unlike those of industry, were not primarily chemistry-pharmacology screening collaborations. Only in a very few cases were such collaborations seen in universities (*see* cyclophosphamide, succinylcholine, and naloxone; interestingly, all three of these contributions took place in the 1940s). University contributions were both preclinical and clinical, and were investigative in nature: 57% were composed of pharmacology, biochemistry, and physiology, as well as other preclinical disciplines, and 43% were from diverse clinical specialties (*see* propranolol, captopril, chlorothiazide, azathioprine, chlorpromazine, imipramine, iproniazid, L-dopa, D-penicillamine, methotrexate, cyclophosphamide, albuterol, chenodeoxycholic acid, and ursodeoxycholic acid). In some instances clinical contributions came from specialties completely unrelated to the ultimate areas of clinical utility (*see* chlorothiazide, chlorpromazine, and iproniazid).

It is very clear from the previous paragraphs that, subsequent to the 1940s, a major distinction between the contributions to drug discovery coming from industry and those coming from universities (primarily medical schools) is the lack, in the latter, of significant interaction with organic (medicinal) chemists. Whereas university pharmacologists were once actively involved in defining the actions of new chemicals as possible therapeutic agents, this type of collaboration with chemists appears to have largely ceased in the 1950s. It seems a strange parting of the ways to have occurred, since drugs, by and large, are organic molecules, and drug discovery seems to have been of genuine interest to university pharmacologists, or pharmacologically oriented investigators, in the 1930s, 1940s, and early 1950s (e.g., Leake et al., 1933; Merritt and Putnam, 1938; Konzett, 1940; McCawley et al., 1941; Paton and Zaimis, 1948; Krantz et al., 1953; see also Leake, 1970). Schwartzman (1976) pointed out that, at the time of his writing, academic researchers would not desire to search for a drug systematically by synthesizing a class of compounds suspected of having desirable pharmacologic properties, because it was their perception that the university's function of expansion of basic knowledge (and education) would not be furthered by such efforts. As noted by Swann (1988), such a perception of basic knowledge as essentially distinct from practical knowledge is based on the late nineteenth century German concept of Wissenschaft as "...a dedicated, sanctified pursuit" of phenomena, "...not the study of things for their immediate utilities...." This concept strongly influenced the development of science, including biomedical science, in American universities during the early twentieth century. An associated negative attitude developed toward the patenting of information that might be of help in the relief of human ailments. Some of these sentiments apparently lingered well into mid-century, especially in preclinical departments in medical schools. Cuatrecasas (1983) felt that, over the past 25 years, the independence of academia from economic forces in the private sector as a result of the generous support of biomedical research by the federal government, and the "grant ethic" that evolved, had isolated university research from the industrial community. Other factors undoubtedly played a part in diminishing the interest of university researchers in drug discovery. Leake (1970) felt that drug-discovery efforts were hampered by the regulatory actions taken by local, state, and federal agencies, which generated the need for a vast organization and tremendous amounts of money to develop a chemical compound to the point of effective delivery.

The practical upshot of the attitudes and events ennumerated above seems to have been a considerable diminution in the close interaction of university preclinical biomedical scientists—particularly pharmacologists or pharmacologically oriented researchers in medical schools—with organic chemists on drug-discovery projects. Interestingly, within the decade of the 1980s, a trend of increasing university-industry collaborations has been established, fueled in some significant part by the dwindling of federal funds for the support of university research (Bearn, 1981; Varrin and Kukich, 1985; Swann, 1988).

Hospital

Not surprisingly, 11 of 12 hospital entries were clinical. Moreover, of the eight drugs that had hospital entries in Table 1, half had these entries appear as initiators of lines of research via a serendipitous clinical observation (*see* chlorpromazine, iproniazid, hydroxychloroquine) or via a serendipitous preclinical observation (*see* lithium). For three other drugs, hospital entries provided the necessary proof that compounds had an important pharmacological activity (imipramine, L-dopa, and beclomethasone dipropionate), and one hospital entry provided a rationale for the clinical testing of one compound (D-penicillamine). It would seem that the importance of hospital experimentation in drug discovery lies in unearthing unexpected activities and in supplying proof of the presence of activities that cannot be reliably measured in animals.

Government and Private Institutions

Government research contributions were part of the scenario of discovery for only three drugs (cyclophosphamide, succinylcholine, and albuterol). The first two agents represent work carried out in the 1940s; the third, work carried out in the 1950s. There seems to be no common pattern to these contributions. The same can be said for the contributions of private research institutions in the discovery of three drugs (hydroxychloroquine as an antirheumatic agent, chenodeoxycholic acid and ursodeoxycholic acid as treatments for gallstones) and for hospitals (VA), which were also involved in the discovery of the use of chenodeoxycholic acid and of ursodeoxycholic acid. The contribution of government to drug discovery in the USA may increase in the wake of the Federal Technology Transfer Act of

1986. This act revised patent policies so as to enable, and to encourage, government scientists to collaborate with industry, thus reversing a long-standing aversion of government laboratories (NIH) to the private sector (Culliton, 1989).

The impact of nonindustrial contributors, taken in the aggregate, exceeded that of its component members taken individually. Thus, lithium (as an antimanic agent) was the only drug discovered solely by way of a single nonindustrial institution (hospital), but, collectively, nonindustrial institutions yielded another seven innovative drugs without entries from industry (*see* succinylcholine, iproniazid as an antidepressant, L-dopa as an anti-Parkinson drug, D-penicillamine and hydroxychloroquine as antirheumatic agents, and chenodeoxycholic acid and ursodeoxycholic acid as treatments for gallstones). The lack of industrial involvement is mirrored in the fact that, with the exception of succinylcholine, there was no active participation by organic chemists in any of these discoveries.

The discovery of agents without scientific contributions from industry probably reflects on industry's part:

1. A lack of interest in substances, especially naturally occurring substances, for which significant information was prematurely put into the public domain, therefore rendering the discovery unpatentable (*see* comments in section III of the chapters on lithium, D-penicillamine and chenodeoxycholic acid);
2. A perceived limited market;
3. Uncertainty as to the significance of early findings; or
4. The lack of valid animal models in which to conduct preclinical work.

These rationales probably hold also for industry's lack of scientific contributions to the discoveries of the useful actions of ursodeoxycholic acid, hydroxychloroquine, L-dopa, and iproniazid. Industry, however, was involved with succinylcholine and, indeed, was in the foreground of research with this agent (*see* the work of Phillips and of Castillo and de Beer in section II of succinylcholine chapter). Industry's interest in iproniazid as a model compound for MAO inhibitors was shown in the proliferation of "me-too" agents that followed its discovery.

Industry has been criticized for its lack of interest in important but unpatentable substances and in compounds with small market potential. The lack of interest is generally defended on grounds of the high costs of drug discovery and development, and the need for return on investment in order to ensure survival (*see,* for example, section III of carbamazepine chapter). Whatever the reasons, this lack of interest has acted as a deterrent to drug discovery by effectively removing the contribution of the organic chemist from the process.

National Origin

Although 67% of all entries in the tables were from the USA and the UK (47 and 20%, respectively), the remaining one-third of the entries came from 12 additional countries. In addition, the discovery of a full 40% of the innovative drugs involved more than one country—usually two, sometimes three. These facts suggest strongly that innovative discoveries frequently depend on contributions from widely dispersed sources and that the national locations of these sources are not easily predictable.

A very interesting observation regarding the interactions of the various research institutions is that, other than some of the drugs that were discovered solely by industry via chemistry-pharmacology collaborations, none of the 32 drugs appears to have come about from planned, integrated research programs, either within a single institution or among institutions. The predominant pattern was for an observation made in one laboratory to be extended, or capitalized on, by other laboratories—sometimes in widely divergent fields or institutions (*see* propranol, captopril, chlorothiazide, azathioprine, chlorpromazine, imipramine, iproniazid, D-penicillamine, hydroxychloroquine, methotrexate, cyclophosphamide, succinylcholine, naloxone, albuterol, chenodeoxycholic acid, ursodeoxycholic acid). In some cases before a chemist was brought into the research path, the orientation of the work was not necessarily drug discovery (*see* captopril, chlorothiazide, chlorpromazine, albuterol). We suggest that the nearest approximations to planned, rational, collaborative drug discovery programs, other than some of those consisting of a single industrial contribution, are arguably those of L-dopa, beclomethasone dipropionate, and cimetidine.

The above discussion indicates that it is not often possible to predict the sources from which pertinent information will come in the discovery of truly innovative drugs. Therefore, such information may not be forthcoming via preplanned, orderly research programs within an institution or across several institutions (with the always potential exception of chemistry-pharmacology screening collaborations). It is conceivable that relatively large, formal collaborations, such as those now occurring between some industry and university laboratories (Varrin and Kukich, 1985; Williams and Neil, 1988; Swann, 1988) and between industry and government laboratories (Culliton, 1989), could yield truly innovative drugs, but probably only if the collaborations brought the pharmacologically oriented scientists in medical schools and in government laboratories into significantly greater direct contact with the output of organic chemists. Without this contact, however, such a result is uncertain, judging from past history, in which (as already noted) innovative drugs do not seem to have sprung from purely investigative research carried out by collaborating teams. Vane and Cuatrecasas (1984) felt that even in the currently glamorous area of genetic engineering, "...in most spheres of activity, the genetic engineering approach to the biosynthesis of specific [protein] molecules is a prelude to (and will encourage) development of superior and less expensive alternatives by organic chemists and biochemists."

II. Routes to Discovery

The Basic/Rational/Planned/Ideal Approach

Since scientists have a predilection for logical progressions, perhaps the ideal method for the discovery of drugs would be to carry out the following scenario via an organized research team(s):

1. A workup of the physiology and biochemistry of the normal state of the system of interest;
2. A workup of the physiological and biochemical pathology of the system;
3. A logically determined augmentation of, or interference with, the deranged system via an agonist, antagonist, metabolite, anti-

metabolite, transport augmenter or inhibitor, or the like, as needed, to correct the problem, based on detailed knowledge of receptor sites, enzyme structure, and so forth.

It is safe to say that such an integrated, planned approach was not in evidence in any of the 32 drugs we reviewed. As noted earlier, although the semblance of such orderliness occurred in some cases, on close examination the work usually was seen to come from several laboratories that were not true collaborators or, on occasion, were competitors. More realistically, a planned collaborative approach directly aimed at producing a drug, if it occurred, was initiated relatively late in the "ideal" scenario. Integrated rationality usually appeared as the logical, often multistep, followup by a given research group, or collaborating research groups, on physiological or biochemical observations first made by one or more other independent groups; the followup was spurred on if the findings were perceived as being amenable to pharmacological manipulation, especially if the manipulation had potential therapeutic application. Examples of such programmed rational activity occurred in the discovery of the following drugs after certain facts became known:

- Propranolol—beta blockade was possible, as demonstrated with DCI, and potentially useful in angina;
- Captopril—ACE inhibition was possible, as shown with the peptide BPF and had potential usefulness in hypertension;
- Azathioprine—as shown by 6-MP, antiproliferative, anticancer agents inhibited the immune system and had potential therapeutic use in transplantation of organs;
- L-Dopa—dopamine was important in motor function, as shown by reserpine-induced depletion of dopamine and by the unique localization of dopamine in the striatum; disturbances in dopamine metabolism might be involved in motor disorders;
- Methotrexate—folic acid was an antianemia agent and growth factor; antagonists of folic acid might have therapeutic potential in preventing cell proliferation.

With only one exception (L-dopa), the discoveries of all of these drugs were intimately involved with the contributions of organic chemists and involved a considerable amount of screening.

Screening

Screening as an approach to drug discovery, especially in untargeted form, is often considered not to be a "rational" approach. It is clear, however, that screening, even untargeted screening, *is* a rational procedure; it does not represent some form of illogical reasoning. The problem with untargeted screening as a modus operandi is that it has only chance probability of succeeding. In addition, untargeted screening is not intellectually satisfying to many scientists, since it may not be related to any logically ordered information regarding the system being used as a test object and, furthermore, the compounds being screened are not analogs of the known structures of substrates, agonists, or antagonists of the system. However, screening, either untargeted or targeted, offers a trade-off for these shortcomings by bringing to bear at the discovery frontier the power of the organic chemist to take the drug-oriented biomedical scientist "beyond the limits of knowledge." Beyer (1978) used this phrase to mean going "...beyond the limits of what is accepted as factual."

Very significant drugs have come from lines of research that had important components of untargeted screening (propranolol, verapamil, nifedipine, diltiazem, cyclosporine, haloperidol, imipramine, chlordiazepoxide, diazepam, indomethacin), as well as from lines of research that had significant components of targeted screening (propranolol, captopril, chlorothiazide, furosemide, azathioprine, chlorpromazine, imipramine, diazepam, carbamazepine, methotrexate, cyclophosphamide, succinylcholine, halothane, fentanyl, naloxone, albuterol, beclomethasone dipropionate, cimetidine).

Targeted screening might be considered to be more "rational" than untargeted screening, because it is more directed than untargeted screening: positive information exists regarding the way in which compounds that, chemically, are closely related to the one being screened influence the system under study (e.g., a substrate, an agonist, an antagonist). Modification of these structures often, but not always, has a considerably greater than chance probability of producing a compound with some desired effect (e.g., *see* methotrexate, azathioprine, and propranolol chapters). Targeted screening is appealing to chemists because it gives them a starting point for the synthesis of active analogs; this fact is also the basis for the profusion of "me-too" drugs that many medical scientists find offensive. However, a negative attitude toward "me-tooing" needs to be softened, because it must be remembered that genuinely innovative drugs have come from lines of research that can be considered to have had a component of "me-tooing" in them (*see* propranolol, haloperidol, imipramine, fentanyl, naloxone, albuterol, beclomethasone dipropionate). Furthermore, new pharmacological concepts often grow out of the study of available drugs. For example, the concept of alpha- and beta-adrenergic receptors depended on the availability of a series of "me-too" agonists, as did the further division of beta receptors into beta$_1$ and beta$_2$ subtypes. Moreover, both concepts were materially substantiated via the availability of a group of alpha and beta blocking agents (*see* chapters on albuterol and propranolol).

It is very obvious from our analyses that screening, in one or the other of its forms, appears to be all but indispensable to the discovery of innovative drugs, having been involved in the discovery of 25 of the 32 case histories covered by us. There seems to us to be three reasons for this:

1. The effects of structural changes on the biological activity of a molecule are often unpredictable.
2. Compounds are "smarter" than the scientists studying them, in that they will exert their activity whether or not *we* understand the mechanisms that they employ in doing so. Digitalis acted on Na$^+$/ K$^+$ ATPase for centuries before the enzyme was described. Aspirin knew all about arachadonic acid pathways 70 years before Vane (1971) discovered that it did, and it managed to do very well for itself during the years of our ignorance. Verapamil blocked Ca^{2+} channels quite satisfactorily for years before Fleckenstein et al. (1969) found out about what it was doing. Cyclosporine, with its ungainly, fungus-designed physique, happily inhibited production of interleukin-2 by T-helper lymphocytes as soon as it made contact with them, quite some time before Borel et al. (1976) knew that it was doing so. Important, new pharmacological, and potentially clinically useful, activities can be detected in relatively poorly understood systems if the researcher is alert, open-minded, and methodical enough to do so.

3. Organic chemists make novel compounds and thereby open the door to new pharmacological discoveries.

In this vein, Leake (1970), in discussing his role in developing divinyl ether as an anesthetic, commented: "It is gratifying, but also puzzling, to realize that one may devise a chemical compound to relieve the certain pain of surgery without knowing what pain is or how the chemical agent acts!"

Serendipity

Serendipity was a significant event in the drug-discovery process, since it was involved in the initiations of eight of the 30 lines of research reviewed by us (preclinical serendipitous initiations: propranolol, haloperidol, captopril, lithium; clinical serendipitous initiations: iproniazid, chlorothiazide, chlorpromazine, hydroxychloroquine). Serendipitous observations occurred in the histories of drugs discovered in the 1940s (lithium), very often in those discovered in the 1950s (iproniazid, haloperidol, chlorothiazide, chlorpromazine, hydroxychloroquine), and less often in those from the 1960s (propranolol) and the 1970s (captopril). Interestingly, serendipity was more common in lines of research initiated by nonindustrial research institutions (captopril, lithium, iproniazid, chlorpromazine, hydroxychoroquine) than in lines of research initiated by industry (propranolol, haloperidol). Moreover, several of the serendipitous leads that had been generated by nonindustrial institutions were picked up and extended by nonindustrial laboratories (captopril, iproniazid, chlorothiazide, hydroxychloroquine) as well as by industrial laboratories (propranol, captopril, chlorothiazide, chlorpromazine). These facts suggest that the particular brand of luck called serendipity can occur in, and command the respect and attention of, all types of research laboratories.

Some Effects of Clinical Specialties
on Routes to Discovery

The analysis of drugs by their clinical groupings indicates that innovations do not follow a uniform progression and that the area of clinical interest may dictate, in part, the form that progress will take.

Thus, the analysis indicates that the psychiatry and rheumatology groups of drugs were much more dependent on clinical studies, and somewhat less dependent on screening and industrial contributions, than were the CV&R and anesthesiology groups. In addition, the psychiatry group had the largest number of drugs with hospital and with serendipitous contributions. The differences between the psychiatry and rheumatology groups on one hand, and CV&R and anesthesiology groups on the other, are most likely attributable to the fact that the events measured in CV&R disciplines and in anesthesiology are objective, and can be measured validly and readily in normal animal systems, whereas psychiatric illnesses, especially, and rheumatoid illnesses, to a significant extent, are less readily and validly measured in animal model systems. It appears that psychiatry and rheumatology have been fairly dependent on hospital and university clinical observations for the initiation and advancement of innovative drug discovery.

It seems clear to the authors that the intellectual histories of innovative drugs rarely fit the ideal of a compact, "rational" approach, but that despite this, drug discovery is a very meaningful occurrence. The intellectual elements that go into discovery are disparate, and they do not, and probably never will, fit predictably into neat collaborations. Indeed, several lines of research that led to important drugs were initiated on the basis of premises that were later shown to be wrong (*see* naloxone, chenodeoxycholic acid, succinylcholine, and penicillamine) and, as already mentioned, eight drugs had unpredictable, serendipitous initiating events. Furthermore, the human impulses to get on with the job, be they dedication, ego-drive, grantsmanship, commercial gain, careerism, or the like, frequently push the process on ahead of codified knowledge. Therefore, people who look toward discovering really innovative pharmacotherapeutic agents (or who wish to be fair critics of the process) cannot afford to disdain these realities, but should adjust to them and encourage their sensible utilization. In so doing, it might be well to embrace, comfortably, both untargeted and targeted screening, as well as serendipity, along with traditional investigative research, as valued methods needed to yield avant-garde therapeutic agents.

III. Attitudes

Attitudes concerning the various methods employed in drug discovery and the institutions employing them, as toward anything else, are determined by the accuracy of the information one has at hand to consider and by the preconceived notions and prejudices that one carries into the considerations. From a scientific point of view, these latter prejudicial components ideally should be kept to a minimum, and the evaluation of accurate information should take precedence. The authors would be grateful to the readers if they would kindly bear this in mind as they read on.

Productivity in the drug-discovery process, in addition to relying heavily on the chemistry-pharmacology screening contributions of industry, was also found to rely heavily on nonindustrial investigative contributions of diverse nature. This latter fact may reinforce the attitude held in some quarters that the industrial contributions in drug discovery, including innovative drug discoveries, simply represent the opportunistic use, for proprietary gain, of the painstaking advances in basic knowledge provided by the nonindustrial research communities on a nonproprietary basis. From our case histories, arguments could be made that, to some extent, such opportunism was manifest in the discovery of several drugs (*see* captopril, chlorothiazide, chlorpromazine, cyclophosphamide, and albuterol), but it is very difficult to support such an attitude regarding the 19 drugs that had one or more industrial contributions, but in which there was no dominance of early contributions from universities (or other nonindustrial institutions). It would seem scientifically fair-minded that the attitude be tempered by this knowledge.

In the course of reviewing the history of innovative discoveries, we found several commonly held conceptions that seemed to us really to be misconceptions; these can serve as examples of erroneous ideas that can distort attitudes concerning the discovery of very important drugs. These examples are:

- Propranolol: The notion that Ahlquist's theory of alpha- and beta-adrenergic receptors was a determinant in the discovery of DCI and, therefore, that it was, in a manner of speaking, ultimately responsible for the discovery of propranolol, is not supportable. DCI was sorted out serendipitously via a screening program aimed at finding long-acting bronchodilators, quite independently of Ahlquist's theory.

- Ca Antagonists: The notion that Fleckenstein's description of calcium-channel blockade by verapamil was involved in verapamil's discovery is unfounded. On the contrary, verapamil (as well as nifedipine and diltiazem) was found by an untargeted screening program, and it was in clinical trial as an antianginal agent some years prior to Fleckenstein's definitive work. Fleckenstein's description of specific calcium-channel blockade (permitted by the availability of verapamil) allowed for successor compounds to be looked for via a known mechanism.

- MAOIs: The notion that the discovery of the antidepressant activity of iproniazid was dependent on the observation of Zeller and associates that it was an inhibitor of monoamine oxidase is also less than clear. The work of Robitzek and associates was carried out independently of the work of Zeller and associates; it was not until the publication of the work of Crane and of Kline, Saunders, and coworkers several years later that MAO inhibition was emphasized in rationalizing the clinical results that brought iproniazid to the fore. It might seem more appropriate to credit Zeller's work with prompting the successors to iproniazid by supplying a mechanism of action that could be exploited via targeted screening programs.

- Beta$_2$ receptor agonists: The idea that beta$_2$ receptor agonists were developed only subsequently to the definition by Lands and associates of the beta$_2$ receptor as distinct from beta$_1$ receptors is not tenable. Isoetharine, metaproterenol, and albuterol were all developed on the basis of other rationales. Isoetharine and metaproterenol were discovered years before the clear formulation of Lands' concept, in the empirical search for agonists that influenced bronchiole muscle more than heart muscle.

All four of these misconceptions tend to perpetuate the idea that an immediately applicable mechanistic or theoretical framework is an absolute necessity (rather than a convenience or a great advantage—or possibly an encumbrance) before important drug discovery can take place. In fact, in several of the above examples, the situation was reversed—the availability of a new and independently discovered drug provided an essential tool that permitted a much-needed verification of some at-risk concept. Indeed, verapamil (and other early calcium antagonists) and iproniazid can be considered to be discoveries that took pharmacologists beyond the limits of knowledge available at the time, and which subsequently permitted significant *new* concepts to be developed.

As an adjunct to the preceding paragraphs, we would like to present other examples of the fact that innovative drugs were often powerful tools in explaining normal and disease processes in humans. The discovery of these drugs played a permissive role for future research that would not have been possible without the drug (in a manner similar to the permissive role of the work described in the "Background contributions" in section II of each case history). Moreover, the discoveries of several of these agents also represented taking science beyond the limits of knowledge, a notion mentioned in the preceding paragraph and earlier, and attributed to Beyer (1978).

- Captopril permitted the detailed exploration of the role of the renin–angiotensin system in essential hypertension and other disorders.
- Chlorothiazide and furosemide, and acetazolamide before them, gave many insights into normal and abnormal mechanisms of renal function. Their discoveries were examples of being taken beyond the limits of knowledge (see section IV of the furosemide chapter).
- Azathioprine and cyclosporine both had a large impact on basic and clinical immunology and on organ transplantation. The discoveries of azathioprine and cyclosporine are additional examples of being taken beyond the limits of knowledge (*see* section III of the azathioprine chapter and section IV of the cyclosporine chapter).
- Chlorpromazine, imipramine, and lithium permitted the development of basic theories about the biologic bases for schizophrenia, depression, and mania, respectively. Their discoveries also are examples of being taken beyond the limits of knowledge.
- Chlordiazepoxide and diazepam permitted opening the door to the research that defined the benzodiazepine receptor and its interaction with Gaba and chloride ion channels.

The above discussion suggests that the discovery of innovative drugs should not be viewed, in the main, as intellectual parasitism of one type of research institution on another. For aside from the many discoveries made solely by industry and the significant discoveries made solely by nonindustrial institutions, much of the discovery of innovative drugs results from interactions of both domains, in which, in the long haul, all of the groups involved give as well as receive on an intellectual level. Certainly, clinical medicine and suffering patients have been the real recipients of the fruits of these interactions, which, although rarely collaborations in the true sense of the word, have served the public interest well.

References

Bearn, A. G.: The pharmaceutical industry and academe: Partners in progress. *Am. J. Med.* **71:** 81–88, 1981.

Beyer, K. H.: *Discovery, Development and Delivery of New Drugs,* SP Medical & Scientific Books, New York, 1978.

Borel, J. F., Feurer, C., Gubler, H. U., and Stahelin, H.: Biological effects of cyclosporin A: A new anti-lymphocytic agent. *Agents Actions* **6:** 468–475, 1976.

Cuatrecasas, P.: *Contemporary Drug Development—Dilemmas,* Publication Series, Center for the Study of Drug Development, Department of Pharmacology, University of Rochester, New York, 1983.

Culliton, B. D.: NIH, Inc.: The CRADA boom. *Science* **245:** 1034–1036, 1989.

Fleckenstein, A., Tritthart, H., Fleckenstein, B., Herbst, A., and Grün, G.: A new group of competitive Ca-antagonists (Iproveratril, D600 prenylamine) with highly potent inhibitory effects on excitation-contraction coupling in mammalian myocardium. *Pflugers Arch.* **307:** R25, 1969.

Konzett, H.: Neue broncholytisch hochwirksame Körper der Adrenalinreihe. *Arch. Exp. Pathol. Pharmakol.* **197:** 27–40, 1940.

Krantz, J. C. Jr., Carr, C. J., Lu, G., and Bell, F. K.: Anesthesia XL. The anesthetic action of trifluoroethyl vinyl ether. *J. Pharmacol. Exp. Ther.* **108:** 488–495, 1953.

Leake, C. D.: The long road for a drug from idea to use, in *Discoveries in Biological Psychiatry.* F. J. Ayd and B. Blackwell, eds., J. B. Lippincott, Philadelphia, 1970.

Leake, C. D., Knoefel, P. K., and Guedel, A. E.: The anesthetic action of divinyl oxide in animals. *J. Pharmacol. Exp. Ther.* **47:** 5–16, 1933.

McCawley, E. L., Hart, E. R., and Marsh, D. F.: The preparation of *N*-allylnormorphine. *J. Am. Chem. Soc.* **63:** 314, 1941.

Merritt, H. H. and Putnam, T. J.: Sodium diphenyl hydantoinate in the treatment of convulsive disorders. *JAMA* **111:** 1068–1073, 1938.

Mossinghoff, G. J.: *Facts at a Glance,* Pharmaceutical Manufacturers Association, Washington, DC, 1987.

Paton, W. D. M. and Zaimis, E. J.: Curare-like action of polymethylene *bis*-quaternary ammonium salts. *Nature* **1:** 718, 719, 1948.

Schwartzman, D.: *Innovation in the Pharmaceutical Industry,* Johns Hopkins University Press, Baltimore, 1976.

Swann, J. P.: *Academic Scientists and the Pharmaceutical Industry,* Johns Hopkins University Press, Baltimore, 1988.

Vane, J. R.: Inhibition of prostaglandin synthesis as a mechanism of action for aspirin-like drugs. *Nature* (New Biol.) **231:** 232–235, 1971.

Vane, J. and Cuatrecasas, P.: Genetic engineering and pharmaceuticals. *Nature* **312:** 303–305, 1984.

Varrin, R. D. and Kukich, D. S.: Guidelines for industry-sponsored research at universities. *Science* **227:** 385–388, 1985.

Wardell, W. M. and Sheck, L. E.: Is pharmaceutical innovation declining? Interpreting measures of pharmaceutical innovation and regulatory impact in the USA, 1950–1980. *Ration. Drug Ther.* **17:** 1–7, 1983.

Williams, M. and Neil, G. L.: Organizing for drug discovery. *Prog. Drug Res.* **32:** 330–375, 1988.

Appendix

Analyses of Table 1*

I. Analysis of 30 Lines of Research†

Columns 1 and 2—Sequence and Orientation

Col. 1 (sequence)			
Total no. of entries	94		
Col. 2 (orientation)			
Total initial entries	30	Total no. of entries[a]	97
Preclinicial	73%	Preclinical	67%
Clinical	23%	Clinical	33%
Preclinical +			
clinical	3%		

[a]Three double entries in this column (*see* cyclophosphamide and cimetidine).

*For ease of display and comprehension, all percentages have been rounded to the nearest whole number; therefore, minor discrepancies occasionally may appear, e.g., totaling percentages may yield 99 or 101%, instead of 100%.

†All double entries were handled as two separate entries throughout this analysis except where noted. Double entries were made when two forms of the variable described in a given column occurred in the research contribution being analyzed (e.g., preclinical and clinical studies occurring in the same publication). A comma was used to separate double entries in the chapter tables. Please note, however, that a pharmacology/chemistry entry or a chemistry/pharmacology entry in the column labeled "nature of study" represents a single entry.

In the absence of double entries, the number of initial entries for each of the columns would be 30 and the total number of entries for each of the columns would be 94.

Column 3—Nature of Study

Total no. of entries[a]	97		
Biochemistry	10%	Oncology	1%
Chemistry	3%	Pharmacology[b]	17%
Chemistry/nutrition	1%	Pharmacology/	
Chemistry/		chemistry[b]	8%
pharmacology[b]	32%	Physiology	4%
Dermatology	2%	Psychiatry	5%
Gastroenterology	5%	Pulmonary	2%
Neurology	2%	Rheumatology	5%
		Surgery	2%
No. of chemistry/ pharmacology + pharmacology/chemistry entries	39		
Chemistry/ pharmacology	80%	Pharmacology/ chemistry	21%

[a]Three double entries in this column (*see* D-penicillamine, cyclophosphamide, L-dopa).

[b]Chemistry/pharmacology + pharmacology/chemistry + pharmacology = 57%; other = 43%.

Column 4—Research Institution

Total initial entries[a]	32	Total no. of entries[b]	99
Government	6%	Government	4%
Hospital	13%	Hospital	12%
Industry	53%	Industry[c]	41%
Private	0%	Private	3%
University	28%	University[c]	38%
Hospital (VA)	0%	Hospital (VA)	1%

[a]Two double initial entries in this column (*see* methotrexate, cyclophosphamide).

[b]Five double entries in this column (*see* L-dopa, methotrexate, cyclophosphamide, cimetidine, chenodeoxycholic acid).

[c]University and industry: total entries are almost equal and account for 79% of all entries.

Column 5—National Origin

Total no. of entries	94		
Australia	2%	Spain	1%
Austria	2%	Sweden	5%
Belgium	2%	Switzerland	5%
Brazil	1%	Tunisia[a]	1%
France	5%	UK[b]	20%
Italy	1%	USA[b]	47%
Japan	2%	West Germany	4%

[a]French naval hospital.
[b]UK + USA = 67%; others = 33%.

Columns 6 and 7
Nature of Discovery and Screening Involved

Col. 6 (nature of discovery)

Total initial entries	30
Serendipitous initial entries[a]	27%

Col. 7 (screening involved)

Total no. of entries[b]	94
Percentage of entries involving screening	46%
No. of entries involving screening	43
Targeted	74%
Untargeted	14%
Untargeted, targeted	12%

[a]All serendipitous entries were initial entries.
[b]Double positive entries (e.g., untargeted, targeted) were counted as one positive entry; "no" entries represent negative entries.

Comparisons across Columns 4 and 2
Research Institution and Orientation

Incidence of clinical entries for:	
Government	20%
Hospital	92%
Industry	7%
Private	100%
University	43%
Hospital (VA)	100%

Comparisons across Columns 4 and 6
Research Institution and Nature of Discovery

Total initial entries[a]	32
Institution–serendipitous linkages	
Government	0%
Hospital	13%
Industry	6%
Private	0%
University	6%
Initial serendipitous entries[b]	
Hospital	100%
Industry	12%
University	22%

[a]Two double initial entries occurred in column 4 (*see* methotrexate, cyclo-phosphamide).
[b]Percentage of each institution's total initial contributions.

Comparisons across Columns 4 and 7
Research Institution and Screening Involved

Incidence of positive screening entries for:	
Government	50%
Hospital	8%
Industry	90%
Private	0%
University	16%
Hospital (VA)	0%

II. Analysis
of 32 Innovative Drugs

Columns 1 and 2—Sequence and Orientation

Col. 1 (sequence)

Total no. of contributions	99
Mean ± SE, contributions/drug[a]	3.1 ± 0.4
Mean ± SE, years between initial contribution and establishment of scientific basis[b]	5.1 ± 1.0

Col. 2 (orientation)

Total no. of innovative drugs[c]	32	
Having preclinical contributions only	53%	Propranolol, captopril, verapamil, nifedipine, diltiazem, furosemide, azathioprine, cyclosporine, haloperidol, chlordiazepoxide, diazepam, carbamazepine, indomethacin, succinylcholine, halothane, fentanyl, naloxone
Having clinical contributions only	16%	Iproniazid, D-penicillamine, hydroxychloroquine, chenodeoxycholic acid, ursodeoxycholic acid
Having both preclinical and clinical contributions	31%	Chlorothiazide, chlorpromazine, imipramine, lithium, L-dopa, methotrexate, cyclophosphamide, albuterol, beclomethasone dipropionate, cimetidine

---

[a]Range: 1–8 contributions.
[b]Range: 0–20 yr.
[c]The figure 32 was used throughout this analysis of 32 innovative drugs.

Column 3—Nature of Study

Drugs with at least one contribution from:

Biochemistry	16%	Pharmacology	31%
Chemistry	9%	Pharmacology/	
Chemistry/nutrition	3%	chemistry	28%
Chemistry/		Physiology	6%
pharmacology	56%	Psychiatry	13%
Dermatology	6%	Pulmonary	3%
Gastroenterology	6%	Rheumatology	13%
Neurology	3%	Surgery	3%
Oncology	3%		

Column 4—Research Institution

Drugs with at least one contribution from:

Government	9%
Hospital	25%
Industry	75%
Private	9%
University	53%
Hospital (VA)	6%

Drugs with contributions solely from:

Government	0%	
Hospital	3%	Lithium
Industry	38%	Verapamil, nifedipine, diltiazem, furosemide, cyclosporine, haloperidol, chlordiazepoxide, diazepam, carbamazepine, indomethacin, halothane, fentanyl[a]
Private	0%	
University	0%	
Hospital (VA)	0%	

(continued)

[a] 11 of these 12 agents, the exception being diazepam, were defined by a single contribution; all 12 resulted from screening, with eight of the 12 having untargeted screening.

Column 4—Research Institution *(continued)*		
Drugs with contributions solely from:		
Combinations of nonindustrial institutions	22%	Iproniazid, L-dopa, D-penicillamine, hydroxychloroquine, succinylcholine, chenodeoxycholic acid, ursodeoxycholic acid

Column 5—National Origin		
Drugs with contributions from:		
1 country only	59%	
Australia	3%	Lithium
Belgium	6%	Haloperidol, fentanyl
Japan	3%	Diltiazem
Switzerland	6%	Cyclosporine, carbamazepine
UK	9%	Halothane, beclomethasone dipropionate, cimetidine
USA	22%	Iproniazid, chlordiazepoxide, diazepam, indomethacin, D-penicillamine, methotrexate, chenodeoxycholic acid
West Germany	9%	Verapamil, nifedipine, furosemide
2 countries	31%	Propranolol, chlorothiazide, azathioprine, chlorpromazine, imipramine, L-dopa, hydroxychloroquine, succinylcholine, naloxone, ursodeoxycholic acid
3 countries	9%	Captopril, cyclophosphamide, albuterol

Columns 6 and 7—Nature of Discovery and Screening Involved

Col. 6 (nature of discovery)		
Drugs with at least one serendipitous contribution	25%	
Preclinical	13%	Propranolol, captopril, haloperidol, lithium
Clinical	13%	Chlorothiazide, chlorpromazine, iproniazid, hydroxychloroquine
Col. 7 (screening involved)		
Drugs without screening contributions	22%	Iproniazid, lithium, L-dopa, D-penicillamine, hydroxychloroquine, chenodeoxycholic acid, ursodeoxycholic acid[a]

[a]None of these drugs had any industry contributions.

32 Innovative Drugs by Decades

	Decade			
	1940s	1950s	1960s	1970s
No. of drugs discovered	3	8	13	8
Drugs involving serendipitous observations, %	33	63	8	13
Drugs involving screening, %	67	75	85	75
Drugs involving untargeted screening, %	0	25	39	50
Drugs having at least one contribution from various institutions, %				
Government	33	13	8	0
Hospital	33	50	15	13
Industry	33	75	85	75
Private	0	13	0	25
University	67	63	46	50
Hospital (VA)	0	0	0	25

III. Analysis of the Innovative Drugs Taken as Groups

In the CV&R, psychiatry, rheumatology, and anesthesiology groups, there were an adequate number of drugs (six or more) to permit separate analysis. The neurology, pulmonary, and gastrointestinal groups were not analyzed because of the small number of drugs involved. The drugs in each group were as follows:

- Cardiovascular and renal (including renal transplantation): propranolol, captopril, verapamil, nifedipine, diltiazem, chlorothiazide, furosemide, azathioprine, cyclosporine
- Psychiatry: chlorpromazine, haloperidol, imipramine, iproniazid, lithium, chlordiazepoxide, diazepam
- Rheumatology: indomethacin, D-penicillamine, hydroxychloroquine, azathioprine, methotrexate, cyclophosphamide
- Anesthesiology: succinylcholine, halothane, fentanyl, naloxone, propranolol, diazepam
- Neurology: L-dopa, carbamazepine, diazepam
- Pulmonary: albuterol, beclomethasone dipropionate
- Gastrointestinal: cimetidine, chenodeoxycholic acid, ursodeoxycholic acid

Please note that azathioprine, propranolol, and diazepam appear in more than one group.

Column 2—Orientation

	Cardiovascular and renal	Psychiatry	Rheumatology	Anesthesiology
No. of drugs[a]	9	7	6	6
Preclinical contributions only	89% Propranolol, captopril, verapamil, nifedipine, diltiazem, furosemide azathioprine, cyclosporine,	43% Haloperidol, chlordiazepoxide, diazepam	33% Indomethacin, azathioprine	100% Succinylcholine, halothane, fentanyl, naloxone, propanolol, diazepam
Clinical contributions only	0%	14% Iproniazid	33% D-Penicillamine, hydroxychloroquine	0%
Preclinincal + clinical contributions	11% Chlorothiazide	43% Chlorproma-zine, impira-mine, lithium	33% Methotrexate, cyclophosphamide	0%

[a]These figures for numbers of drugs were used throughout this analysis (section III).

Column 4—Research Institutions

	Cardiovascular and renal, %	Psychiatry, %	Rheumatology, %	Anesthesiology, %
Drugs with at least one contribution from:				
Government	0	0	17	17
Hospital	0	57	33	0
Industry	100	71	67	83
Private	0	0	17	0
University	44	43	67	50
Hospital (VA)	0	0	0	0
Drugs with contributions solely from:				
Government	0	0	0	0
Hospital	0	14 Lithium	0	0
Industry	56 Verapamil, nifedipine, diltiazem, furosemide, cyclosporine	43 Haloperidol, chlordiazepoxide, diazepam	17 Indomethacin	50 Halothane, fentanyl, diazepam
Private	0	0	0	0
University	0	0	0	0
Hospital (VA)	0	0	0	0

Column 5—National Origin

	Cardiovascular and renal, %	Psychiatry, %	Rheumatology, %	Anesthesiology, %
Drugs with contributions from:				
1 country only	56 Verapamil, nifedipine, diltiazem, furosemide, cyclosporine	71 Haloperidol, iproniazid, lithium, chlordiazepoxide, diazepam	50 Indomethacin, D-penicillamine, methotrexate	50 Halothane, fentanyl, diazepam
Australia	0	14	0	0
Belgium	0	14	0	17
Japan	11	0	0	0
Switzerland	11	0	0	0
UK	0	0	0	17
USA	0	43	50	17
West Germany	33	0	0	0

(continued)

Column 5—National Origin *(continued)*

	Cardiovascular and renal, %	Psychiatry, %	Rheumatology, %	Anesthesiology, %
Drugs with contributions from:				
2 countries	33 Propranolol, chlorothiazide, azathioprine	29 Chlor-promazine, imipramine	33 Hydroxy-chloroquine, azathioprine	50 Succinylcholine, naloxone, propranolol
3 countries	11 Captopril	0	17 Cyclophosphamide	0

Columns 6 and 7
Nature of Discovery and Screening Involved

Cardiovascular and renal, %	Psychiatry, %	Rheumatology, %	Anesthesiology, %
Drugs with at least one serendipitous contribution:			
33 Propranolol, captopril, chlorothiazide	57 Chlorpromazine, haloperidol, iproniazid, lithium	17 Hydroxychloroquine	17 Propranolol
Drugs with no screening involved:			
0	29 Iproniazid, lithium	33 D-Penicillamine, hydroxychloroquine	0

No. of Innovative Drugs by Decades

	Decade			
Group	1940s	1950s	1960s	1970s
Cardiovascular and renal	0	1	4	4
Psychiatry	1	4	2	0
Rheumatology	1	2	3	0
Anesthesiology	1	1	4	0
Neurology	0	0	3	0
Pulmonary	0	0	1	1
Gastrointestinal	0	0	0	3

Index